Damocles' Wife

Damocles' Wife

the inside story of
cancer caregiving
& long-term survival
in the midst of
motherhood,
marriage &
making life matter

by Shelly L. Francis

Foreword by Clarissa Pinkola Estés, Ph.D.

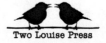

Two Louise Press

Two Louise Press
Lafayette, CO 80026

Published 2012

Cover and book design by Shelly L. Francis.
Cover photograph © 2012 All rights reserved, Shelly L. Francis
This book is set in Palatino Linotype and BernardMod MT.

"Stories of Damocles" Foreword by C.P. Estés, © 2012
All Rights Reserved. Permissions, ngandelman@gmail.com

"Music in the Morning", from FACTS ABOUT THE MOON by Dorianne Laux.
Copyright © 2006 by Doranne Laux.
Used by permission of W. W. Norton Company, Inc.

Publisher's Cataloging-in-Publication Data
Francis, Shelly L.
    Damocles' wife: the inside story of cancer caregiving and long-term survival in the midst of motherhood, marriage and making life matter / Shelly L. Francis; foreword by Clarissa Pinkola Estés, PhD
p. cm
    ISBN 978-0-9855665-0-0
1. Cancer-Popular works. 2. Cancer-Patients-Home care. 3. Caregivers.
4. Brain-Tumors-Popular works. 5. Cancer-Psychological aspects. I. Title.
    RC266.C338 2012
    616.99'4--dc22

Ebook ISBN 978-0-9855665-1-7

For Scott. Thank you for the gift of your courage
so that I could find my own.

For Wil. Thank you for being your true self.
Always remember our heartstrings.

For Julie Hayes, you were our trailblazer,
Mike Luparello, our inspiration, and for all our cancer heroes.
You lived!

**Damocles is pronounced
DAM-uh-kleez**

*(The author would like you to know this because
as a little girl she once read a storybook about mosquitoes
and the whole time thought the strange word was MOSS-kwee-toes.)*

Contents

Foreword
Damocles' Stories

The story of the Damoclean Sword is told by the Roman pundit and philosopher Cicero. It opens with a tyrant having taken the throne, Dionysius II. One of his courtiers, Damocles, asks for what he sees as pure happiness, that is, to be seated on Dionysius' throne, having the same perceived abundance, beauty, majesty, untroubled life.

The tyrant Dionysius II asks Damocles, that since this royal life delights him, does Damocles wish to taste it for himself...secretly meaning, to test what it is like to have such seeming fortune?

Damocles says Yes! and thus Dionysius causes to be brought in a golden couch covered with a soft rich rug for Damocles to lay upon, and all manner of feasting foods and servers of great beauty to attend to Damocles' every wish. As it was written in the ancient manuscript of Cicero, the perfumes were burning and the most beautiful music being made. And, Damocles thought himself ultra fortunate.

But, Dionysius also ordered that a shining sharp sword be fixed to the ceiling, dangling over Damocles' neck by a single horse hair. And thus was complete the picture of 'the fortunate man,' not just Damocles' fantasy, but with a hard reality added in.

Damocles, alert then, did not gaze at all the sumptuous beauty all around, nor feast from the delicacies brought to the table just for him, but instead, he worried and worried about in what wind, or even breath of conversation, that sharpest sword might fall upon him. And he begged Dionysius that he be allowed to leave the bed and table, that he had had enough of being 'fortunate.'

Though one could understand this as a moral legend about 'being careful what you wish for,' I think that is the least of it. Far more so, it is a story about how delicate happiness is for we humanlings on earth, how 'fantasy' happiness can seem like a state that is without any whisper of lethal concerns...at least until we meet a significant challenge of life and death...one that 'hangs over our heads' and calls on our most warrior-like, most pure child self—for that is the creative self—to engage and to charge toward fullest Life possible.

Here, in her book Shelly Francis details several lives, her own, that of her husband, and her young son, as her husband Scott suddenly is brought under the sword hanging by a horsehair...for Scott has been diagnosed with a brain tumor. Their happiness is startled. The adults are called to step into harness and to pull. And pull. And pull. Toward health, yes. But also, to a different form of happiness than before. One based on growth of self, truth telling. One that winds through many stages of fear, help, support, frustration, abject tiredness, upticks in hope and love. Here, in this work are detailed how one woman, a creative woman, a woman as a young mother and wife, came through it all.

There is a fairytale also called The Damocles Sword. In that version told by "peasant" people in my own family, the wine runs out at a wedding, and the groom is sent to the wine cellar to bring more. But he sees a sword hanging from the ceiling and weeps that one day his children, yet to be born, will have a wedding feast, come to the cellar to bring more wine, but the sword will fall on them and kill them and...the groom cannot bear this.

Soon comes the bride looking for her groom who is found weeping in the wine cellar. He tells her the terrible story of the fate of their future children and she too is overwhelmed with the grief of it all, and collapses down beside her weeping groom.

One after another, wedding guests come to the wine cellar to find the missing bride and groom, and they too are told the story of the future, and they too are overwhelmed and begin to weep.

Finally an old old woman comes down the rickety steps to the wine cellar. Everyone cries out the terrible story to her. She looks at them with compassion and with mercy. She tells them to take the sword down so it does not fall on them nor on their future progeny, that we can do what we can do.

And they do take the sword down, and the wedding feast resumes. But not without the sense that there is a sword in life, and that insofar as we can, we strive to focus on life, life, life...even though we know the sword is still in the world.

All these stories are true in a psychological sense, in a spiritual sense about our souls. Life brings harms to the body, hurts to the heart. But also life brings many helps to the soul, both in travails and in triumphs. There's the place to focus, on the helps, not on the harms only. It is true as in the first legend of Damocles, that happiness is fragile, but too, that contentment, coming to terms with, having a life that does not solely revolve around perfection nor around illness, frees us more and more during hard challenges, even as we lay tired, even as we lay feeling we might be dying very soon ourselves from the overwhelm and pressing down of it all.

It is true that as in the second story told in my immigrant/refugee family who tell stories that lifted them during their own egregious travails in wartime, that striving to focus on one's own life, as well as on the lives of hurt loved ones, protecting them as best we can with our own bodily cloak of realness and compassion and spiritual warmth, has to be ever planted in the soil of Life, Life, Life, not in the soil only of "what if...."

Many of us have had close conversations with Death down at the River of Life, and most of us know that Death is always sitting in the alcove there, folding and unfolding her gloves. It's just that there are times when we see Death near and clearly, and other times not. I think the truthfulness of this book by Shelly Francis will help identify the many emotional, mental, and spiritual phases of walking with another soul on earth whose body has been struck by deep challenge. It's the truth telling that I think readers in similar situations will resonate with.

Isn't it those who have gone before us, who tell the truth, who often offer us the most, not solutions, but rather critical latitude and longitude points that show much to us...those points that are not written on most popular culture maps? Yes, I think many of you know so too.

May you who have chosen—and been chosen—to walk with another in challenge, be blessed and guided always.

Clarissa Pinkola Estés, Ph.D.
Rocky Mountains, Spring 2012

Part One:
Crescent Moon Coping

I wish you didn't need to find this book. I wish you didn't find yourself one day in a new role, needing to know how to survive as a caregiver while your loved one fights cancer. I wish cancer was a thing of the past, but until it is, we're going to be busy.

If you suddenly find yourself wondering how in the world you're going to manage all this—finding the right doctors, the right treatments, taking care of your kids, plus your household and the rest of the family, paying the bills, moving one foot in front of the other, keeping the faith, needing peace, and ensuring when it's over you're still standing strong—you're going to need help. Please know you're not in this alone. I hope our story will encourage you with glimmers of light, both practical and, let's say, spiritual, to add to your own inner strengths that I know you can summon.

If you're wondering how someone survives brain cancer, here's the story of how my husband did it—and how he could not have done it without me and the rest of our caregiving crew. If you wonder what happens inside the caregiver as she learns to see how courage and fear coexist, to imagine a way beyond worry, to let go of the past and have faith in the future, to become a survivor herself, here's my story.

Once upon a time, not so long ago, a young family lived...

ॐ

Let choice whisper in your ear
and love murmur in your heart.
Be ready.
Here comes life.
—Maya Angelou

1
Setting Intentions

Three days after surgery, on that Tuesday night, I was sitting next to Scott's bed in his private room on the neuro ward. I was near the end of Richard Bach's book *Illusions* where the Messiah's Handbook concludes: Everything in this book may be wrong. I said out loud, "I love this part."

Just then the neurosurgeon came through the door. I moved to the wide window ledge as the doctor examined Scott's head, unwrapping, peering, poking, and rewrapping the bandage. Then he pulled up a chair and sat down. Realizing he was here to give us Scott's pathology report, I pulled out my bookmark to write on, an empty purple envelope from a get-well card.

"It's a slow-growing astrocytoma," he explained.

The brain tumor had been named—astrocytoma—and I rolled the sound around in my head. Astrocytoma. Then I heard him say that the tumor was malignant, but only a grade two, two out of four, where grade four is the most aggressive.

"That's good news," he tried to reassure us. "There's a big leap between grade two and three. Of course, it could degenerate into a more aggressive tumor at any time. This type of tumor can never be cured completely, but we can keep it in check with radiation, perhaps chemotherapy, and it likely won't recur for years. My recommendation is that you have radiation, which can start as soon as we remove the staples from your scalp, in a couple of weeks."

He named a few specialists to contact as our next assignment. The neurosurgeon left the room, with a backhanded wave saying he'd check on Scott the next morning and decide when to send him home.

Alone again, Scott and I just looked at each other. I turned to a blank page in my big spiral notebook, dated the page "Tues 11/17/98—6 p.m.", and transcribed my notes in clear handwriting onto our permanent record. With that we realized that Scott's brain tumor treatment had barely begun.

Not long after that, I left Scott alone to sleep for the night—or to not sleep and consider the words of the neurosurgeon and the pathology report. "No cure...can manage the disease for two to five years, maybe ten." After that moment, I never recalled "maybe ten."

I can't recall walking down the hall, into the elevator, across the large hospital lobby, or through the parking garage. I must have been on autopilot to maneuver the car past the ticketing booth and out onto the streets. My guardian angel, who made sure I survived driving at night and through crying jags, was surely on duty, clicking the traffic lights to green and clearing the roads for me until I arrived at my parent's house. The trip might have lasted all of ten minutes. Once parked, I gathered my purse, my spiral notebook, and my backpack of all-day-at-the-hospital necessities, and I stepped out of my car, looking up at the second story windows of the welcoming house that had been home most of my life. The front bedroom lights shone, meaning Wil was still awake inside.

I took a deep breath of cold November night air and glanced up and down the block. Our house at 360 South Corona was six houses from the corner of the tree-lined street, two blocks northwest of Washington Park. The neighborhood was a mix of Craftsmen bungalows and post-Victorian homes spaced no more than fifteen feet apart—kitchen windows looking into dining rooms next door. Our 1917 Denver Square was a clay-red brick with a deep front porch that spanned the full width of the house. The porch swing was empty now, of course, but full of memories of summer evenings, Sunday mornings, and countless afternoons talking with neighbors, reading alone, or swinging with best friends while planning our futures or weekends. We moved here a week before Christmas in 1970, halfway through my kindergarten year, and here I was, just shy of full circle, 360, coming home that night to my own son, who would soon start kindergarten himself.

Glancing up at the sky, I hoped to see some of the meteor showers that the newscasters explained came once every thirty-three years. Despite the dark of the moon, Denver's lights were too bright to see any shooting stars. I wondered if thirty-three years ago, when Scott was born, if the meteor showers were visible above the Michigan farmland where he grew up—but then I realized that no, he was born in Chicago and the city lights even then might have been too bright for stars. I sent a mental note to the sky, *Thanks for the meteor showers even if I can't see them. It's nice to know they're there.* I walked up the wide concrete porch steps and entered the house with a sigh. Home.

Sure enough I heard splashing bathtub water, Wil's giggles, and my dad's soft voice spilling down the oak staircase. I could picture Wil's bubble beard matching Dad's white one, their round cheeks giving credence to genetics. Wil's face at four looked just like the tinted sailor-suit photo of Dad at that age, the difference being Wil's blond widow peak wasn't black and his eyes were bright blue, not hazel. The saucy grin was the same.

I unloaded my armful onto the third-step landing and checked my eyes in the narrow antique mirror. Pure exhaustion stared back at me. As much as I hungered for a hug from my son, I was relieved that Dad had him occupied for now. The living room on my right was empty, but the kitchen light was on. Mom stepped into view and said, "I'm making hot tea. Would you like some? Did you eat dinner?"

"I'm not hungry. Tea sounds nice, but no caffeine. I want to sleep tonight."

I sat down on a kitchen chair at the yellow Formica table with curved metal legs that had been in her mother's kitchen, and I leaned against the wall. For a minute I soaked up the sounds of a happy boy getting cleaner upstairs and the comfort of my mom's kitchen, the safest place on the planet. *Thank goodness I'm not driving home to Highlands Ranch tonight*, I was thinking. *It will be nice to sleep upstairs in my old bedroom, snuggle with Wil, and let someone take care of me for tonight. And it will be a much shorter drive back to the hospital in the morning.*

Mom put an empty flowered mug in front of me, a plate of sliced banana bread, and her bright red teapot full of hot water. I had a choice of decaf Constant Comment, Celestial Seasonings mandarin orange, or chamomile. As usual, I picked mandarin orange and she poured hot water. Mom sat down across from me and reached her hand over to mine.

"How is Scott doing tonight? You?"

"He's okay. I'm tired," I said, dipping my teabag in and out of the water, watching the water seep darker. Without looking up, I said, "We got the pathology report back tonight." She squeezed my left hand and waited.

I repeated Scott's prognosis, having already memorized the words of the neurosurgeon. "He said this type of tumor can never be cured completely, but they can keep it in check," and I spat out that phrase, "for two to five years. Keep it in check? What does that mean?" I felt my anger beginning to boil like the tea kettle that had been whistling minutes before.

"Oh, Shelly," Mom said, emotion welling up and spilling out her brown eyes. "Oh, Shel." She took a deep breath before continuing.

"It means you have options for treatment—radiation, chemotherapy—lots of options that your surgeon might not even know about. Those numbers are only statistics. They don't necessarily define what is going to happen to Scott."

I looked at her and knew she was right. I sipped my tea and took a bite of banana bread, not tasting either. I was too overwhelmed to consider Scott's survival options just then. All I could think of was the deadline on his life, our life together. I burst into tears and in between blubbers I uttered, "I don't want to be a widow." Sob, gasp. "I don't want to be a single mother." Sob, sob, gurgle. "I don't want him to die." Sob, sob, sob, snort. "I...need...a Kleeeeenex."

"Oh honey." Mom scooted her chair around the table to be closer, then stepped in and out of the bathroom to hand me a roll of toilet paper. "It's going to be all right," she said, patting my leg while I unrolled a long piece, folded it, and blew my nose. I leaned into her shoulder and cried for several more minutes, while tears streamed down her face, too. Upstairs, Wil was still splashing in bubbles but the sound seemed more muffled, as if Dad had put up a protective shield to protect Wil from my fears.

When I stopped crying and started breathing again, my mom took the plates to the sink. I felt an energy swirling around the kitchen, this kitchen full of our lives for almost twenty-nine years. This kitchen held all the magic of eating sourdough pancakes with chokecherry syrup on Saturday mornings, sisters and neighbor kids standing on stools to wash dishes so we could hurry up and play after dinner, sitting on counters kicking the cupboards below waiting for popcorn to finish exploding in the pressure cooker on the ancient gas stove, walking around twirling the cord of the wall phone while giggling about boyfriends and haircuts, bumping elbows with aunts, uncles, and cousins as we filled our cups and plates for Easters, Christmases, and graduations, lingering talking as grown-ups at this same kitchen table on weekends home from college or on vacation back home when we lived in Tennessee. My whole life of being fed in this kitchen was spiraling into a storm, funneling all our dreams and hopes for the future into a raging tornado.

Mom turned around and said with a catch in her voice, whispering her greatest wish as a mother, "I wish with all my heart you didn't have to go through this."

If mothers could protect their children with a wish, it would have come true right then and there without any more pain. Instead, something caught inside me like a hook in a trout and I felt myself standing up from the chair, pushing it back, defiant, and flipping out like that fish deciding to live.

"No! If I have something to learn from this, I'm ready for it. We're not going to just give up without a fight. Scott is not a statistic. There must be a reason for all this shit. So let's figure it out. Bring it on, I say!"

Bring it on. Fighting words to the gods. If somewhere in the universe you can hear a noise when someone shouts an intention like that, it might have sounded like a high-pitched squeal and the echoing CHUNK of a monstrous metal cog settling into gear, locking into place your new direction. Something in me shifted then, refusing to be a victim before the battle had begun.

Mom stepped closer for a tight hug and affirmed, "Okay, bring it on."

I went upstairs to kiss a prune-skinned Wil goodnight. He and Dad were waiting, snuggled under the covers reading from my childhood pages of Richard Scary's *Busy Town*. Then I tiptoed into the small study off of my parent's bedroom where, by the light of a desk lamp, I caught up on incoming email. One announced baby-cousin Jack's happy arrival on Earth (okay, Minnesota). Another was from my friend Julie, reporting that after only two chemo treatments, the tumor in her breast had shrunk by an amazing fifty percent! I scanned the subject lines of the many emails awaiting and left them marked as unread until I had more time and energy. It was enough to know they were full of good wishes.

With what I had left, I typed my day into words and sent them through cyberspace to be heard.

Sent: Tuesday, November 17, 1998 8:45 PM
Subject: Pathology Report on Scott

Dear Everyone, (and please forward the message for us)

I am at my parent's house tonight, 10 minutes from the hospital, to get a long, snuggly night's sleep with Wil and then return to the hospital to be with Scott tomorrow. I wanted to let you all know that the neurosurgeon gave us the results of the pathology report tonight.

Here's the news. Scott's tumor is called an astrocytoma, which is made up of the "support cells" of the brain (as opposed to the thinking cells). Of the possible 4 grades of such tumors, where 4 would be rated as the most aggressive, Scott's rates as a 2. (The surgeon's first impression from the MRI 10 days ago was that it

was certain to be a 4—nice surprise it wasn't.) As further comparison, he says
there is a large difference or leap between a 2 and a 3, so 2 is pretty good. On the
down side, however, this type of tumor is not completely curable and could become
more aggressive (a 3 or 4). HOWEVER, it can be "kept in check" for YEARS through
radiation, possible more surgery someday much later down the road. And that is
good news.

So, our next step is to seek opinions and select a team of oncologist, radiation oncologist and also a gamma knife specialist (this is a newer, different type of radiation that MIGHT be appropriate in Scott's case). Scott will start some type of radiation treatment in the next week or so. One scenario if we can't have the single-
dose gamma knife treatment would be 6 weeks of radiation, 5 days a week. That
means we might be done right around Xmas.

Soooooooooo, we're not done yet but are content that we now have passed through
another waiting period and are on to the next phase. Scott and I KNOW that your
positive thoughts, prayers and massive doses of love sent our way helped us
through the surgery on Saturday and will keep us going as we continue to battle
whatever remains of this dragon.

I would like to share a dream Scott had in recovery, which he told me today. The
first part was of himself "slaying" and killing whatever was left inside after surgery,
and the second part was of him inside his brain repairing the damage caused by
surgery, "hoisting the girders back into place." He is so confident in this imagery,
believing that whatever remains are simply remnants and carcasses that need to
be vaporized. :)

Wil came to visit Scott at the hospital today. From now through the radiation
treatment, we want Wil to know that Daddy will be having a healing light shining
on his head to finish making him all better. As a near-5-year-old, that's all he
needs to be told. Beyond that he needs lots of hugs and reassurances.

Scott is regaining his strength and is starting to catch up on two weeks without
sleep. Scott will come home from the hospital either tomorrow (Wed.) or Thursday.
Because we are all EXHAUSTED and emotionally worn out, we will not be answering
our phone much nor having visitors for awhile yet. But we sure do welcome your
emails, cards and more than anything, continued loving thoughts and prayers.

Thank you again for accompanying us on this hard journey. It would be a lot lone-
lier and much harder without you—thanks for lightening our load. We love you and
appreciate you SO SO much.

Talk to you soon,
Love, Shelly

Home, home on the range
Where my dear son and the neighbor kids play
Where seldom is heard a discouraging word
And the skies are not cloudy all day

2

Foreshadows on a Periwinkle Wall

I can tell you the actual moment I knew, deep down, that life was about to change. Hazelnut coffee wafted on a Saturday morning October breeze. The Indigo Girls were multiplying life by the power of two on my CD player. And the color was periwinkle. More precisely, it was probably something like Martha Stewart Hydrangea Frost in washable satin finish. Just a shade lighter than the color you'd find in Van Gogh's bedroom. If I were in charge, my particular shade of periwinkle would be known as "clear sky overhead twenty minutes past sunset before the first star."

But what really matters is that I was finally painting the vaulted wall behind my bed, having waffled over paint chips in my purse for months. I was done waffling because my friend Julie found out Monday that the lump in her breast was malignant.

What if the universe prepares us for change through the life-changing disaster of somebody else? I'm all for wake-up calls, but what if we wake up from a life we thought was already happily ever after? What if we're not as wide awake as we think?

I had been happily getting to know Julie for two years through our local chapter of FEMALE (Formerly Employed Mothers at the Leading Edge—or at Loose Ends), a national organization for stay-at-home moms. When I saw Julie at the very first meeting with her short brown curly hair, her rosy smiling face, and her talkative confidence, I thought, *Ooooh, I want to be friends with that woman*. We did become close friends through playgroups, book club, gourmet dinner nights, newsletter and website committees, and the monthly chapter meetings. We spent several nonstop-talking weekends with women-friends at her mountain cabin.

Irony was everywhere: Julie found the lump herself after a mammogram missed it. And the day before her diagnosis was Denver's annual Susan G. Komen Race for the Cure, for which she had already raised money to honor her mother and two aunts as long-term survivors. She skipped the race due to overwhelming worry about her test results. I skipped it, too, but only because Scott and I had the weekend to ourselves—Wil with Scott's parents—so we could celebrate our eighth anniversary.

The phone call spreading Julie's news came Monday afternoon. Hanging up the kitchen wall phone, dazed, I grasped for something to do to offer support. I turned just a foot to my left and opened the folding doors of my pantry, which held art supplies instead of canned food. Staring at the shelves full of paper, paints, plastic boxes full of my raw materials, I decided to fabric-paint a white sweatshirt for Julie's friends to sign with fabric-paint pens. I wanted to create a tangible way for our love to wrap around Julie anytime she needed a hug and we weren't there in person. When I was done, the words on Julie's sweatshirt sang their own tune: "Anything you want, you got it; anything you need, you got it, anything at all, you got it! We love you, Julie."

I took the sweatshirt next morning to a Me & Moms meeting (Julie was the group leader that year and had arranged for our guest speaker; understandably, she choose to stay home). Me & Moms met at First Presbyterian, which was known then and now to me and my friends as Julie's Church. The red-brick Gothic Revival structure was built in 1929, became a historic landmark in 1996, and by providing its grounded divine energy on that day, it became a landmark in my memory. A dozen women soon filled the "bride's room" next to the sanctuary, while church ladies entertained our preschoolers in the basement. I spread out Julie's sweatshirt and a handful of fabric markers on the table next to the Styrofoam coffee cups, paper napkins and store-bought cookies—and a Kleenex box. With the sweatshirt's pale pink checkerboard design surrounding the hot pink words, it looked like a fun birthday surprise.

"What's that?" each woman asked upon entering, happy to have an hour without toddlers in tow.

"It's for Julie," I would say, unable to soften the brunt of the news. "She found out yesterday she has breast cancer. We're signing this sweatshirt for her, as a way to send her our love."

With each explanation, I watched faces fall, mouths twist, and suddenly the sweatshirt idea seemed really stupid. Tears, shock, and indignation at the injustice of motherhood interrupted boiled over and spoiled the air like burnt coffee grounds. Yet we didn't allow enough time (not that any amount would be enough) to soothe each other or release our tension, because the meeting had to begin.

We gathered in a small circle of soft chairs, loveseats, couch, and a few folding chairs. Then, to this audience of crossed arms and red eyes, our wise-woman-healer guest speaker guided us through what she intended as an inspirational talk about embracing life's changes. Beth had inspired us the previous May on the topic of motherhood, so perhaps that allowed and excused the group's general rudeness. As sunlight poured through the beveled glass windows, I don't recall Beth's exact words, just a permeating sense of peace. Most of the moms exuded anger, interrupting with so many "Yeah, but..." remarks, too shocked over Julie's news to hear any message of hope.

Later that night was our monthly meeting of FEMALE and as chapter leader it would be my job to inform the 60 or so attendees who didn't already know about Julie and set in motion our official support network. While our kids stayed at home with the dads, we women converged on the lower south wing conference room of Mission Hills Church, a megabuilding on the corner of Orchard Road and University, where we set up folding chairs in a large circle, trying to avoid the posts that held up the low ceiling.

Our Highlands Ranch/Littleton chapter began with 25 women and was nearing the 100-member mark. Douglas County was the fastest-growing county in the United States in the late 90's, attracting young families to Colorado's high-tech mecca, and plenty of former career women were now set loose on the suburban prairie south of Denver as stay-at-home moms.

Like the prairie dogs, coyotes, and antelope trying to survive in the midst of suburban sprawl, these former executives found themselves wondering how in the heck to adjust to spending full days with kids on a tight budget, managing single-handedly while husbands flew away during the week and golfed on weekends, and grasping to maintain their identity as women beyond mothering. FEMALE was our lifeline to sanity. Though we met in a church, the organization was strictly secular, by charter avoiding discussions of politics and religion.

"Okay everyone, let's get started," I said, sitting down in my chair and flapping my papers up and down on my knees. "Since we have a guest speaker tonight, who is going to help us organize our lives" —I waited for the cheers to subside—"let's skip introductions tonight and I'll put most of the announcements in our email minutes. I have some news I'd like to share with everyone. As many of you already know from the email loop and each other, Julie found out yesterday that she has breast cancer."

I waited for gasps and whispers to sweep the circle like "The Wave" at a baseball game.

"The short version is that she is researching the best doctors in Denver, along with clinical trials and new treatments. If anyone has information for her, you can send it by email. Please don't call her at home, though. Once she has a plan for surgery and chemotherapy, I propose we get the Care Committee involved to help with meals, as well as babysitting and play dates for her son, Cameron. He's only two, so he might not understand what's happening, but he'll need friendly faces and his same old routine."

I nodded at Pat, one of the Care Committee co-leaders, who raised her hand and spoke.

"Since helping Julie might be more long-term than our meal deliveries for moms with new babies, I am passing around a sign-up sheet for anyone who wants to participate on an ongoing basis."

Pat came prepared with a sign-up sheet for name, phone, email, and "willing to...." duties. Heads nodded in agreement, pens poised to start volunteering. I pointed toward Julie's sweatshirt on a table off to the side of the room and explained my intent. "So please sign the sweatshirt after the meeting if you haven't already."

Then I introduced our cheerful guest speaker woman who switched gears to invigorate us to organize our files, utilize one central desktop or wall calendar, and follow other handy tips to manage our households, husbands, and kids' activities. As she spoke, everyone listened intently. Julie's sign-up sheet traversed the circle, nearly everyone adding her name—even three visitors who decided to join on the spot—each of us thankful in our own private hearts that we could be of service, yet guilty with relief that we weren't on the receiving end, like Julie.

Wednesday and Thursday I rode a rollercoaster of tears, worrying how Julie was coping, wondering what she was thinking, projecting how hard she would fight to survive, reluctant to call her and ask. Friends in FEMALE stepped up within days to answer Julie's email requests for physician recommendations and notable treatments. I forwarded an email from *my* mother who recommended her own local gynecologic oncologist who believed in aggressive treatment and helped her survive stage-four ovarian cancer.

Friday I bought a gallon of paint.

Life is short and precious, I was thinking as I drove to The Great Indoors store at Park Meadows Mall while Wil was at preschool. *Do not waste another moment without color! Paint at least one wall periwinkle! White walls are not about resale value anymore,* defying Scott's argument against colored walls. While I watched the man behind the counter squirt exact amounts of blue and magenta into the white base paint, pound on the lid and strap the can into the shaking machine, I continued my internal ranting rationalization. *I plan to live in this house forever! I will not go another day without my periwinkle wall!*

So on Saturday morning, October 10, 1998, I woke up early, determined to paint my tall bedroom wall. I had a morning's reprieve from mothering while Wil played in the cul-de-sac with the two girls from next-door-north. They doted on Wil and he adored them in return, better than sisters. Smiling at their silliness, I picked up two overdue library books from Wil's floor. As I walked back to my bedroom to begin paint preparations, I set the books on the top stair so I would remember later to return them to the library

Scott was downstairs, logged in remotely to work on the computer in our main-floor office. Whistling, whiz-kid workaholic that he was, my husband wanted to check on his software projects that morning. I didn't want to interrupt him to ask for help moving furniture or give him a chance to talk me out of my painting. If he dared, I would threaten to paint all four walls plus the ceiling.

I dragged our unmade queen-size bed into the center of the room and stretched several old sheets over the carpet. On the west wall of windows, I raised the white fake-wood blinds to reveal a cloudless turquoise sky over Colorado's Front Range and foothills. The three largest "fourteeners" — Pikes Peak, Mount Evans and Long's Peak — were already snowcapped. As a rare Denver native in the midst of so many transplants, I considered these *my* mountains and felt personal pride in how stunning they looked as backdrop to the endless gray rooftops and short young trees of Highlands Ranch. Every day I wondered what weather would pour over those peaks, and each evening I stopped to watch as they became black silhouettes and played second string to the sunset.

After blue-taping the baseboard and cutting in all of the corners, I opened my gallon of periwinkle. I cranked the soundtrack from *Boys on the Side,* humming and singing along, memorizing all the words without realizing it. Each song seemed written for Julie.

The CD was playing for a second time and I was half done rolling on periwinkle paint, standing on the aluminum ladder five rungs up, when Scott came into the room. Cupping a bowl of Total cereal in both hands, he sat on the bed. "I think I just had a seizure," he said.

"What?" I asked, looking down from the ladder as if out of my body. "What are you talking about?"

"I think I just had a seizure," Scott repeated, pushing his glasses sideways to rub his eyes. Then between slow bites, chewing, he explained. "Something really strange just happened. I was on the computer, you know, and all of a sudden my right hand wouldn't move the mouse. I was telling it to, and it wouldn't. I felt kind of dizzy, so I went to the kitchen for a drink. I looked at the faucet, then at the cupboard, and I didn't know how to get a glass of water. So I just stuck my head under the faucet. And then it passed, and I got myself of bowl of Total. I think I'm okay now. But it seemed like a seizure."

Still on the ladder, I dove into denial. "No way. You've been drinking how many cups of coffee this morning on an empty stomach? That's probably what made you dizzy." I was thinking, *even though Scott is ambidextrous...right-hand, left-brain, hand not moving...that was a brain thing*.

"Hmmm...I don't know," he answered.

I had swiftly discounted his alarming experience, not having the guts to analyze it further. *If I stop painting now, I might never finish*, I thought. Part of me wanted to jump off the ladder and circle him with my arms, or have him hold me and tell me it was nothing. The rest of me couldn't move. I could only grip the ladder with one hand, balancing the weight of my dripping paint roller with the other, and try to keep breathing. I noticed that thick fuzzy dust coated the ceiling fan blades, slow-spinning from the breeze, like my mind.

Silent and alone, Scott ate his cereal, brown head bent, until it was gone and he slurped the last of the milk from the bowl's rim. "I'm going to lie on the couch for awhile," he said and disappeared downstairs. On my CD player, the Indigo Girls gave way to Stevie Nicks, who demanded "I need someone to *stand* by me, just one time." Now I didn't know if she was singing for Julie or Scott, or for me.

I allowed myself one numb thought as I climbed down to soak my roller in more periwinkle. *All week I've been crying about Julie. But if something is wrong with Scott...* I couldn't even finish my own silent sentence. I did finish painting my wall.

A few hours later, tools and furniture back in place, paint drying, Scott and Wil cuddling on the couch watching *Toy Story* yet again, I went to the library to return Wil's overdue books and pay the 50-cent fine. I ran into my friend Kathy Matsey on the shady sidewalk outside the strip-mall library. Her blue eyes glowed behind her blue eyeglass frames, perched on her adorable pixie nose that I covet. I met Kathy for the first time at a FEMALE Christmas party at Julie's house. Kathy and Julie met at swimming lessons for their boys.

"I painted my wall today," I said, one periwinkle fan to another. "And, well, Scott is feeling kind of strange today." I went on, changing my tone. "He had something strange happen this morning where his right hand wouldn't move for a minute, even though he was telling it to. I think he was having a caffeine buzz, that's all. He's lying down now, taking it easy."

Kathy was the first person with me on this cancer-caregiver trip I didn't even know yet was coming. She had her suspicions, but allowed my denial for now. I felt a certain comfort to tell Kathy about Scott that day; she would become an indispensable confidante on my journey.

Scott's second episode happened on a Friday night, October 23, two weeks after the "too much coffee" day, when Scott and two buddies went out for beers on Old South Gaylord Street. I picture a dark, smoky nightclub full of yuppies in denim shirts and khaki pants, sipping from bottles of Fat Tire. I just can't picture what types of women were there. A guys-night-out was a rarity. Scott knew Kevin since high school—they roomed together some during and after college and Kevin was in our wedding. Kevin recently returned from a long stint in Japan teaching English to children and wishing a Japanese woman would fall in love with him. Scott worked with Alex at Lockheed Martin Aerospace, both of them as subcontractor computer programmers.

After three beers in as many hours, Scott felt dizzy but not drunk. Kevin and Alex were busy scoping chicks and Scott didn't want to ruin their fun. Not a big talker anyhow, his silence didn't seem out of place. Scott sat on a bar stool thinking *Have I become a three-beer lightweight...or is this THAT?* He sat there waiting, listening to trivial bachelor banter until his dizziness passed.

Long after midnight, feeling somewhat stable, Scott stood, said "Later" and walked alone to his white Geo Tracker parked down the block. Seatbelt in place, he started the engine and used his left hand to place his right on the stick shift. Scott drove the ten miles home to Highlands Ranch, never removing his hand until he pulled into our garage. His hand wasn't numb and he could move his arm just fine. But if he had let go of his grip in the dark, he would no longer have known where his hand was.

Scott kept Friday's episode a secret, but on Monday made an appointment with a doctor, any doctor, just a doctor he found in the insurance-coverage notebook. Scott never established a primary care physician, not in the two and half years since we moved back to Denver from Tennessee. He confessed at the dinner table to making the appointment, trying to look nonchalant with his left thumb wiping the condensation on his water glass.

"The doctor didn't have an opening for two more weeks, but that's fine. I told them it wasn't urgent," Scott said in response to my exasperated expression. "It's just a pinched nerve or something like that."

Wil pushed his peas around the plate and looked from Scott to me, as if trying to gauge the truth. Referring to our recent family trip in September, he said "I wish we were still in Disney World."

Still clinging to the safety of denial and ignorant of Scott's second seizure, I tried to overlook the implications of his appointment and just swallow my salad. I suppose I knew in my gut the big change was closer. It's like the weeks after conception where it's too soon for a pregnancy test so you stock up on those supplies and you don't listen when your body whispers, *You aren't going to need those for awhile.*

A few days before Halloween, I took Julie to her first chemotherapy appointment. She opted for a then-controversial clinical trial that would postpone a mastectomy and instead deliver a new drug first, aiming to shrink the tumor before surgery and preserve as much breast as possible. A tiny titanium clip was inserted into the tumor to mark where it started. I was surprised Julie asked *me* to take her to chemotherapy instead of another of her close friends or her husband. Was it the good luck of my mom's twelve-year survival of cancer, that I would be a quiet companion, or was she spreading out requests of each friend? Always practical, Julie said she didn't want Tim to take any time off work to go with her. No matter what, I was honored.

From not witnessing my mom's cancer treatment (she insisted I finish my last year at college), my mind was stocked with horror stories about nausea, hair loss, and nurses who couldn't find a vein. I never went to mom's chemotherapy, so my mind filled in the blanks.

You have to understand: Julie was facing *my* worst fear. I was twenty-one when my mom was diagnosed, she age forty-one, and ever since, I was convinced it would happen to me. You see, I just *knew* it was genetic, despite the fact that none of our vast matriarch of Irish-immigrant relatives ever fought ovarian cancer. My genes felt doomed, despite the fact that it was my sister who looks like Mom with their brown hair and eyes, and skin that tanned. I, on the other hand, with my honey blond hair, blue eyes, and all the other recessive genes, am the one who inherited my mom's same droopy left eye that winks when we smile, the same thin lips, and the same love of Fiestaware plates. Plus my dad swore I scolded and summoned my son in the exact same voice as Mom. "Scary," he'd say, shaking his head and pretending to shudder. I was becoming my mother! Except that she never had trouble getting pregnant. It took me six rounds of an ovary-stimulating drug called Clomid to get pregnant with Wil, but nothing I tried after Wil was born ever helped bring him a sibling. A Chinese herbalist (who failed to reverse my infertility but did cure my springtime hay fever) once tried to ease my irrational expectation of cancer by holding my gaze and my hands, saying, "You are *not* your mother." She offered a sliver of hope I couldn't accept, and so in 1998 I was obstinate in believing that someday a doctor would tell me, "You have cancer."

I thought sure ovarian cancer would strike me, and I was equally sure the odds were I'd crumble, too chicken to fight, much less win.

Then I found myself witnessing Julie face cancer with resolute courage. Already she was a heroine in my eyes. That first day of her chemo, I was scared on Julie's behalf, but I didn't want to scare her. I suggested bringing along a few snacks for her stomach. We agreed she would drive there and I would drive home.

Chemo had changed a lot in a decade. First was a brief appointment in the doctor's office, him behind his big oak desk, asking Julie did she have any last-minute questions? She did. I have no recollection of taking notes in her spiral notebook, but Julie told me later how the pages of answers I wrote down for her were invaluable as she tried to remember everything the doctor had said.

We then walked into the chemo room, cozy with soft chairs and blankets, and other women in headscarves hooked up to IVs who smiled and welcomed Julie as newcomer. Julie held my hand, just a few tears in her eyes, while the gentle nurse connected an IV needle through a plastic mediport that a week before was surgically implanted under the skin of Julie's right upper arm. She was wearing the white "We love you, Julie" sweatshirt, which she and her mother had altered by cutting a hole in the armpit so the IV could reach her port. "That wasn't so bad," Julie said to the nurse. She talked to her fellow cancer patients while I sat by her side like a shadow, reading a magazine for the duration of her chemo drip, offering Oreos midway through the hour.

No, that wasn't so bad, I thought. In the dim, enormous parking garage, I was shocked when Julie approached the driver's side of her SUV, keys in hand, and said she felt good enough to drive home. After a quick stop at the King Soopers pharmacy for her anti-nausea meds, she dropped me at my house.

That night while watching the ten o'clock news in our family room, I told Scott how impressed I was with Julie's attitude. "Cancer just didn't look that scary today," I said. "I was amazed and so relieved for Julie. She even drove home."

"Here, let's watch the lotto drawing and if we win big, we'll split it with Julie," Scott joked, oblivious to the significance of my day and Julie's bravery. As an early birthday present to himself, he rushed to Safeway before dinner to buy 33 lotto tickets in time for the drawing, along with a gallon of milk.

"Hey, we won!" he laughed after the numbered balls rolled onto the screen and he scanned the lotto printout. "On one row at least. We didn't get all six, but we win something with four."

As it turns out, we won $40, a whopping seven-dollar profit. Since it wasn't the jackpot, sharing half with Julie didn't even occur to us. But still, it *was* winning. The odds of winning four out of six numbers in the Colorado Lottery are 1 in 556; the odds of winning all six are 1 in 5,245,786. The odds of a man getting a brain tumor are 1 in 171. Scott didn't know any of those odds back then, but he always said, "You gotta play to win."

The day after winning the lotto our neighbors next-door-south decided *not* to move. Diane and Scott (he said to call him Scoot) had been entertaining a job offer that would mean moving to Illinois.

"The guy called me today," Scoot said as we stood in their driveway watching our boys chase each other on the grass. "He wanted an answer, now or never. It just didn't feel right, so I said 'No' and I'm so relieved. It just wasn't right."

"Well thank goodness for us you're staying!" I said hugging Diane and wanting to dance, remembering the day that we met.

When we were house-hunting in March 1996, Desert Willow Way was the last street we saw, a long curved block still under construction. Scott drove twenty-two hours straight through from Tennessee to Denver to make sure I didn't jump the gun and buy a house without him. I telephoned him with excited updates on potential homes all week that I'd been in Denver doing reconnaissance. On that Sunday morning, Scott and I had already walked through several home models in various stages of construction when we found *our* house.

Walking through the open studs on bare plywood floors, we fell in love with the ten-foot ceilings, the curved arch between living and dining room, the big kitchen that opened onto the family room with its fireplace, the mountain views, and the large walkout basement. We only wished the house had a full front porch.

As we wandered back to the front yard with the realtor, we saw a young couple with a new baby walking through the frame of the house next door. The woman was a brunette beauty in running shorts and a t-shirt, and the man was a tall freckled redhead wearing a button-up oxford and Levis. I asked the woman from the builder's office who was speaking to our realtor, "By any chance is that woman's name Diane?"

"Why, yes it is. How did you know?" she replied. "They just bought that house."

"I went to broadcast-news summer camp with her one week back in high school. We both attended Colorado State, but I never saw her again. Wow, now we could be neighbors." I breathed, in awe of synchronicity. "Scott, we *have* to buy this house. We'll already know our neighbors."

"What are the odds of that?" Scott laughed, "Small world."

So we stepped over construction debris and dirt clods to introduce ourselves, and Diane recognized me, too. "Oh my God, Shelly!" She gave me a hug, saying, "This is my husband, Scott."

"This is *my* husband, Scott," I replied with a grin.

Over the next two years we became close friends and spent countless happy afternoons on *her* big front porch, watching our sons grow up. Her first son, Drew, and her second son, Noah, born a year after we moved in, were like little brothers to Wil. We put a gate in our shared side fence so the kids could run back and forth between backyards. To think of Diane leaving had just been too sad, and now I didn't have to worry. She was staying. What luck!

October had been my month of denial about Scott. Taking Julie to chemo and witnessing our friends swirl their feminine intelligence and energy around her began to heal for me a long-standing fear about cancer. Winning four numbers in the lottery passed in a flash but our next-door neighbors not moving was a big prize. In retrospect, I now know, the Universe blessed me with a grace period to sleep well beneath my new periwinkle wall and reflect on my good fortune.

Like textured walls needing second coats of paint, it took one more of Scott's seizure-like episodes before I *knew* that not only was life about to change, but I would never return to a white-wall existence. When I woke up to reality in November, I was primed to pay attention to the moments that mattered.

The big question is whether you are going to
be able to say a hearty yes to your adventure.
—Joseph Campbell

3
D-Day (Denial Ends with Diagnosis)

My denial ended on Monday, November 1. Scott left for work that morning by seven, as usual, in his suit and tie—his business-dad outfit as Wil always said. Wil was watching *Little Bear* on Nickelodeon while I caught up on incoming email. "You've got mail" chimed AOL.

A friend in Tennessee sent me a message depicting a guardian angel typed in Courier X's and O's. I marked it unread so I could reply later. But was it really an omen?

Feeling restless, I called Scott at work. I wouldn't usually bother him at work on a Monday morning but something kept urging me to dial the phone. No answer. Thirty minutes later, after reading more email and paying bills, I tried calling again; no answer. I made macaroni and cheese with frozen peas for lunch, getting Wil's backpack and snack together for afternoon preschool. Scott must be at lunch, I thought. At 12:15, I went back to my office phone, pushed redial, and he answered.

"Hey, how are you doing?" I asked, "How's your Monday?"

"It happened again," he said, and I knew what he meant. "I was in the cafeteria for lunch. All that stainless steel for the trays to slide across—I couldn't focus on it. I couldn't count out the money. I could hardly walk back to my office."

"Oh, shit," I said, glad Wil was in the family room. "Get your butt home. I am taking you to the walk-in clinic. Can you drive?"

"I think so," he said. "Let me close down my computer and I'll be home in 20 minutes."

I hung up the phone. "Time for school, Wil," I said, trying to sound cheery. I was calculating how long it would take me to drive the few miles to Little Luke's Preschool, wondering whether Scott would be home when I got back. We'd have about three hours to go to the doctor before I would have to pick up Wil again.

"Let's get in the car, kiddo," I said, scooping up Wil's backpack and shuffling him into the garage, my hand on his back. I poked the open button for the garage door, impatient while Wil climbed in the back of our Civic so I could strap him into his car seat.

Drop-off complete, I was back home in a blur, confident Wil hadn't caught on to my urgency. Scott's Tracker sat on the right side of the driveway. I found Scott sitting in the family room, now wearing his Levi's. He looked up at me with a grim smile, and all I said was, "Ready?"

Outside again, I got into the driver's seat. Scott leaned back, began repeating what happened that morning. I wound east and uphill through our suburb, listening without looking at him, as if part of me was already in the future. Ten minutes and three stoplights later, we came to the clinic.

The physicians of the new walk-in clinic in Highlands Ranch were listed in our insurance book as accepting new patients for family practice. I saw a young woman doctor in September for an annual check-up and liked her direct style, her openness to my questions. If it hadn't been for that, I would not have known where to take Scott. Instead, I felt sure this place would give us some answers. (Somewhere in the universe, I'm certain, a chime ting'd to keep track of good luck.)

The nurse who checked Scott in was Doug, a wiry young man who chatted about his wife being ready to deliver their first baby soon. After blood pressure and weight measurements in a closet-like room, we went into the expansive triage room. Another man was finishing his ankle x-ray, but otherwise it was a quiet afternoon at the clinic; we had the staff's full attention.

Our assigned doctor came into the room and shook our hands. She was a petite woman with long brown hair that wasn't styled. Not the doctor I'd seen in September, but also in her early thirties or younger, it seemed like this whole walk-in clinic was run by brand new doctors. First test, safety pins poked up and down Scott's arm. Blood draws to test for low blood sugar and who knew what else. She asked many questions, taking notes, and Scott related the episodes of October and offered his own diagnosis of a pinched nerve. That's when I first heard about Scott's beer-night episode.

"Why didn't you tell me?"

"I didn't want you to worry," he said. "Besides, I made an appointment that Monday."

The doctor shrugged aside our argument and concluded, "It doesn't seem like a nerve path. Let's send you for an MRI. And until we find out more, no driving."

In fact, the notes the doctor made in Scott's chart said "Suspect multiple sclerosis or brain mass." That she didn't share her suspicion was a good thing. No news is good news...that is, until you get the news.

Scott didn't return to work the next morning. I sent a short email to a few friends and cousins living in Denver: "Scott is having an MRI of his head today. We don't know what's wrong, but please keep us in your thoughts. I'll keep you posted."

I asked my next-door neighbor, Kathy Wucherpfennig, if she could take care of Wil for the afternoon, if he could play with Rachel and Andrea. I gave Kathy a brief explanation of our doctor's visit and she said yes, of course. Then we drove to Swedish Hospital. The same Swedish where my mom went through chemotherapy and surgeries. The same hospital where, when I was two years old, I had surgery to repair a leaking artery in my tiny right thigh. My mom once told me the story of leaving me alone in the hospital. She would have been twenty-two back then.

"I had to leave. In those days, they didn't let anyone, not even the mother, stay past visiting hours. I was feeling so guilty, so awful about leaving you there. You stood up in your little hospital gown and screamed, 'Don't leave me alone!' but I had to go. I didn't want to. They wouldn't let me stay. I was too young to think of asserting myself." My mom's voice could hardly say the words out loud, her anguish thirty years later still piercing her heart.

"It's okay, Mom," I had said, putting my arms around her shoulders. "I survived, didn't I?" My adult self was over it, but in the coming months of Scott's treatment I wondered if my two-year-old energy was still stuck in that hospital, panicking with separation anxiety.

On the way to Swedish Hospital, I asked Scott to predict his MRI outcome. "What do you think it will show?"

"It'll be nothing," he lied. "We'll be back to more tests." What he couldn't say out loud, not yet, was that he was damn sure it was going to be something. Something big.

"I guess it's like Schrödinger's cat," he added. "We won't know til we know."

To be or not to be? That is Hamlet's question. We asked Schrödinger's question instead. *Is the cat dead or alive?* In his 1933 Nobel-Prize-winning thought experiment, scientist Erwin Schrödinger asks us to imagine a cat locked in a box. Also inside the box are a radioactive atom and a vial containing a deadly poison. If the atom decays, it triggers a hammer to smash the vial, releasing the poison to kill the cat. Until we open the lid of the box, we cannot know if the atom has decayed or not, thus whether the cat is dead or alive. The potential exists for either situation — until the box is opened.

Will the MRI show something in Scott's brain or not? Does a brain have a disease when it has its first symptom? When its image is captured on an MRI? When the radiologist sees the image and writes a report? When you hear the diagnosis? When your mind believes the diagnosis? (How ironic is this that the brain can and must contemplate its own fate?)

During the MRI, I sat alone in the small waiting room listening to the pounding clatter of the machine through the walls and ignoring a soap opera on the TV hung from the ceiling. Scott's keys and coins were in my pocket, his wallet in my purse, his wedding ring on my thumb. He had to empty his person of anything metal due to the magnet's 15,000-gauss force resonating inside the machine, 30,000 times stronger than the Earth's own ambient magnetic field of 0.5 gauss. Metal objects could become missiles, credit cards could be erased. I would have emptied my own pockets to be able to go into the technician's room and see what they were seeing, real-time. On the other hand, I'm glad I wasn't allowed.

In about forty minutes, the MRI was done. On our way out, the technician told us, "It could be a few days before you hear from your doctor. She'll give you a call."

We drove home in silence. Picked up Wil from Wucherpfennig's house. At four o'clock the phone rang. The primary care doctor said, "We have your MRI report back. Can you come into the office right now?"

Obviously, you can get good news by phone, but bad news is delivered face to face. Trying to be nonchalant for Wil's sake, I called my neighbor. "Can you keep Wil again? We have to go back to the doctor."

It took so long to drive to the clinic that afternoon. We hit every red light, delayed, delayed, delayed. "Shit, shit, shit," I kept saying, trying to drive straight, stop at the lights, and not start crying, not yet.

Scott put his hand over mine on the gear shift, "It'll be okay," he said. "It'll be what it is." He was thinking, *No matter what the doctor says my life will never be the same after today.*

We held hands as we walked into the clinic, again deserted in the afternoon. Doug took us to a back hallway, past triage, turned left, end of the hall, last door on the left. "She'll be with you in a minute," he said, as he tucked Scott's chart on the door.

"Do you think they stuck us way back here in case we start screaming?" I tried joking, actually wondering if the news would make me scream.

Scott sat on the exam table and I sat in the chair, facing the door. Such a small room, I was thinking, seeming narrow enough for my hands to push out on both walls, left to right, as if reality was already squeezing in. We didn't talk. I kept clicking my ballpoint pen, poised over my brand new five-subject spiral notebook, and I turned to the third blank page, as if leaving room for a title and preface. It's a habit I have with all my new notebooks.

The doctor opened the door, stepped in and leaned back against it, as if reluctant to enter the room. Scott got off the table and stood up beside me, his hand on my shoulder. I wanted to laugh, she looked so young and scared. Then I wanted to throw up.

"The technician called me today, right after your MRI. He said, 'Did you know this gentleman has a large mass on his brain?' I'm glad he called—they don't usually take the initiative. I haven't seen the films myself or the radiologist's report, but I've called a neurosurgeon who can see you tomorrow morning. Call his office first thing, and they will get you right in. Before you go, you'll need to pick up the films at Swedish, in the Radiology file room."

I didn't scream. We didn't cry, not in front of her. My inner executive knew business came first. I took notes. "What do you think it is?" a stoic Scott asked.

Scott's new primary care physician didn't want to worry us in advance that Scott's "mass" could be the worst type of tumor. Even with an MRI image, nobody can say for sure what the mass is until the neurosurgeon delivers a biopsy slice on a slide for the pathologist to examine. We didn't know then that the radiologist wrote on his initial report: "Impression: Probable glioblastoma, left parietal occipital brain, with extension towards the corpus callosum, and probable extension across the posterior corpus callosum."

"Well, I don't know. The neurosurgeon can show you the MRI and tell you more."

That was all she would say, but then she gave us her pager number, offering immediate access to her, day or night. She printed it herself on my notebook page, to be sure it was correct. It felt like a special hall-pass given only to favorite students. That's when we began calling her by her first name.

So we knew that much. I have to believe it was the appropriate amount of knowledge for us at that moment. A large mass in Scott's brain was telling us, "En garde! Your new life has just begun."

SHIT.

"I shouldn't be driving," I said as we got in the car. Tears had begun. My hands were shaking. But what was I going to do, spend the next nine months crying in the parking lot of the walk-in clinic? I had to drive—from now on. I pulled out of the parking lot, heading west into the sunset.

It's a grand sight near the intersection of University and Highlands Ranch Boulevard, with all of Metro Denver and the Front Range in view. My entire life was laid out on the plains like clothes on a bed—from our home in the rolling suburbs below, to the four Park Lane Towers by Washington Park a few blocks from my growing-up house, to the cluster of skyscrapers downtown where Scott and I lived before getting married, to the peaks above Fort Collins, one-hundred miles to the north and eleven years in the past when I met Scott on my birthday, the last semester of college. The brown cloud of pollution and pre-winter rush hour was settling over the city. The sun and my heart were sinking behind the mountains.

I handed Scott the cell phone and dictated Kathy's phone number. He dialed, then gave it back to me. I asked Kathy if Wil could stay a bit longer. "Yes, it's bad news, but can I please tell you later? We need to call our family and have them come over in person."

When we got home, just ten minutes later, it was dark.

During the worst of all my crises, friends appeared.
Since then, the first thing I do is ask for help.
—*Paulo Coelho*

4

Party Time

Knowing I needed both hands on the wheel for the rest of the drive, I waited until I parked the car in our garage and we were inside to call my mom and dad. "Mom. It's me. Bad news. The doctor called us in to tell us the MRI results and she said Scott has a large mass on his brain," I kept talking, not giving her a chance to respond, though with her quick intake of breath I knew she was hearing me. "She made an appointment for us with a neurosurgeon tomorrow morning.

"Can you come over right now?" I asked, steeling my voice to get through the logistics. I would have preferred giving her our news in person, but I needed my parents to pick up the MRI films for our appointment in the morning. Swedish Hospital was halfway between their house and ours.

Scott called his dad, then his sister, Amie, saying the same thing both times. "We have something we need to talk about. It's important and we need you to come over tonight. No, we'll explain when you get there."

Everyone arrived within the hour; they all had thirty-minute drives across town. We answered the front door with solemn tear-swollen faces and asked them to come straight to the family room. Amie and her husband, Lance, and Scott's dad, Bill, sat on our couch. Amie leaned into Lance, holding hands with Bill. My mom and dad sat on the big chair and ottoman. I hid the big envelope of MRI films behind the door of my office, unopened. Scott and I already agreed not to look, knowing our untrained eyes would not know how to interpret the images. Moreover, we weren't ready to know how big of a mass we were dealing with. Tomorrow would be soon enough for details like that.

Scott and I stood up facing our family, with our backs against the half-wall separating us from the kitchen sink.

Scott took everyone through his symptoms of the past month, concluding with the day's MRI and news from the doctor. They all just sat there and gulped, tears welling up in their eyes, being strong for us. Bill stood up and hugged Scott. "We better call your mom," he said, his gruff voice breaking and catching in his throat.

Scott's mom was in Palm Desert, California, beginning a kitchen renovation on a condo that would become their winter getaway. She and Bill drove the seventeen hours to Palm Desert only the week before, and she planned to stay all winter. Bill flew home the day before to keep building custom homes. My parents had been visiting my sister in Cincinnati, also flying home on Sunday. It was as if the gods made sure most of our family was in town to get the bad news.

One day years later while walking our poodle-mix dogs, Maggie and Mia, around Crown Hill Lake by her house, I asked Scott's mom if she remembered that phone call. "Of course I do, every detail," she said, scoffing at the idea she could possibly forget. Her grip tightened on the leash and she didn't look at me, but straight ahead as if focusing on that night alone in California.

"When I answered, Scott said he had something important to tell me, then another call came in and he put me on hold. I thought 'oh no, they're getting a divorce.' But of course, it was much worse than that."

My brain skipped a step wondering why she guessed at divorce, but I was more interested in what else she would say, so I never asked.

"I couldn't believe it. My kitchen cabinet doors were laying all over the patio, ready to paint, and I had to find Maggie a pet carrier for the plane."

Linda's voice raised and her pace quickened at the memory. "I had to go to Petsmart. I couldn't find the right size carrier for the airplane, and nobody would help me. I was standing at the counter, saying 'this is an emergency!' I was shaking, and I couldn't drink enough water. I drank bottles and bottles of water."

It was one thing for my husband to have a brain tumor, but if it had been Wil—I often found myself thinking—could I have coped? For Linda, even with her son an adult, it was overwhelming to think of him facing brain surgery. Theirs was a never-been-sick-in-my-life kind of family with no experience facing cancer, like my family had. Linda flew home the very next morning after our phone call, with her faithful companion Maggie in tow. I think of Maggie's white downy fur, her soulful dark eyes, and her cheerful pink tongue offering solace all the way home on the plane and every day and night after, and I know Maggie's presence made a difference.

Bill picked his girls up at the airport and drove straight to the neurosurgeon's office. They arrived minutes after our appointment ended (my parents came with us to take notes and help us ask questions), and we ran into them at the revolving doors of the medical building. Scott gave Linda a hug without words. He looked so tall holding her, and Bill leaned in to support them both. For several minutes, they didn't let go.

The neurosurgeon we met on Wednesday didn't tell us he thought the tangerine-sized tumor was malignant. He explained that surgery was needed to drain the fluid-filled cyst and remove as much mass as possible, gaining a sample for pathology to determine its type. It's a good thing we hadn't looked at the MRI at home because when I first saw the film on his wall, I thought the big rounded X of white ventricles in the center of his brain was the tumor. Actually, his tumor was off to the side, looking like the crescent moon when you can still see the full outline. We saw the black, fluid-filled cyst edged by a lower crescent of white cottage cheese that was the tumor mass itself.

Brain surgery was scheduled for Saturday. Suddenly I wanted everyone who ever knew Scott to know what was happening. I wanted their prayers, though I couldn't say then I believed prayers worked, absolutely, for sure. Mostly, I didn't want us to face brain surgery alone. My inner technical writer teamed up with my heart to send out this email, like laying out ground rules:

Subj: Scott Vickroy needs your prayers
Date: 11/4/98 9:56:41 PM Mountain Standard Time

Dear Everyone,

Hope you're sitting down. Just this week, Scott was diagnosed with a large brain tumor in the left rear portion of his brain. In the past three weeks, he had three "episodes" of right-sided "malfunctioning" and disorientation, each lasting about an hour but getting worse. Monday we went to a great walk-in emergency clinic, had an EKG and blood work to rule out the easy stuff, then we went on Tuesday (yesterday) for an MRI. Within a few hours, we had the results back that showed a tumor. We met with a neurosurgeon today for explanation. It appears to be the size of a small tangerine, a round cyst filled with fluid, as well as another tissue area adjacent. It is located in the parietal region of the brain, which happens to be the "silent region"—and that explains the overall lack of symptoms. The size of the tumor is causing significant swelling, however. The episodes are seizures, which are now being controlled by some medication called Dilantin.

The good news is that the location IS operable and the doctor is confident. We've heard from more than one source that he's the best and we were impressed with his professional manner and good listening skills. We are breathing again after a long and scary Tuesday night.

Although we haven't received final confirmation, surgery to biopsy and remove the tumor will probably be on Saturday. Until the biopsy is done, we don't and won't know any more details as to the type of tumor or follow-up treatment needed, but will keep you posted as well as possible. The surgery will last 4-6 hours, followed by 4-5 days in the hospital, then recuperation at home.

Wil is doing pretty well, although his empathy vibes are picking up what's happening. We've told him that Daddy has an owie in his head and that the doctors are going to get it out and take good care of him. Wil has been staying with our wonderful next-door neighbors on both sides of us, and we're sooooooo so lucky to have both sets of parents, Scott's sister, Amie, and her husband, Lance, plus lots of extended family here to support us, as well as our neighbors, my network of stay-at-home moms, and Scott's coworkers. My sister, Jenéne, is waiting in the wings to fly in from Cincinnati when necessary, maybe for some of the recovery period at home.

We are very concerned that Wil understands he is loved and protected, and want his daily life to continue as normal as possible with preschool on MWF afternoons and play dates with buddies. It's okay for him to be afraid and to cry, since we all might be doing that. Having fun kids to play with will be a great help. When we know more after surgery, we'll let you know what help we need. What we need from everyone now are your prayers and positive energy -- only thinking the best most possible outcomes. Imagine hearing "We got it all—it wasn't malignant." And then imagine old-man Scott talking about this as that strange brain sucker that nearly ruined his 33rd birthday (this Friday 11/6), then gave him a new lease on life. :)

We're exhausted, but hopeful. Please don't call us at home, as we need to conserve our energy. Cards and emails are most welcome. We'll keep you updated. THANKS!

We love you,

Shelly & Scott & Wil Vickroy

p.s. Feel free to pass on this message, or the gist of it, to whomever else you know that we know in Tennessee, Denver, Michigan, wherever. We need all the prayers we can muster.

Next day, we discovered that surgery would be a whole week away, not in two days as we first expected. The neurosurgeon wasn't able to schedule a surgery suite with his choice of team until the following Saturday, which still was a favor to us to squeeze it into a weekend. The squeezing-in made life feel urgent, so it was hard to be patient for seven more days of limbo. What can you do with a grace period? We decided to have a birthday party to fill our house with well-wishers. If it hadn't been his birthday that week, we could have had a "bon voyage to Scott's tumor" party before surgery to fill our house with friends who would be willing enough to dance the limbo.

Subj: Latest Update on Scott
Date: 11/5/98 5:40:16 PM Mountain Standard Time

Hi Everyone,

We have an update on the surgery date. It is NOT this Saturday as mentioned before, but NEXT Saturday, November 14th.

DETAILS: Friday the 13th (my lucky day, really!!) at noon we meet with the surgeon for an hour to hear the complete description about the surgery. At 1 p.m. we go for the Pre-Op, which means physical exam, health history and briefing from the nurses. Saturday morning at 5:30 we arrive at the hospital, 7:30 the surgery begins. It should last 4-6 hours, and then he'll be all better!!!!! Hopefully the tumor will be removed, and the biopsy will have been taken, results read, and we'll know then what the tumor consists of. We'll be in the hospital 4-5 days afterwards.

Why the delay? There were no operating rooms available this weekend, and the surgeon wants to ensure he has the specific team members all together for Scott. We also have to trust that if the doctor doesn't mind waiting 7 more days, neither should we. Turns out he usually doesn't do surgery at all on Saturdays and this is a favor to us. Scott is taking Dilantin for the seizures, which should stabilize him in the meantime, and we'll keep the doctor informed in case we feel he's getting worse.

We are disappointed a little at having to wait, but also trying to view this as a gift of another week to take a breath, collect our thoughts, get organized, and spend time with each other as much as possible, not to mention taking time to build up a huge positive-energy force of prayers and love for Scott, our family, and the doctors, too.

Also, our primary doctor spoke with the neurosurgeon today and gave us some more good news. Because of the location of the tumor, we're expecting that Scott will wake up good as new, with no loss of function.

Thanks for all your love. We ARE getting the vibes, or should we say "brainwaves." And it's nice to get the emails and feel connected. We are still and always will be computer geeks at this house. :)

Love, Shelly

PS - Please come to an open house birthday bash for Scott tomorrow (Friday) night at our house from 6-8 p.m. Scott wants to see everyone he knows to say hello -- and to see the faces of people who will be supporting me and Wil, as well as him. We'd LOVE it if you could come, even for a few minutes.

My sister, Jenéne, debated about a quick trip from Cincinnati to be there for the party, already planning to come for the surgery whenever it was. Lucky for us, Cincinnati is a Delta hub and there were frequent special weekend rates to Denver during that year. I remember our phone conversation. "I can come if you need me to be there," she offered.

"No, I'd rather have you here for Scott's surgery than his birthday party." But less than an hour later, feeling very much like a little sister, I called her back.

"I changed my mind," I said between sobs. "Can you come tomorrow?"

"I am. I already booked my flight," Jenéne replied, and it felt like she hugged me over the phone.

Friday morning, she and Amie ran errands for us, buying helium balloons, some food, soda, beer. It's a family joke that our sisters look more like each other with their dark brown hair and brown eyes than they look like either of their blue-eyed siblings. Something about taking care of us together made them soul-sisters for the first time. Scott and I basked in the sun and their caretaking that afternoon, with Wil still at preschool. Wil was thrilled when they picked him up and he got to introduce both of his aunts.

At six o'clock, a steady stream of people began to arrive, and kept coming and coming. We gave up answering the door and just left it open, looking outside to wonder how far down the street they were parking. Food, presents, drinks, and two extra, unsolicited birthday cakes (cheesecake and chocolate) piled on the tables as our house became full of the people we love. I later found a box of Marie Callender's macaroni and cheese in my freezer that someone stashed. Eyes were red, hugs were prolonged, small groups formed around the main floor with whispers, but laughter too. It was just what we needed. Wil hosted his own party upstairs with all the kids piled into his room and in, under, and on top of his bunk bed, overflowing into the Jack-and-Jill bathroom and guest bedroom.

My friend Sue brought a gray sweatshirt and fabric pens, which we put on the dining room table for people to sign—just like I did for Julie a month earlier. Sue called earlier in the day to get Scott's shirt size, asking for ideas for a design on the sweatshirt. "Does he have any special hobbies or interests?" All I could think of was his computer and who wants that on a sweatshirt? With fabric paint Sue wrote "Friendship Makes a Difference" above bright red, yellow, and blue squares. And around those designs—front, back, upside down—people wrote lots of We love you's, God bless you's, We're with you's, and these positive thoughts and affirmations:

"All our love—anything for you guys!—Julie and Tim

"Soak up all the positive energy sent to you" —Boggs

"P.U. I love you" with an arrow at the armpit, from Amie

"Look back here! [upside down on the back] May your farts smell like roses! I love you , buddy," —Kev

The sentiments, both heartfelt and hearty laughter invoking, were a way to wrap up Scott in the energy of that night and those people, keeping him warm with reminders that he wasn't alone. On the dining room table, alongside the sweatshirt, someone placed a jar and tiny squares of paper, with a sign directing guests to write encouraging thoughts for Scott to unfold during the next days and weeks. With photos taken that night, my cousin sent us a big collage on a poster board as further reminder of everyone who came from near and far to support us that night.

Friends brought birthday gifts: books and some stylish funny hats. Our friends were there in solidarity to say we love you, but I know, in the back of everyone's mind, they were wondering if they'd ever see him again.

Wearing my denim overalls and black turtleneck, laughing when one of my friends showed up in her matching stay-at-home mom's outfit, I wandered from dining room to crowded kitchen, to hallway, to living room, squeezing hands with best friends, dipping into the small talk, receiving encouragement.

"I knew a man who had a brain tumor. They got it all out with surgery and he went back to work two weeks later. He's been fine ever since," said one of our neighbors.

"Our friend, the doctor, said that from what he knows, the type of brain tumor with a fluid-filled cyst is a good kind to have," said someone else. "He also knows your neurosurgeon and said that if he needed brain surgery, that's who he'd go to."

The hopeful attitudes I really needed to hear, regardless of their accuracy. In my mind, only positive statements were allowed—no horror stories. But inevitably one well-meaning party guest broke my rule, assuring me, "No matter what happens, we will be here for you. If the worst should happen, God forbid, we're here for you."

It felt like a stab to my heart. I held up my hand as if shielding myself from her words. "Please don't—I can't even think like that now. The worst isn't going to happen."

"Yes, but if it does, we're here for you."

NO! I felt like screaming. I wanted to say *Stop it!* and shake her shoulders. But I didn't. I just walked away. I spent my energy keeping on a positive face for our guests, not hugging too long else risk bursting the dam of tears. I was Pollyanna personified. I had to be strong. I had to demonstrate to my friends and family that *this* was the way we were going to fight this battle, with strength and positive attitude. And I meant it.

In the end, it was a good, good night. My cousins stayed late to clean up and vacuum, then settle on the couch for a few more minutes of easy company, soft words, lingering hope. We went to bed that night, exhausted but fulfilled. Next night, I sent this email:

Subj: Keeping you posted re: Scott
Date: 11/7/98 9:02:03 PM Mountain Standard Time

Dear Lifesavers,

Thank you so much for your thoughts, prayers and positive energy that you are sending to Scott. We are overwhelmed by the many messages we've received and by the messages that have been forwarded and forwarded some more. We're even receiving messages from people who don't know us, or who've met Scott once, or whom he helped over the phone once. A few messages are coming from overseas, too. I just know that all this love and prayer directed toward Scott (and our family and the doctors) is going to pull him through safely. I envision this protective web of good thoughts now encircling the globe, visibly glowing toward us in Denver and John Glenn up in space wondering what on earth is happening down there. :)

We had a great birthday celebration for Scott on Friday night, filling our house not only with people, balloons, and wonderful presents, but also giving us the gift of your presence. Our house was so filled with positive energy that we all slept very well. Coming downstairs this morning to the 40+ helium balloons and countless presents was like having both Christmas and New Year's Day early. The balloons danced on the ceiling all day by the fireplace.

Please continue keeping Scott in your thoughts all week, imagine the tumor shrinking significantly between now and surgery next Saturday, and send us more energy so we can make it through, day by day. Wil and I both need extra energy from you too, as do our immediate family.

I'll continue keeping you posted if anything changes, but may not be answering many more emails. We are printing every one off and making a big notebook. We've started a scrapbook, too. Lots for Scott to reflect on in his old age someday.

We love you and thank you for your love, too.

Shelly

A half-foot of snow greeted us the next morning. Wil and I rolled and patted a snowman to life in our backyard. Jenéne came out with a camera when we were done. She framed a snapshot for me, of mother and son in the snow, facing each other, tossing handfuls of snow in the air. *Come on, life! You can't stop us now!! We're still gonna make time for joy, dammit!*

One way we used the grace period between Scott's party and his surgery was to schedule a massage to help Scott relax. I drove him to the home of Beth, the same Beth who spoke to Me & Moms on embracing life's changes the day after Julie was diagnosed with breast cancer.

Scott and I stood in Beth's cozy, dim basement, holding hands. After a minute of small talk, Beth said to Scott, "Not only am I a massage therapist, I consider myself a healer. I can work with you to heal yourself, if that's what you wish."

"Of course," Scott laughed, not sure if she was serious. Beth lit a small bundle of sage and herbs (all legal), wafting it around the room as she prayed a blessing over Scott and their upcoming work. While Scott went into her studio, she left me to sit on a couch, where I started a new journal in which to document our personal brain tumor journey (not the doctor appointments). An hour later, they emerged. Scott looked more relaxed.

"Did you get rid of the tumor?" I joked.

"I don't know," he shrugged. "But the massage was nice. Thanks, Beth."

We drove home to wait out the rest of the week and finish getting our affairs in order. We used software to draft a will, a durable medical power of attorney, and a medical directive about life support and do-not-resuscitate orders. Scott said he didn't care and I could decide if it came to that point, but at least we touched the edge of that conversation; we could always revise the documents later if we changed our minds before Scott lost his mind.

We asked our next-door neighbors, Kathy and Diane, to sign the forms as our witnesses. Before signing, Kathy and Diane asked if they could hold our hands and say a prayer, as if cementing a soul-pact to keep loving and praying on each side of our house, with us in between, from that moment forward.

Have you ever had a prayer feel like someone throwing a lasso of love over your roof, anchoring it from one porch to the next, from front yard to back, as if weaving a web of protection? As if cinching down the corners so that the house and everyone in it would be safe, even from acts of God?

We signed the forms ourselves in front of the notary guy at our bank. It felt eerie yet powerful to be so efficient.

On another day before Scott's surgery, I booked my own massage with Beth. By that point my shoulders had moved up to my ears. "My neck is as hard as an oak tree," I observed, while Beth worked out the kinks. She offered a different image.

"It's funny how often we equate an oak tree as the epitome of strength. I'd rather think of myself as a willow, you know, that can bend and sway in the wind."

She continued releasing the stress from my muscles, and I tried to relax under the warmth of the oil and her firm hands, picturing myself like the old weeping willow in my grandmother's back yard. I told myself to book massages more often, for both me and Scott. It was well worth the money. Before I left that afternoon, Beth gave me a bit of advice.

"Don't get swept away caring for Scott," she said. "I can tell you love taking care of people—it gives you energy. But don't go overboard thinking you are responsible for his outcome. Whatever happens to Scott is between him and God. It's none of your business. You're only responsible for your own survival. So take care of yourself. Promise?"

I gave a blithe promise. I couldn't know then how hard it would be to keep.

During that week while driving here and there to get our affairs in order, I heard a new song on the car radio. The song cradled me in a voice so deep and a beat so strong that I could feel it pumping my heart. *Everything's gonna be all right, rock a bye, rock a bye.* I kept the words in my head, especially at bedtime when it was hard to fall asleep, keeping my ears open for everyone else in the house to make sure they were breathing. The song's popularity kept it on the radio so that everywhere I went, I heard Shawn Mullins' personal reassurance over the airwaves, and I chose to believe him.

5
Our Mothers' Dreams

A brown-haired little boy sits up in bed in his starlit room. He looks deep into my mother's eyes, and in his solemn midnight-wide pupils she sees the glint of a laughing old soul looking out. Cicadas are chirping on the lawn below. The cotton-woods crinkle in the wind, tossing moon-glow and shadow puppets on the boy's bedroom walls. He giggles and the cicadas fall silent. Through the open window glides the crescent moon, not large as the sky but toy-size and pale, like a slice of honeydew melon. The crescent's silhouette weaves past the other shadows on the wall, encircled with a hint of full moon. The crescent moon moves gently through the little boy's head, as he sits amid his pillows and pets his soft cotton bunny. Without stopping, but slow like a saltwater wave, the crescent moon reappears above his left ear. It pauses. The little boy smiles as if he's been blessed and sinks back on his pillow, turns over, and sleeps. The moon swoops to the sky. The cicadas sing again.

If you could see what I see in my own mind's eye, that is how you would picture my mother's dream. That is the way I imagined it, instantly and over months and years, adding details and sounds as if her dream were my own. She and I sat on my family room futon as she told me her dream the after-noon after Scott's birthday party.

What Mom actually said was, "I had a dream last night about a little boy, with brown hair and blue eyes," and I knew her dream had been a vision of Scott, not Wil. "The boy sat up in bed and looked straight at me, like an old soul. Then a crescent moon came in through the window and moved through his head. And I knew, I just knew, it was a healing."

"It was a lucid dream," she continued, as if trying to explain or affirm its magic. "It gave me a sense of such peace that I was able to sleep for the first time all week. I just wanted you to know."

Mom hugged me with a kiss to my forehead, choking back tears, shy at sharing her dream like a silly, superstitious omen. Mom is a poet at heart, a writer and artist, with two green thumbs, manifesting as an inner-city kin-dergarten teacher. She raised me reading fairy tales, singing songs, sewing dresses, playing dolls, planting peach pits, sampling after-school classes and summer camps, helping me and my sister search for our gifts and passions.

Twelve years earlier, in 1986, as my sister graduated from college and started her chemical engineering career in Cincinnati and I left for a summer magazine internship in Boston, Mom was diagnosed with stage-four ovarian cancer. Though the symptoms had gone on for years, she learned on St. Patrick's Day that a large tumor was growing inside her. She waited for both of us to embark on our adventures in June before undergoing her hysterectomy, which revealed the cancer throughout her abdominal cavity, including her abdominal aorta. She didn't tell us the extent of her diagnosis. She wanted our lives to continue, though hers had a deadline of less than six months.

In the fall, I returned to college for my senior year at Colorado State University, an hour north of Denver, and Jenéne commuted from Cincinnati to Winter Haven, Florida, learning the intricacies of orange juice engineering. Mom fought for her life with eight rounds of extreme chemotherapy. Dad was her caregiver, never asking for my help or my presence, though buoyed by the help of his and Mom's sisters. Dad drove her to every appointment, spent nights sitting next to her bed in the hospital, and as often as possible, took her on mountain picnics to find wildflowers or watch the snow. Bloodwork in January hinted her cancer was gone. By St. Patrick's Day of '87, a second-look surgery confirmed that none of the cancer remained—she was all clear, everywhere. Her silent, introspective nine months of treatment had succeeded. But how she really survived—in her psyche—was a mystery to me.

I suspect Mom's survival had something to do with paying attention to messages from her soul. And now, a dozen years later, she was sharing a bit of her soul's wisdom with me.

"The greater part of mankind gets its knowledge of God from dreams," said Tertullian, the ancient Christian Latin writer, on the page of Mother's Day week in my 1998 desktop calendar. I would amend Tertullian's words with "… and from our mothers."

That same day, we encouraged Scott's parents, Bill and Linda, to rest at home but come over later for lasagna and cheesecake to celebrate Scott's birthday again. Linda told us about her nap as we sat around our oval wooden table in the kitchen after dinner.

"I was lying there, too tired to sleep. The panic kept coming, wouldn't stop. So I decided to pray, 'God, please give me peace. Send me strength and energy,' and all of a sudden I felt myself growing lighter and lighter. It seemed a voice was saying 'everything is okay,'" Linda shivered, reliving her amazement. "I looked at the clock and it said one-fifteen. I was thinking, in one week exactly Scott's surgery will be over.

"I just know everything is going to be all right," she added, choking up but adamant.

If a mother believes it, then it must be so.

A week later on Saturday, November 14, 1998, Scott and I woke up at 4:30 a.m. and showered together. Mental note: More showers together. At 5:10 we woke up Wil to say goodbye. It was a 40-mile trek from our house in the suburbs to Rose Hospital. At least it wasn't rush hour. My parents stayed with Wil for the early morning until they could deposit him safely with our next-door neighbors. My sister, who'd flown home for the second weekend in a row, came with us in our Honda Civic, a dent in its left rear door mimicking the location of Scott's tumor. Jenéne drove, with Scott in the passenger's seat, and I in the back with Scott's duffel and our backpacks full of books, journals, snacks, and water for the long day.

I saw the crescent moon rising with its faint outline of the full. My heart lurched at recognizing not only my mother's dream but the moon's rendition of Scott's tumor that we'd seen on the MRI films, the curved growth of tissue with a fluid-filled cyst. "Scott, there's our lucky moon," I whispered, leaning forward and squeezing his shoulder. Breathe, breathe, I told myself.

Scott's parents, plus Amie and Lance, met us for the early morning check-in. A young couple holding hands said as we passed from one room to the next, "How lucky. I wish our family could be here today." We went with Scott into a prep room where he donned long, white tight socks and a short cotton gown. We tried to stay lighthearted by taking silly photos, but when the film was developed I noticed that everyone's eyes were red from crying.

Only Linda and I were allowed into the curtained pre-op holding area. By then, Scott was hooked up to an IV, under a sheet on a bed that was cranked at an angle for sitting. The anesthesiologist came in to say hello and find out details of Scott's life, such as Wil's name, so he could talk personally as Scott slipped in and out of consciousness. Scott's fear about the dangers of general anesthesia was relieved when the anesthesiologist told us how he would be using a piece of equipment on loan to the hospital for only that month. It would enable him to control the depth of Scott's sedation with as little drug as possible.

The neurosurgeon came in next, "How are we all doing today?"

"We're good. Did you stay out late partying last night?" asked Scott.

The surgeon held out his hands, palms flat down, "See, not a quiver." It was the single sliver of humor we ever saw in him. "Okay, I'm off to scrub. I'll see you soon." He left after patting Scott's leg and my shoulder. The anesthesiologist followed.

Linda had arranged for a minister from her Presbyterian church, Shepherd of the Hills, to come pray with us. Jane arrived, a tall old woman with a graceful presence. She held both of our hands as she introduced herself. "I find it special to be here today," she said, "My husband had a brain tumor over twenty years ago. He's still living strong." Those words were more memorable to me than her prayer.

It was time for Scott to go. I gave a twist to his wedding band, taped to his finger, practicing our secret handshake the pre-op nurse suggested for after surgery. I gave him a long, tight hug around his neck, crying and whispering, "I love you. I love you." Linda did the same. It was 8:00 a.m. when they wheeled him away. Linda and I left the room, but stopped in the middle of the hallway to hug, both of us sobbing for an instant in shared fear.

"I'm so glad we get along," I said between sobs.

She laughed and looked at me funny. "Of course we do, Shel."

"I mean I'm glad we're not dealing with family dynamics."

We walked together to the hospital's main floor waiting room, which was just one huge lobby at the hospital's front door. There we found Jenéne, Bill, Amie, and Lance waiting for us. "Come on, let's get breakfast" I said, and we took the elevator to the basement cafeteria to put scrambled eggs, donuts, and coffee in our nervous stomachs.

Throughout the day, we waited in a lounge on the same floor as surgery, which the surgeon arranged for us to occupy since it was Saturday. Friends came and went through the day, piling up like extra pillows in the room, bringing us food, laughter, and distraction.

The phone in the waiting room rang at 1:15. It was a nurse saying the surgery had ended and that the surgeon would come speak to us soon. An hour and twenty minutes later, he did. The surgeon was startled to see all the faces. "Is everyone family?" he asked before revealing his report. I said yes, tacitly daring him to send anyone from the room. He looked only at me when he shared the news.

"The surgery went very well. The cyst has been drained, and I sent a frozen section of tissue to pathology. We'll need three to four days for a final report. The brain tumor cells appeared very similar to normal brain tissue, so it was difficult to see the precise edges and I couldn't remove it all."

"I couldn't remove it all" was all I heard, even though I kept writing as he kept talking.

"It is consistent with a tumor type known as an astrocytoma. After we get the pathology report, we'll know for sure what it is and how aggressively it's growing. Then we'll discuss follow-up treatment, such as radiation."

The surgeon looked around the room as if for a reaction. We were silent, all muttering "Thank you." I couldn't think of any questions, so he left. I wrote down some details in my spiral notebook, then pushed through the heavy door into the hallway alone. A few minutes later, Mom joined me.

"Are you okay, honey?" she asked, putting her arms around me and pulling me into a hug.

I was numb, realizing most of Scott's tumor remained in his skull, and wondering What Next. I wasn't sure whether to be happy that Scott had come through the surgery or sad-scared-mad that the surgery was only the first step.

Truth be told from years of hindsight, I was irrationally mad at my mom. I'd spent years being scared of her cancer, unclear how she survived or how long she would live, or if I would get ovarian cancer, too. I hate being scared. And here I was facing cancer again, as a wife, a woman, a mother myself. On the verge of exhaustion already, I didn't know how I was going to cope.

But Mom had given me a hint by sharing her dream, and that was the notion of hope in the midst of a mystery. I wasn't thinking about her crescent moon then, the one I had glimpsed that day before dawn. But over the next nine months, her dream moon became my lucky moon. It reappeared in the sky, waxing or waning, at every next step of Scott's treatment, giving us faith that all shall be well and healing would come.

The only way to live longer is to sleep less.
—*Scott Vickroy*

6
Waiting Room Wondering

I was standing in the hallway outside the waiting room in my mom's embrace when a surgical nurse came round the corner. "Shelly? Scott is awake now and in the recovery room. You can come see him for a few minutes, if you'd like."

I disengaged from Mom with a quick smile and followed the nurse down the hall. She held the heavy door open for me, and I walked into a dim room where Scott lay propped up in a bed. Another nurse by his side fed him ice chips from a paper cup with a plastic spoon, which she handed to me. His arms had IV tubes, his eyes looked sticky and red, and from under the turban-like bandage around his head came another tube hooked up to a machine, which I learned was a drain and the intracranial pressure monitor, or ICP. I held his hand over the metal rails and twisted his wedding ring as my secret entry code. Scott opened his eyes and grimace-smiled.

"How did it go?" he asked me, and I was glad to hear him speak.

"Good. He drained the cyst and sent off the biopsy for a pathology report. We won't know more for a few days. How are you feeling?"

"Like I was hit by a truck. My throat hurts."

"Here, have some more ice chips," I said. He closed his eyes. "So where did you go during surgery," I teased him, referring to our joke that he would have an out-of-body experience.

"Tahiti," he said flatly, opening his mouth for another spoon of ice.

The nurse came back to the bedside. "We'll be transferring Scott to the intensive care unit in a few minutes. Once he gets settled, we'll come find you."

I kissed Scott on the cheek, "See you soon, honey. Sleep if you can and get some rest."

I walked back to the waiting room where family and friends were gathering their coats, books, bags, loitering a little, wondering whether they were excused or needed to stay. "Scott's awake," I said with my last bit of cheerfulness. I could feel myself crashing physically and emotionally, so I sent them home.

While I went to dinner with my parents at a nearby cheap Japanese bistro, Scott's parents went home to rest for awhile but promised to return later. Linda was going to spend the night with me in the ICU waiting room so we could take turns checking on Scott. I don't know what we thought would happen to him overnight, but neither of us wanted to leave him alone.

When I got back to the hospital, Linda had already found a stack of flannel blankets and the least uncomfortable blue vinyl couches where we could stretch out to sleep. "I just saw Scott," she said, then added with a quizzical smile, "He keeps calling me Mommy."

It wasn't clear whether he was saying so to soak up all the mother-love she was there to offer, or if something had happened to his brain in surgery and he might be regressing mentally, permanently. We didn't know whether to laugh or be worried. It didn't occur to us to ask the ICU staff for an answer.

"Your Healing Touch girl is in there with him now," Linda added. "Pam, right?"

"Oh good," I said. "Yes, it's Pam. She'll work on him for an hour or so. I guess I'll get settled."

I went to the women's restroom to take out my contacts and put on my glasses and sweatpants. I took a little pill that my doctor had prescribed for me, saying the Ativan would take the edge off my anxiety and let me sleep, but also let me wake up anytime without feeling groggy. *Better living through chemistry*, I said to myself as I swallowed it with a handful of water from the faucet. Then I walked back to the waiting room to wait for Pam to finish her Healing Touch session with Scott, wondering what she would be able to do.

I knew that Healing Touch could make a difference in Scott's pain tolerance, although I was still trying to figure out how. My sister was first to introduce me to this energy medicine modality after she had taken a Level 1 class. I knew it had something to do with our chakras, those centers of energy—sometimes closed, preferably open—that spin from our feet, knees, sacrum, solar plexus, heart, throat, forehead, and top of our head, connecting us to the universe.

I was open to the concept and curious, so I decided to see for myself whether it was real. For Wil's spring break from preschool earlier that year, he and I visited Jenéne in Cincinnati and had dinner at the home of her friends, Joan and Don, who were scientists, and as Healing Touch practitioners were working their way through five levels of classes and 100 hours of client sessions and case studies to achieve certification from Healing Touch Program. (Healing Touch was developed by a registered nurse and the HT Program is endorsed by the American Holistic Nurses Association.)

After dinner, Jenéne and Wil sat on the floor of the vaulted-ceiling living room under a tall banana tree with a variety of toys and books, thanks to the grandparent-preparedness of our hosts. Don brought out a massage table and set it up in the center of the living room. "Jump up," he said, patting the table.

I was wearing my black turtleneck and blue denim overalls and kicked off my clogs before lying flat, face up, on the table, a pillow under my head. Joan, who is six feet tall, stood on my right and Don stood on my left. They faced each other, holding their palms over and under each other like they were about to play pat-a-cake.

"We're balancing our energy, tuning into each other," Joan explained. "We do this as a team, but it's common to have only one practitioner, too."

As I lay there, listening to Jenéne and Wil chatting, Joan and Don began by putting one palm on the bottom of each of my stocking'd feet, the other on my ankle. Their touch was barely-there light and warm. In a few minutes, their hands moved to ankle and knee, then after a few more minutes their hands were on my knees and hip bones. "This is a chakra connection," Joan said. I closed my eyes, trying to see if I could feel any energy pulsing or moving. I couldn't, but didn't mind imagining it happening anyway.

About twenty minutes into my treatment they moved their hands over my right thigh. "Do you feel that?" Joan asked Don.

"Yes, it's cooler," he said, giving her a curious look. Their hand movements changed to a stitching motion, then a waving or brushing movement. "You've got a leak," he said to me.

"Huh?" I responded, raising my head to see what they were talking about and where. "Oh, that's my scar," I said, putting my head back on the pillow, surprised that they found it because I hadn't said a thing. Then I decided to sit up to watch their movements.

"It keeps popping open," Joan said, her hands seeming to pantomime a drama of surgical sewing, figure-eight drawing, and simple mommy-motions we've all used to mend a boo-boo. "We patch it up, then it bursts another leak. But we're getting it now."

"That's my scar," I repeated. "I've had it since I was two years old. It's a bunch of scar tissue from a surgery I had to fix a leaky artery that I was born with, a hemangioma. I guess it looked like a big bruise all the time. You can feel it," and I motioned for Joan to feel the lump in my quadricep.

"It hurts almost all the time, and gets worse when the weather changes. Wil can't even sit on my lap on that side, most of the time. Back in high school we asked a plastic surgeon if he could fix it so it wouldn't hurt. He said he could only improve it cosmetically, to make the scar less noticeable, but that I'd have to stay off of it for six months to make that work. So of course I didn't bother. I don't care what it looks like. But it's always sore."

"Hmmm," they said together. "Isn't that something. I guess those were the days before they knew about deep-tissue massage." In another minute or so, they took a step back, apparently feeling that my Healing Touch session was over, my leg-leak as plugged as possible.

"Wow, I can't believe you found my scar," I said again. I was so amazed that I hopped off the table and dropped my overalls then and there in a fit of total disregard for my modesty. I hopped right back on the table, pulling my turtleneck down to conceal my undies, saying, "Here, you gotta see this."

Don and Joan laughed, looking startled, and Jenéne and Wil came over to see the scar, too. Everyone inspected the three-inch wide scar intersecting my right thigh. The scar is shaped like an unsmiling mouth with fuller lips than mine, a pencil-eraser size bruise on the left end.

"Well, they went right through the muscle instead of parallel to it," Don said, "No wonder it hurts. There's a lot of scar tissue in there. Well, maybe the Healing Touch will help. Let us know how you feel in a few weeks."

"Yeah, I'll be interested to see." I said, while I hooked up my overalls again, returning to my modest self. We went to the kitchen for dessert, conversation returning to normal everyday things.

Funny thing is, in days, not weeks, I noticed a significant difference in the tightness and tenderness of my scar. I could touch it without wincing and plop Wil on my lap without worry, and the improvement was permanent. It seemed as if Healing Touch had helped. In the months that followed, I asked Jenéne more questions about Healing Touch and learned that it can help with many aspects of healing, including a speedier recovery after surgery. And that is why, when Scott's brain surgery was scheduled, I was convinced I had to find a local Healing Touch practitioner who could help Scott.

Healing Touch Program and the Colorado Center for Healing Touch were both headquartered in Denver then, so when I asked nurse Doug if he could help us find a practitioner, he knew where to start. In a few days, he called me with the name of someone named Carol who lived in Highlands Ranch, plus another woman named Ruth. I left a message on Carol's machine and got through to Ruth and explained the situation, giving her Scott's surgery date.

"I'm sorry, dear," she said, "My grandson is battling meningitis right now and I need to be with him. I'm sure you can find someone else. Call me back if you need another name. And please, tell me you husband's name again. I will pray for him."

It was sometime during the week between Scott's birthday and his surgery that the phone rang, when I had just about given up. It was a young woman named Pam, who said. "I heard you were looking for a Healing Touch practitioner. Can I help you?"

We arranged for her to come over to our house on Friday night, before Scott's surgery, to do a preparatory session and meet us so we could get comfortable with each other. Then she agreed to come to the hospital after surgery. "I can help move out some of the anesthesia afterwards," she suggested.

When she rang our doorbell on Friday night, we had just finished dinner and were sitting around trying not to be nervous. She set up her portable massage table in our bedroom upstairs and worked with Scott for an hour before coming back downstairs alone.

Friday night's session had gone fine. Scott said he felt relaxed for the first time since his diagnosis and expected to sleep pretty well. Jenéne spoke to Pam on her way out and told us that Pam had performed a "Spiral Connection." I don't know what that meant, but it sounded good. I decided to have faith that something good was happening.

And so that surgery-Saturday night, after an hour of waiting, I walked into the ICU and found Pam leaving Scott's darkened room, zipping her parka.

"Hi, Pam. Thanks for coming. How did it go?"

"You're welcome. It went fine. Both of us could actually smell the anesthesia coming out as I was working on him. Strange, but that's what Magnetic Clearing is supposed to be doing—clearing out the gunk. Should I come back tomorrow? Or you can call me next week or when he comes home, if you want some follow-up sessions."

Pam hung her purse on her shoulder and left. I went into Scott's room.

"Hey there," I said, "Are you okay?"

"Yeah, I guess. My head doesn't hurt as much as it did before."

I stood there a few minutes, wondering if Pam should come back the next day. I looked for clues as Scott closed his eyes. He didn't want to talk any more. I sat by his bed for a few more minutes, until a nurse came in. "We need to limit his visitors. Why don't you get some sleep? You can check on him later. I'll let you know if anything changes."

I returned to the waiting room, down the hall and around the corner. The TVs were off. Linda was lying under a white flannel hospital blanket, reading. Another woman across the room was sleeping, sitting up in a reclining chair. I climbed under my own blanket and was asleep in a matter of minutes.

The waiting room was darker when I woke up, Linda touching my shoulder.

"Scott wants to see you," she said, her tired voice shaking a bit. "He can't sleep."

The ICU was darker, too, the nurses' station in the center of the round room glowing from a desk lamp and the computer monitors. A machine in one room was beeping and several nurses and a doctor were conferring inside that door with some family members. I entered Scott's room. He looked worse. "I can't sleep," he said in an angry-scared tiny voice. "I keep hearing alarms. Am I okay?"

"Yes, you're fine. Those aren't your alarms. That's the guy next door. You're okay. You're fine. I'm here. I'll stay."

"When I close my eyes, I disappear."

I sat in the stiff chair next to Scott's bed, holding his hand for as long as I could. It was going to be a long night.

For health and joy,
For love and friends,
For everything Thy Goodness sends,
We thank Thee.

7

Thanksgiving Leftovers

Scott came home on Wednesday after four days and nights in the hospital. It was much sooner than I expected. I mean, who knew you could have your head opened up, some brain scooped out, and be back in your own bed half a week later? I didn't know if Scott would have the stamina, strength or balance to make it up the stairs to the bedroom, much less back down again. After a brief assessment by a hospital physical therapist, however, Scott was released with a prescription for a few more visits by a physical therapist at home to help Scott figure out how to navigate the stairs and the shower. A nurse went over the complicated medicine instructions with me and then we were dismissed.

Our two cats were purring at the front door along with Amie and Lance, and the gas fireplace was lit, as if the entire house were welcoming us home. Scott basked by the fire, with a simple, "Aaaah."

Soon after dinner, Scott was ready to go upstairs for bed, so Amie and Lance went home. "I better try to sleep before the alarm goes off at eleven for meds," he said to excuse himself. "It's not like I slept in the hospital." My parents were spending the night so I wouldn't be the lone nurse, wife, and mother.

"I will tuck you in," said Wil, racing up the stairs into his own room before Scott even started the climb. My dad stood ready at Scott's elbow, but Scott managed the hike by himself just using the railing, and I followed behind. Wil met him at the top of the stairs, clutching an armful of things and impatiently wiggling his hips in his thick zip-up pajamas.

"Whatchya got there, Wil?" I asked.

"Tuck in toys," he answered, zooming into our room to start his preparations. Scott made it up the stairs and sat on the end of our bed for a minute to rest.

"I'll go help your mom load the dishwasher," said my dad.

Scott went into the bathroom to brush his teeth and change into softer sweatpants to sleep in.

When Scott came back out, Wil patted the bed. A stuffed polar bear was next to Scott's pillow, along with a tiny Barbie-sized lace pillow, a larger toy pillow, and a polka-dotted cotton baby blanket that Wil was never attached to but kept on his bed for his bunnies.

"Here, Daddy, climb in bed."

Scott obliged, pulling the turned-back triangle of quilt over his stomach, saying, "Wow, you're taking really good care of me."

"Yes," said Wil, all business. "Now, here is the baby monitor," pointing to the bookshelf an arm's length away from Scott's side of the bed with a seriousness that belied his almost-five years. "The other part is in the kitchen downstairs, so we can hear you if you call.

"Sleep tight," he added with a kiss on Scott's cheek. "I'm glad we're all home."

"Me, too," Scott answered. "Thanks for tucking me in."

If only it could have stayed that easy for Wil. After breakfast the next morning, I had to unwrap the bandage on Scott's head to make sure the incision wasn't oozing. First we took happy photos of Wil in his gray and green pajamas standing on the bed hugging his daddy, his head tucked under Scott's chin and his arms stretched across Scott's grey "Friends Make the Difference" sweatshirt. The camera captured the bliss of that hug and their matching blue eyes, as well as the small red hole in the third-eye spot on Scott's forehead where a screw held his head steady on a frame during surgery. Wil was curious to see the big owie, and so without a second thought, I let him see the suture and twenty staples. The red, scabby incision curved like train tracks to nowhere, and Scott's four-day shadow of re-growing hair looked like little burned trees in a war-torn field.

"Eew! Does it hurt?" said Wil, climbing down from the bed.

"Nope, it's not too bad," said Scott, meaning it, but Wil looked at him skeptically.

"I think I'll go downstairs now," Wil said, padding away in his pajamas.

"Hmmm, maybe that wasn't such a good idea," I said. Scott didn't answer. His incision was clean, so we left the bandage off.

Later that afternoon, Wil went to play at the house of my friend, Elaine. He stayed for dinner and didn't return until nearly bedtime. Elaine and her husband, Mike, and I had worked in the same government building in Oak Ridge, Tennessee, and we were pregnant with our sons at the same time. In a neat coincidence of career moves, they moved to Highlands Ranch earlier that year and bought a house a few streets away. We thought it would be a fun diversion for Wil to play with Mitch and his younger sister, Chloe, that day but instead Wil was cranky when my friend brought him home.

"He was a good boy," Elaine said. "I hope he had fun. Hey, did I tell you that your email updates are making the rounds in Oak Ridge. Mike Hill contacted us and said to tell you he's sending good thoughts for Scott."

"Tell him thanks," I replied. "I had an email from an editor I used to work with there who lives in Ohio now and she said she's received our emails from more than one source. It's amazing how email gets forwarded." We both paused to reflect on that fact. "Well, thanks again for today."

As Elaine walked down our steps and I closed the front door, I marveled yet again at the connections of friends all over the country. It was as if Elaine brought with her to Colorado a giant elastic band of energy that stretched from Tennessee, acting as a conduit for prayers and positive thoughts from everyone who knew us back there. Ironically, the Frames moved back to Tennessee the next year, as if the universe no longer required their proximity once our crisis subsided.

"Let's get you into a bath and then bedtime, buster," I said, shuffling Wil from the front door directly upstairs where Scott was already in bed.

"No, I don't want to," he said, like a typical tired-out kid.

"Oh, come on, the bath will feel good. We'll add extra bubbles," I cajoled, not up for a battle. Bathtub time was one of my favorite activities, loving to make Wil giggle in the bubbles. I didn't mind sitting on the fluffy bath mat, reaching over the tub to lather Wil's hair, because bath time was when we seemed to laugh the most.

"No!" Wil yelled back, "I...don't...want...to! I hate you!" He ran downstairs into the family room, where he sat on the futon, arms crossed, face pouting.

"Hey," I said as I walked into the room after him. "Don't say that. It hurts my feelings."

I sat next to him and tried to pull him closer into a hug.

"Go away," he said, pouting and pulling away, "I hate you."

With a heavy sigh but wanting to cry, I decided to let him cool off and give myself a time out. I wasn't used to temper tantrums from my usually sweet, silly boy. I walked into the kitchen a few feet away, with Wil still in view, and decided to empty the dishwasher. He used the remote control to turn on the TV.

"Oh, let's not turn on the television," I said, turning my back to put plates in the cupboard. "How about finding a book we can read?"

"No. I don't want to. I want to watch TV."

"There's nothing good on right now," I said, still in the kitchen, "It's really almost bedtime."

"I'm watching TV," he said again, turning up the volume on a stupid cartoon.

"Hey, keep it down. Turn it off. Dad is trying to rest upstairs." I tried being reasonable but I was running out of patience.

"You hate me!" he yelled, throwing down the remote and heading down the hall. I intercepted him and we sat on the floor in the narrow hallway in a gripping hug.

"I don't hate you, honey. I love you. I love you lots. And I know you don't hate me."

He started to cry, then to sob, hanging on to me. His story seeped out with his tears.

"I'm scared about Daddy." More sobbing.

I could only hold on, whispering, "I know."

"I don't like the Band-Aid on his head.

"I didn't like seeing the cut from his surgery. Those staples are scary.

"I'm afraid Daddy is going to die," and he said this with a wailing cry, sobbing even harder.

"Oh, honey, I'm so sorry you're afraid," I said in his ear, "I believe Daddy is going to be okay. He is all done with his surgery and he's healing now. He doesn't want to leave us."

I couldn't bring myself to say Scott wasn't going to die. I was afraid of it, too, and I didn't want to be a liar. I started to cry, too, and Wil looked up at me, startled.

"I'm so sorry you're afraid," I repeated, trying to stop my tears. "I don't want you to be scared. I wish Daddy didn't have a brain tumor, but he does. And the doctors are helping him get better. We just have to take good care of each other and give each other lots of love."

Wil would do anything to make sure I didn't cry, so he turned off his tears and disengaged from my arms. "Maybe we could read my body book some more," he said, changing the subject. He walked to the family room and picked up the extra large *Human Body* book we purchased the week after Scott's diagnosis. It portrayed the human brain with clear graphics and labels, with words meant for children to understand. Wil found it fascinating that certain stuff in your head would determine your thinking, your feelings, your memory. He was more fascinated, however, by the pages on reproduction.

"Our family is too small," he said, handing me the book to read to him. "I think we should adopt me a brother or sister."

"You do, huh?" I said, taking the book and sitting on the futon so Wil could climb onto my lap. I wasn't alarmed at his suggestion, because it was something we had discussed before as a family. I marveled at his chain of thought, thankful that our trauma had ended, at least for that night. "Well, let's just take it one step at a time. What pages should we look at?"

The next week went by in waves of deep, shattered exhaustion and little, quiet pleasures. It was still warm enough outside that Wil and I could take a bike ride around the neighborhood, me on my mountain bike pulling Wil on his Tag-Along. It was a blue contraption I bought for myself on Mother's Day, a half-bike that hooked under my seat and let Wil hang onto handlebars of his own and peddle behind me. On the long uphills that didn't look steep until you were riding, I would yell back to Wil over my shoulder, "Peddle like you mean it!" Bicycling was a good workout, pumping me full of endorphins and burning off stress.

Thanksgiving was easy that year. Scott's sister offered to come over all day and do the basting and mash the potatoes, while my mom offered to make most of the other fixings. I only had to bake pumpkin pies the day before and set the table. Scott's parents had flown to Palm Desert to close up the condo for winter and drive Linda's car back to Colorado. Thanksgiving Day was blue-sky beautiful, so Wil played outside with the neighborhood kids. At dinner we toasted Scott's courage and spoke of our awe for the love and support streaming toward us. His tumor gave us new gratitude for life.

We held hands while saying our new family prayer which I had combined from a few sources. Before Scott's tumor I planned to paint it on the edge of my old antique table so that in case we forgot to say grace out loud, we would still be covered. After Scott's tumor I didn't have time to paint, plus we made it a new habit to say grace before every dinner.

We thank Thee, Lord, for happy hearts,
For rain and sunny weather.
We thank Thee, Lord, for this our food
And that we are together.
For health and joy,
For love and friends,
For everything Thy Goodness sends,
We thank Thee.

The day after Thanksgiving, three of my cousins came over with their families for leftovers. I had mailed the invitations on the first Monday of November, just hours before Scott's final symptom at work when I insisted he come straight home and go to the walk-in clinic. I could have cancelled since I mailed the invitations before his diagnosis, but instead I decided to have the "Leftovers Party" as planned. It seemed easy enough, since the leftovers were ready and one of my cousins had flown all the way in from Kentucky. I hoped it would be a low-key way to connect and give Wil time to play with five cousins close to his age who he rarely saw. The food part and visiting was easy.

The men sat outside on our deck, enjoying the afternoon sunshine and our mountain view, talking about the holiday football games. Scott enjoyed and endured the company. He could not have cared less about the football, but he missed sipping beer. Scott tried to hide being tired and foggy, having over-exerted himself on Thanksgiving, and he was coming to realize that group conversations were harder to follow since his surgery. It was as if his brain had static, making it hard to filter out voices and meaning.

I was sitting on the family-room floor, talking to my women cousins sitting around the room and on the carpet in front of the fireplace. After our entire childhoods of sharing Thanksgivings together, it was relaxing to be talking now as adults while our kids played all over the house. In the midst of our conversation, Wil came up behind me, but I kept on talking, not meaning to ignore him, just not paying attention. Then I felt a tug on my hair. I turned around with half grimace, half smile.

"Oooh, why'd you do that?" I said to Wil as I turned. In his right hand, pointing up at the ceiling, were his purple-handled round-tip scissors. In his other hand, a long chunk of my hair. In his eyes, anger and not a little bit of fear. He threw the handful of hair and his scissors in my lap and ran back upstairs.

I sat there, my mouth hanging open, not knowing whether to laugh or to cry, stunned.

"What was that about?" I said, deciding to laugh but embarrassed at the same time. I'm sure my face was red. Everyone hovered over me to see how much hair was gone. The amputated clump in my lap, once I squeezed it together, was no thicker than a crayon.

One cousin asked, "Do you have some different scissors? I can blend your hair into more layers to make it less noticeable until you can get to a salon."

I nodded, caring less what my hair looked and more about what I should say to Wil.

"Do you want me to go check on him," asked Dawn.

"Yeah, I think that would be a good idea," I said, because I didn't know if I should be mad at him or worried at his outburst or scared of the deeper meaning behind it.

Later she told me he burst into tears when she walked in the room. She hugged him until he stopped crying. Then he said, "Sometimes I just get scared."

When everyone went home, I sat with Wil on his bedroom floor, his eyes downcast. "I just want you to know that I love you," I said. "I wish you hadn't cut my hair, but I love you no matter what."

Wil leaned into me, wrapping his arms round my waist, his head on my belly. "I'm sorry."

Scott's brain tumor was changing everything and causing Wil's world to wobble off its axis. His silly, playful mom, always ready to draw pictures or paint or make messes, had transformed into a teary-eyed, tired stranger who kept sending him on sleepovers to someone else's house.

One day, in the car, our eyes connected in the extra rearview mirror that had been suctioned to the windshield ever since he was a baby, focused on his car seat instead of traffic. "You have sad eyes, Mommy," he observed, not even a question.

"I'm just a little tired. I'm okay," I answered, trying to rearrange my features to hide some of the truth from his insightful old soul.

The next day when I got in the car by myself, I removed the kid-view mirror and I never put it back. Wil never asked where it went.

A few nights later, I took a long hot bath all alone. Before Scott's diagnosis I would dust the white-plastic soaking tub more often than I ever filled it with water for myself. Most of my friends in this new subdivision of designer homes had their soaking tubs full of rubber duckies, spongy non-slip mats, squirting water toys, and baby shampoo, and we all lamented the fact that the homebuilders thought carpet next to bathtubs was luxurious. At Scott's birthday party, Julie gave me a few packets of lavender/green-tea bath salts, just like she had received in October after her breast cancer diagnosis. She was passing along the idea of self-pampering.

While soaking that night, I thought more about me and Wil and how we would cope on this brain tumor journey. I imagine that if Wil could have found grown-up words and a degree in child psychology to explain his recent outbursts, he might have stood up from where we sat in tears and ticked off a list of bulleted points on his fingers:

1. First, I am sick and tired of everyone asking me how my daddy is doing. They never did that before! What am I supposed to say? He's fine? He's sick? I don't know!

2. Second, I wish adults would stop telling me that their kids are saying bedtime prayers for my dad. That's weird for me to hear, and I feel embarrassed. I don't pray for their dad.

3. I know I used to like this, but now I do not enjoy having so many sleepovers. I want you to read me bedtime stories and to kiss me goodnight and to snuggle with me until I fall asleep. I want to wake up in my own house.

4. All my friends have brothers and sisters to play with. I'm lonely.

5. All you ever talk about any more is Dad's brain tumor. Let's change the subject!

6. I want my life back to normal, when Daddy went to work and you played with me.

7. It scares me to see you so sad.

8. I feel sad, too, but mostly I'm angry. I'm supposed to be a good boy so I can't be angry. So now what are the boundaries for me and my behavior?

9. I'm afraid that if Dad can get sick and maybe die, you will, too.

10. When will all this be over?

While children don't have the words to explain their feelings, most of us parents don't either. Wouldn't it be nice if we could instantly tap into the divine perspective of our souls and understand all the issues, and then address each one with logic and eloquence? But life happens, and we can't really control the process, much less the outcome. We can only muck through it moments at a time and hope for grace periods along the way. (And read books on helping kids cope when a parent has cancer, find a support group, or call a child psychologist...or our mothers.)

Over that month I had visions of sitting knees cramped in a motorcycle sidecart with Scott driving too fast, me feeling scared and out of control, barely trusting his skills to maneuver the curves in the road. I needed a different metaphor. That night in the tub, I steered my inner vision to that of a slower, meandering bicycle ride.

We're in this together, our family, I thought, *but Scott's on his own bicycle. I'm riding a separate bike, alongside of Scott, with Wil behind me on the Tag-Along. Sometimes Scott will go off on his own trail, up a steep cliff and through narrow dark tunnels, while Wil and I take a parallel route, catching up later. Sometimes Wil and I should stop and have a picnic just for two, or a party with friends, and sometimes we'll simply sit on the grass in the sun and wait. Sometimes I need to let Wil get off the bike and go do his own thing. And I will keep pedaling; sometimes I'll coast, but always with the Tag-Along attached to my bike, always a mother, always a wife. Sometimes I will put down the kickstand and have my own diversions. We'll need endurance for this long bike ride. But we can stop to watch sunsets or meet new people along the way. I hope we ride together for a long, long time.*

I wrote those thoughts in my journal after the bath and before falling asleep. I didn't ride my bike again until springtime, but in my heart I pedaled through the metaphor more than once. And it helped.

God doesn't send catastrophes to wake us up.
But to say that God doesn't initiate or cause
these things is not the same thing as saying
that God doesn't speak through them.
—*Ron Roheiser*

8
Why?

Why did you get a brain tumor? What caused it? How did this happen? Why me? When we get bad news, we want to know why. Many nights we lay awake in bed talking about why. Seeking the origins of Scott's brain tumor was like doing a life review.

Was it from the time, when he was three and playing with an electrical train and water spilled and he was shocked unconscious? He woke up with black hands, but didn't tell his mom to avoid getting in trouble.

Was it from the time when he was eight and riding his bike along the gravel driveway on his grandparent's farm, how he was distracted by a bird and rode head-on into the mailbox. His mom saw it happen, how he was knocked out for a few minutes, and she drove him to the emergency room for a broken collarbone.

He didn't do drugs in college, so it couldn't be that. He liked his White Russian vodkas and his black and tan beers, which surely hastened the demise of some brain cells, but we couldn't imagine and we've never seen research linking college drinking with brain tumors.

Or did the brain tumor start growing when Scott worked at Rocky Flats, the nuclear trigger processing facility north of Denver, his first job after college? He was a computer programmer and didn't work in a "hot" building. Like all employees there, he wore a dosimeter badge, which was regularly measured to check for radiation exposure. "It was the dust blowing across the fields when I walked from the parking lot to my office, or over to the cafeteria," Scott would say, "The dust is what makes me wonder."

But nobody else Scott worked with at Rocky Flats was diagnosed with a brain tumor, so statistically speaking, it wasn't highly likely. Somewhere along the way, we heard about clusters of people living in Golden, downstream, with an unusually high incidence of brain tumors, but that was blamed on the large radio towers sitting on the mesa above Coors Brewing plant. We've always wondered, though, was there an answer blowing in the wind over Rocky Flats?

And then there was Oak Ridge, where we lived for six years while Scott worked at the building known as K-12, one of the three main facilities in the town that grew out of the atomic bomb's Manhattan Project. While we lived there, glowing green frogs made it into the news. But again, wearing his dosimeter badge and working in an office that didn't come close to dangerous materials, Oak Ridge just wasn't something to blame. I did, however, make a phone call to the Environmental Health office in Oak Ridge, asking if there was someone who collected reports on cancer in former employees. Nothing ever came of that. In the years since Scott's diagnosis, we've had emails from two people whose wives were diagnosed with brain tumors, but we chalk that up to the small-world people-who-knew-us-and-told-them-to-write-to-us more than environmental, statistical significance.

We considered the long list of possible environmental causes, as if using a checklist and a fat red pen to rule out all options. Scott didn't overuse his cell phone, and that causal link was later studied and officially discounted. Of the 150 types of primary brain tumors (ones that originate in the brain and not because another type of cancer spread, or metastasized, into the brain), only one rare type is genetically inheritable—and that wasn't Scott's type. Scott's only (and questionable) exposure to petroleum jet fuel would have been his first six months of life when his parents worked at Chicago's O'Hare airport and they lived in an apartment nearby. There were the farm pesticides to question from his grandfather's soybean farm in Michigan, but if that had been true wouldn't cancer have struck more of his large family of cousins, aunts and uncles, or neighbors?

While we lived in Oak Ridge, Scott earned his Master's degree in computer science (his diploma dated the day Wil was born) with a specialty in artificial intelligence. For his Master's project, he researched and became an expert in genetic algorithms. Whenever he tried to explain it to me, I felt like Ginger the dog in *The Far Side* cartoon where all I heard was my name, "Blah, blah, blah, blah, Ginger. Blah, blah, blah."

Scott's degree in artificial intelligence made us see the irony of his situation. He had become a brain specialist of sorts, expert in the ways our brain—and machines—develop thinking skills and problem solving abilities. This brain tumor could become his greatest research experiment yet.

Seven years later, an article in the January 2006 *Science & Theology News* made sense to me. Written by Richard G. Colling, a biology professor and author on science and faith, wrote this article called, "A random universe: anything is possible in an equal opportunity world," in which the term "random" conveys a positive meaning of the equal probability of occurrence. Maybe that's like saying, as so many friends did when they heard about Scott's brain tumor, "Geez, that could have been me."

Maybe Scott's tumor was simply some random single-cell mutation gone mad, or some other random event that enabled a good brain cell to turn bad and corrupt more rotten brain cells.

Scott's explanation for his brain tumor was that the copious amounts of water he'd been drinking at work, for the sake of improving his health, had caused something small and harmless—that might have always been there—to swell into that fluid-filled cyst that we saw on the first MRI. No doctor ever agreed.

I had my own irrational theory of blame. I wondered if a stint of overtime in 1997 had caused Scott's brain to buzz out on overload. I'm sure I felt this way because part of me was still angry at him for working fourteen-hour days from Labor Day through November, with only one Sunday off in all that time—and loving it. He was leading a project to migrate all of Lockheed Martin's employees to a new email system.

"I'm not saying this to brag," Scott once told me while we were laying in bed in the dark, admitting how much he missed working, how scared he was that he might never go back. "But I was programming more lines of code per day in those months than I know most people could ever do. It was so awesome. I could oversee the project's big picture, explain it to management, help steer the other programmers, program code like a mad man, and keep all the details in my head all at once. It was a piece of cake."

Wow, I thought. *I've always known he was smart.* I know his big brain is partly why I fell in love with him (and his blue eyes). Hearing his view of what he had been, in his brain, broke my heart in a way I didn't know could keep breaking. Like many, he defined himself by his smarts on the job. It was more than that to Scott. It was his gift. And to have it taken away like this, the unfairness of it all, made me want to lash out at someone or something to blame. I needed a target for my wondering angst. There wasn't one.

Programming was such a high for him, doing what he loved and doing it really well. I was proud of him, yes, but wished it hadn't been at the expense of family time for three months. Letting him have his three months of totally fulfilling true-vocation work doesn't seem like such a sacrifice to me anymore.

It was that successful programming effort which landed us on a company-paid congratulatory trip to Disney World in September 1998. It was for three days on the drizzly heels of Hurricane Ivan, and we called it our "Mystery Vacation." We didn't tell Wil where we were going until we arrived at the hotel room. Wil hadn't picked up on the clues at the airport, where posters of Mickey, Cinderella, and Donald Duck hung everywhere — because to a four-year old, why wouldn't you decorate with Disney? He didn't notice the signs as we drove to the tropical resort, and from our fifteenth- floor room overlooking the vast swimming pool below, he thought that was a good enough vacation for him. When we finally sprung the news that we were at Disney World, Wil smacked his own forehead and uttered the only words he could conjure to express such a fantastic surprise, "This is a total disaster!"

Scott's first glimmer of symptom came on that trip on the Log Ride, and Disney captured the moment for us on one of those photos taken as everyone screams in their seats at the final splash-filled descent. "I felt dizzier on that ride than I ever have, like my head was exploding from pressure." He chalked it up to the thrill of taking a ride with his son in Disney World, though a part of him tucked it away for future reference as something to tell a doctor.

Just before our Disney trip, Scott had switched employers to a smaller consulting firm where he was sure his prospects for success would propel him into the future he'd always imagined. Lockheed valued his brain so much, they transferred the last few months of his consulting contract from one firm to the new one, with assurances that the contract could be renewed. But it wasn't long before Scott realized his dreams of having a leadership role, making an impact on client success and the bottom line, were not going to happen, at least not for awhile. The overtime he was expected to give and the lack of decision-making clout, in just the first months, was enough to dash his hopes.

He whispered this to me not long after his diagnosis, "I was ready to call Lockheed and ask for a permanent, full-time position, not as a consultant but as a plain old employee. I knew it would be less money and maybe boring, but I'd have more time with you and Wil."

And then he said it.

"I was ready to turn off my brain in exchange for an eight-hour day."

The blame game is something we always play in the face of disaster. We demand an investigation to determine who is to blame for the heinous event. The armed-to-explode missile of our anger needs an obvious target. Many times, however, there's no one to blame, except maybe God.

Perhaps life is a play and we're cast in our parts, good and bad, to explore all the aspects of the human drama. Perhaps cancer and caregiving are clues to life's mysteries and the answer lies not in the ending but in how well we play our part. If that's the case, perhaps our job isn't to ask why but simply to trust in the process.

At some point, perhaps, you stop asking "why." Sometimes you just need a good comeback line. One of our favorite lines came from the movie *Shakespeare in Love*, which debuted the same year Scott was diagnosed. The wisdom emerged from a conversation between Hugh Fennyman and Philip Henslowe (portrayed by Tom Wilkinson and Geoffrey Rush, respectively).

"Mr. Fennyman, allow me to explain about the theatre business. The natural condition is one of insurmountable obstacles on the road to imminent disaster."

"So what do we do?"

"Nothing. Strangely enough, it all turns out well."

"How?"

"I don't know. It's a mystery."

As Colwell concluded, "Random design has the potential to shape an age by acknowledging that much of what appears random is bursting with purpose and meaning."

If you aren't satisfied with the answer to "Why?" you can move on, like children do, to asking "How do you spell that?" And in learning how to spell, pronounce, and research a word, you step into your power. For us it was spelled *gemistocytic astrocytoma*, pronounced with a hard G, like God.

When the soul wishes to experience something,
she throws an image of the experience
out before her and enters into her own image.
—*Meister Eckhart*

9

Parting Gifts

Speaking of why, why Scott got his tumor, I was asking myself why me, why me as Scott's wife for this part of our life? One of my first thoughts upon Scott's diagnosis was, *Well, at least I've been through this before with my mom. I know some about what to expect. I've seen what it's like to be sick and to become a survivor.* As I began to ponder it more, I began to recall the foreshadowing that I almost call fate.

I thought back to the movies that had become my favorites in the years since I met Scott. It seemed like a cosmic coincidence that the theme-song of *Ghost* (where Patrick Swayze's character dies and leaves his new wife, played by Demi Moore, all alone), that its song *Unchained Melody*, was the most popular first-dance-song at weddings, including our own. Then there was *Always* about the character played by Richard Dreyfus who died in a plane crash fighting a forest fire, leaving his girlfriend Dorinda, played by Holly Hunter, to go on with her life. That movie came out in 1989 when we were still dating, and years later I watched that movie over and over when it was on late-night television reruns one week. My next favorite movie, *Sleepless in Seattle*, as almost everyone knows, is about falling in love after loss and featured a little boy, not just a spouse, opening his heart again.

And then there was *Phenomenon* with John Travolta and his blue eyes like Scott, and his character's brain tumor, like Scott's. When we saw that movie in 1996, the first summer we lived in Highlands Ranch, I cried all the way home in the car because Travolta's character died. I cried on Scott's shoulder for another half hour under the stars on our back porch.

"I don't know why that movie struck me so hard?" I blubbered to him. "Was it because it brought up my fears about losing my mom to her cancer? It's not like I think I'm going to lose you. But maybe that is my fear."

Scott patted my shoulder. "It's not like the movie was all about death. What I liked is how smart he was for awhile, how his tumor seemed to open up the secrets of the universe. He was like an example of how smart all of us could be, how tapped into knowledge, but he was ahead of his time."

"But it was so sad that he died."

It was two years after *Phenomenon* when Scott's brain tumor arrived. Watching our videotape of the movie one night, we gasped at the moment when the character was diagnosed with an astrocytoma.

"God, maybe that's why I couldn't stop crying when we first saw the movie. Remember? What if part of me knew this was coming."

I never thought of those movies as a themed collection before—until Scott's brain tumor. I chose to imagine that my attachment to those movies—movies about losing the love of your life but someday loving again— could mean my soul had been preparing for this frightening brain tumor experience long before it arrived. I also chose to believe that if so, then maybe I did sign up for this role, and if so, then maybe I shouldn't be scared but trust that my soul had a survival plan already in place. My job would be to remember that plan, or make it up as I went along.

Was my role as Scott's wife destiny? What is destiny?

Was it destiny to meet Scott on my twenty-second birthday and find out that my birthday 01-16-1965 contained the same numbers as his 11-06-1965, as if we were born for the same life lesson? If you believe in the theories of numerology, it could be true. Numerology has you add up the numbers from the date of your birth—one plus one plus six and so on. Ours adds up to 38 and if you add three plus eight, you get eleven. So in numerology books, you look up the life lesson description for 38 as well as 11, and 11 reduces to 2, so you read about 2, too.

Was it destiny when we had our first dance at Linden's Tavern the week after St. Valentine's Day? It felt like destiny when I stepped into our very first slow dance, close enough to smell Scott's Polo cologne, our heads thrown back laughing at being only one of two couples dancing. It felt so perfect with my arms round his shoulders, his on my waist. As I tucked my head under his chin, I felt like a key fitting into a lock or a piece fitting into a puzzle. At that moment the universe sizzled and whispered, "He's the man you will marry." Scott felt it, too. We called it our destiny dance (and sometimes our density dance) and I believe that it was. It felt like the moment that shifted our life into gear.

Does that mean I believe in fate, that lives are preordained? I don't believe that fate determines our outcome with no room for choices, but what if our souls choose a theme to explore with our life?

If I explained my What If with a story, it would be a story about the moments before I was born.

Throughout time there lived a soul who loved saltwater and pink seashells so much that, for her next lifetime, she asked the planning team if somehow shells could be part of her name.

"How about Michelle? It's the feminine, and French, for Michael. Translates to who is like God?" offered her tie-dye t-shirted guide.

"Oh, Howard, who told you that?" the girl-soul teased, swinging her bare feet from the stool next to Howard where she sat reading the final orientation tips for Life. "But yeah, I like that translation—sounds like a riddle. Aren't the Beatles singing a song by that name?" she asked, starting to sing the soulful French lyrics. "*Michelle, ma belle...*"

Howard was distracted, reviewing a checklist, stacking papers on a big, waist-high table resembling those found in a high school chemistry lab. Three walls of the planning room were varied shades of blue. On the periwinkle wall, the girl-soul's other guide, Betty, was pushing tacks into earth maps and star charts. The wall of sky-blue framed a movie screen showing only static. The indigo wall had a turnstile where a single red rollercoaster car sat empty, facing sideways into a dark tunnel. The fourth wall was white and it held a frosted-glass door labeled 3811, propped opened to a corridor reminiscent of an eclectic art gallery.

"You won't remember how to speak French when you get there," said Howard rather peevishly because he wished he was going. He wrote her new name in the top corner of the page. "And besides, John and Paul are still working on that song. It won't be recorded down there until November third of this year. Someday you'll like that coincidence."

"Okay, so getting back to the list," he said. "Let me reiterate. Free Will. You can do whatever you choose, but you have to deal with the consequences. That's a big one. You can always ask us for help—that's why they call it guidance—but we can't help unless you ask. Even old souls forget that one," he added, almost as an aside.

"Who do you think I will marry?" the girl-soul asked dreamily, then wheedled, "Come on, give me a hint," as the guide shook his head.

"You know I can't tell you. Free Will, did you already forget?"

"I know, and I agreed to be surprised this time. But you know, don't you? Just a hint, please?"

"Well," said Howard in a whisper, "Just a hint. Look for brown hair and blue eyes. And that's all I'm going to say." The girl-soul grinned, crossing her fingers so maybe she'd remember when she got to Earth.

"So what cards did you draw for this lifetime?" asked Betty, all done with thumbtacks. Betty sported a pink t-shirt touting Chicks Rule, looking good in Levi's and white cowgirl boots. She began jotting down notes in a small spiral notebook. "I'll keep the unofficial journal for you this time, kind of a scrapbook, and we can look at it over popcorn when you get back."

"Still wish you could taste popcorn, don't you?" the girl-soul taunted, cinching the ties tighter on her pink chenille bathrobe. "Let's see…I have the four cards everyone gets, plus Weaver, Artist, and Searcher. I'm excited about those." Then she added with a bit of a pout, "Plus I got Escapist, too. Not sure what I'm gonna do with that card. What's the card for mother-hood? I really wanted that one. Oh well, look in my chart if you want to see the full list."

"You'll have fun exploring that combination of archetypes," said Betty. "Some more fun than others. You can choose lots of minor themes while you're there, for variety. Wouldn't want you getting bored, now, would we?" Betty added, plunking a kiss on the girl's cheek as if for good luck.

"Can I go now? I want to get there in time for my sister's first birthday — January sixteenth," said the girl-soul, excited to start her new life and be with her family again.

"God likes to be here when you leave, to say farewell and all that," said Howard. "Don't be in such a hurry. We have plenty of time from this end. The scar team is making a final check on your new body to make sure the wounds from last time are patched up. You've got a doozy on the right thigh."

"Yeah, yeah, it'll be fine," said the girl-soul, hopping off the stool and jumping from foot to foot, anxious to leave. "Can I have the *Mary Poppins Comes Back* version to travel this time? I love that one, 'I am earth and air and fire and water. I come from the Dark where all things have their begin-ning.' "

"Yes, you can," the girl-soul heard in a James Earl Jones boom. "I like that one, too."

"Oh, come on, use the Audrey Hepburn voice today," the girl laughed, squeezing God's hand then skipping off toward the rollercoaster car. God walked in the room, quoting in the voice of a bright new baby, "'I come from the sea and its tides. I come from the sky and its stars.'" And back to Audrey's adult voice, God said, "P.L. Travers pegged it spot-on with that chapter."

"Oh, God, you're such a good impressionist." The girl-soul, unabashed, dropped her robe to the floor and now sat naked in the rollercoaster car, left hand gripping the release lever that would hurtle her forward. Her eyes grew moist as she took one last loving look around the room. "See ya, everybody. Please send me lots of good signs, and I promise to pay better attention this time. See ya in my dreams."

"Not if I see you first," said the two guides at the same time and quipped, "Jinx joke, you owe me a Coke." Howard and Betty slapped a high five, taking their eyes off the girl for a split second. "Oh shoot, there she goes!"

"There she goes again," chuckled God. "In too big a hurry to get there. They all are. She didn't wait for my parting gift."

Then the two guides leaned together, chanting like a metronome, "It's okay to be angry at God."

"Almost everyone jumps through before hearing more than 'it's okay' and they miss the next part I wrote just for them. Maybe I need to rewrite my send-off," God heaved a sigh but wasn't worried at all. "Her family is full of dreamers, so you'll have plenty of opportunities to send messages. They each signed up for some tough roles this time around. The Bard often asks for troupes who can improvise like this one. They really sink into their characters with an impeccable flair for timing—and costumes and set design. She'll be fine. I can't wait to watch her choices."

"Hey look, there's the full moon, right on cue," said Howard, as he and Betty pulled their stools over by the screen to watch the girl-soul's entry. "Three, two, one…contact!" They jumped up, applauding for a minute, then sat down again and clicked their bottles of Coca Cola in a toast, fizz overflowing to the floor. "But you know, she didn't give the scar team enough time to cauterize her leg. It could give her some trouble, and sooner than later."

"Well, there is a doctor in the family. Let's make sure she reads fairy tales for a clue about the blessings that go with every scar."

And with that, the guides sat back to watch, and God went to the next room where another soul was preparing to embark on Life. God was whistling *Michelle, ma belle*.

So that's my story. After writing it, I sat at my kitchen table where my brown-haired, blue-eyed husband was reading the newspaper and handed him my pages to read next. When he was done and looked up, I laughed and shrugged, "It just feels true."

"I like the part where you crossed your fingers," Scott said, because that's what he does during our conversations when I won't stop talking and he doesn't want to forget his point.

"So if you have two guides, what are their names?" I asked, half joking, half curious to see if he thought my story was at all plausible.

"Howard and Bob," he replied, without a second thought.

Our son walked in the kitchen just then, not having heard my story but drawn downstairs by our laughter. "What are you guys talking about?"

So I asked Wil, without explanation, "Let's say you have two guardian angels. What are their names?"

"Bob and Betty," he quipped without a doubt.

Scott and I looked wide-eyed at each other and said in tandem, "No way!"

If everything seems to be going well,
you have obviously overlooked something.
—Steven Wright

10
The Wonders of Radiation

After Thanksgiving we sought out the next steps in Scott's brain tumor treatment. We thought our appointment with the radiation oncologist was simply a consultation, a chance to ask questions and decide if radiation was a good choice as Scott's first treatment step.

We arrived at 12:30 with our spiral notebook and two pages of questions. First we watched a video in another small room, which portrayed the course of radiation, then we met the radiation oncologist and let loose with questions. Please explain Scott's diagnosis, from your point of view. His prognosis with and without radiation? What are the physical side effects of radiation, short and long term? Is it true that six weeks of radiation is a lifetime dose? Are you the best doctor to treat Scott's astrocytoma? Do you recommend any other brain tumor specialists in Denver for the rest of his treatment?

Those were just some of our questions. None of her answers surprised us, just confirmed that radiation was a standard first course of treatment after surgery, not really a cure. What we didn't expect to hear was Scott's gemistocytic tumor described as "a more deadly, insidious, infiltrative tumor." The neurosurgeon hadn't said *that*. Even though Scott's tumor was technically a grade two (out of four), it was now much more daunting.

And so, when the radiation oncologist told us that over the next few hours Scott would be measured and fitted for his radiation mask so that he could begin radiation next week, we were too stunned to argue. Now I can call it a simple lack of communication, but on that day we felt side-swiped, finagled, tricked into treatment. We felt we couldn't say no.

Scott was whisked away for an x-ray, a CT scan, and mask-making. I was left alone in the waiting room, to read magazines, watch TV…and wait, alone with my worries. I waited for hours.

I never used to make eye contact with people in the doctor's waiting room. Or in elevators, where don't we all lower our eyes, pull in our elbows, avoiding a personal moment and germs. Our excuse is privacy—allowing theirs, wanting our own. But what if we looked up, smiled at someone across the room, and asked, "Hello, you come here often?" After what happened that day, I became more open to making connections.

In the middle of waiting for Scott to return, I looked up to see a middle-aged woman sitting in a chair opposite me. She was filling out forms, a patient herself.

"Are you here for an appointment or waiting for someone?" she asked, not bothering with boundaries.

"My husband has a brain tumor. He's starting radiation next week."

"They've been trying to pin a brain tumor on me since I was nine," she said. "I've had a lot of blackouts lately, so I'm back again."

She came over and sat down next to me. *Oh no*, I thought.

"I've known several people who survived brain tumors. My friends and I prayed for a man with a brain tumor once," she continued, skipping past her own story. "We prayed and prayed. And when they opened him up to take it out, the surgeons couldn't find it. The tumor wasn't there."

"Really? How cool," I answered, skeptical inside, placating outside.

She went on, "Yep, so they sewed him up with a suture in the shape of a question mark."

The nurse came in then, calling her name. As the lady stood to go for her own MRI, she said, "Tell me your husband's name and I'll pray for him."

"Scott" was all I had time to reply before she was gone.

On the drive home that evening, four hours of radiation preparation later, I told Scott the woman's story. He didn't comment on the question mark. "I'm amazed that a stranger would pray for me."

She was our first waiting-room angel, not because she was beyond this world, but because she made our frightening world seem somehow friendlier. I forgot to tell that story when I wrote my next email.

Subj: Update on Scott: 12/6
Date: 12/6/98 8:06:34 AM Mountain Standard Time

Hi everyone,

Sorry for taking so long to send out another update. I hope nobody has been overly worried for not hearing from us. It has been a very rough, emotionally draining week, but also every day has seen a physical improvement for Scott, along with some great happy times with Wil and good, deep talks between me and Scott, Scott and Wil, me and Wil, etc.

On Monday we met our radiation oncologist. Our appointment lasted from 12:30 to 4:15 p.m., which surprised us. We weren't mentally prepared for it being more than a simple consultation. We met with a nurse, then saw a good videotape on radiation treatment, then met the doctor who answered our questions, and then Scott started preparations for radiation.

I think you should all know what we came to realize this week (even though it was explained to us after surgery)—that the surgeon was NOT able to remove ANY of the tumor, but only drain the cyst and take biopsies.

The tumor appears so similar to normal brain tissue that it was risky to remove any of it and possibly cause big neurological deficits for Scott. This was a big realization to us this week that we have the entire brain tumor to battle still. The other letdown was that 6 weeks of radiation is the only first course of action.

We're doing a lot of research on the Internet, with help from several family member and friends, which has just been invaluable (although sobering, too). We're trying hard to focus on one day at a time, really appreciating all the wonderful moments, and even the harder ones.

Tomorrow we are seeing a physical therapist, a nutritionist and a medical oncologist (who our primary care doctor interned with for several months, coincidentally).

We would appreciate hearing from you, as every day words of encouragement, even brief messages, make a world of difference. Don't worry about our email inbox being too full -- there's no such thing.

I'll let you know what time Scott's radiation treatments will be, so if you think of it at the time each day, you can send your collective prayers for tumor shrinking to coincide with the blast of radiation.

All our love,
Shelly

That was a hard email to send and hard to read, as I learned from the email replies we received. But if you ask for replies of encouragement, you'll get them, like a kiss on your forehead with commiseration, perspective, and prayers. I took our inbox to heart—countless emails from friends, family, colleagues, even strangers.

It matters to have life reflected, affirmed, and blessed, and to have it in writing. By sending replies yet again, I reclaimed my own nerve, finding and giving reprieve from our worries.

Subj: Radiation Report/Schedule
Date: 12/9/98 11:31:37 AM Mountain Standard Time

Hi everyone,

Scott's first radiation treatment went off without a hitch this morning. We were in and out in 15 minutes exactly and home again before 7:30 a.m. (Just hope the snow stays away in the early mornings for one more week.) He didn't feel a thing and except for some "hot" ears for a little while, he is feeling fine. So, one day down -- about 32 treatments to go. We will be going at 6:45 - 7 a.m. from today through next Tuesday, then on Wednesday we will start going from 1:00 to 1:15 p.m.

So, set your watches and focus some positive "tumor shrinking" thoughts on Scott at these times, if you can remember. And if not, we'll happily accept your loving thoughts ANYTIME!!!

THANKS,
Love,
Shelly

People are like stained-glass windows.
They sparkle and shine when the sun is out,
but when the darkness sets in,
their true beauty is revealed
only if there is a light from within.
—Elizabeth Kübler-Ross

11

Dark December

Subj: Update on Scott-12/14
Date: 12/14/98 4:43:13 PM Mountain Standard Time

Dear Everyone,

It's hard to believe that a month ago, Scott was having surgery. Time flies whether you're having fun or not! He's had 4 radiation treatments as of today, and so far he is not experiencing any bad side effects, other than fatigue. And that may just be from waking up at 5:30! Some new vitamins, daily exercise, and some amazing Healing Touch sessions are also helping him feel a lot better.

On Wednesday we'll be on the new schedule of 1:00 to 1:15 p.m. treatments, and we won't have to go on XMas or New Year's days. YAY!

On Thursday last week (day 2), I was able to go into the radiation room while Scott was being situated. It was good to be able to watch how the technician precisely adjusted him and the table so that the dosage was in the exact right spot. He's having 3 "doses" to 3 areas of his head -- from the top, side and from underneath. On Friday, I took my camera and snapped a few shots of the setup process. Doing so has taken away the fear for me -- now my imagination can't run rampant.

On Thursday and Friday, Scott experienced the phenomenon of seeing a continuous blue-white light during the radiation. He asked the technician about this, and she confirmed that some people report seeing the light. It's nothing to worry about, just interesting.

This Thursday we are going to see a neuropsychologist. He will help Scott figure out any changes in his thinking as a result of the surgery, and hopefully talk about how to get around any problems. We'll see him again in January for a complete evaluation, but this is a good start. We're looking forward to it! Scott will also do some more physical therapy.

We're also seeing the surgeon again on Thursday (at our request) to ask a few questions and just have closure on that part of this trip. When we see the MRI films (we now have our own copies), we are amazed that Scott is still kicking -- that tumor is not small!!!

For those of you in Denver, I wanted to let you know that my cousins' wives, Jean and Laura, are helping schedule meals to be delivered to us for dinners. They'll be coordinating every other week for friends, coworkers, & neighbors, while my good friend Pat is coordinating the meals from my network of at-home moms and friends in FEMALE (Formerly Employed Mothers at the Leading Edge). We SOOOOO much appreciate this extra help -- words just aren't enough.

Thank you again and AGAIN for your positive thoughts and prayers. It truly makes us feel better to know you're all out there with us. We're gearing up to send out our annual photo collage -- send us your street address if you want one (if you haven't been on our list before). Scott will be the one in the middle! You'll still recognize him.

Love from us all!
Shelly, Scott and Wil :)

Despite my email voice, December grew dark, its dwindling days ever shorter in solidarity with how our life felt shorter and darker, too. Some days seemed to be lit only by the five candles on Wil's birthday cake, the multi-colored twinkle lights on the tree in our front window, and the indigo glow of Wil's bedroom nightlight. Trying to create a bit of festivity, we strung white twinkle lights under the mattress of the top bunk, lighting up Wil's cave below. Otherwise, the moon seemed lost on the other side of the earth, and I missed it.

We left the house at 5:30 every morning in the first two weeks of Scott's radiation treatment, the dark morning streets deserted except for our car, a few lonely commuters, and the dry snowflakes blowing beneath the street lights. Our parents took turns sleeping over so Wil could wake up in his own bed. We'd return home by 7:00 to the cozy smell of coffee and French toast or pancakes, and the sound of cartoons and Wil's laughter.

Days during radiation fell into a quiet, tired repetition—setting our alarm clock for 11 p.m., 2 a.m., 5 a.m. for Scott's medications to control seizures and brain swelling after surgery, driving to and from radiation, reading and replying to email messages, surfing the Internet to research the reality of brain tumors and possible treatments, trying to shop for Christmas and Wil's birthday, and assembling photos for our annual collage and writing the summary of 1998 to send as our Christmas card.

I thought with my letter I was putting a cheerful spin on our year, counting our blessings before the tumor arrived and listing all the happy milestones at my cheery best. I mailed 140 envelopes full of my memories and intentions for a healthier new year. Upon receiving my letter, one friend and former colleague (whose email address I'd been lacking) wrote to say "It was nice to hear of your year, but we were most taken by the news of Scott's illness." Years later when I reread my 1998 Christmas letter, I was taken aback to realize it sounded like a laundry list of all the losses we needed to grieve. I wondered if that's how it sounded to everyone else who read it.

Midway through the month, we decided to drive to the mountains with my parents to cut down our Christmas trees. It was tradition to cut a tree in the National Forest for the price of a $20 permit and the gas money to get there, sometimes knee deep in snow, sometimes on dirt. This year we went to Deckers, an hour away, in a forest that sustained a fire a few years earlier. Cutting trees helped thin the forest that wasn't touched by flames. We borrowed Scott's dad's big red truck so all five of us could fit inside (Scott's mom already decorated her tree), and we packed our hand saws, mittens, a thermos of hot chocolate, and some homemade apple cake. Dad drove, since Scott wasn't supposed to anymore.

We took Highway 285 into the mountains, past Evergreen where Scott's parents lived when he was in college, past Conifer where he lived from junior high through high school when his family moved to Colorado from Michigan, past the restaurant shaped like a hot dog that everyone called The Big Weenie. It was a typical Colorado winter day, clear blue sky with just a dusting of snow.

Then we drove into Deckers, following signs for tree cutters, passing hand-painted signs for a chili supper fundraiser at the volunteer fire department. We parked along the dirt road, with a slew of other families out to seek the perfect Christmas tree, and we headed west on foot into the sparse pine forest, all of us spreading out a bit for our search. "Here's one," we'd yell to the others. "How about this one," pointing up high. "That's too tall," someone would answer. "Hey, over here," we'd yell. It seemed the hunt must follow certain rules, not finding our tree too soon. The tree must be tall and well shaped, and my family preferred the short-needled blue spruce with room for ornaments to hang down, rather than the thicker trees on which ornaments just lay. We called them our "Charlie Brown" trees, like the sapling Linus wrapped with his beloved blue blanket so that it blossomed into a bigger, beautiful tree.

Having hiked maybe half a mile in, close to a hillside of red rocks from which the vast city was visible on the hazy plains below, Scott found our tree. He sat on an outcropping of rocks for awhile, listening to our tree-finder calls, raucous as blue jays. He told me later it kind of felt like sitting in heaven, all alone among nature. Scott was wearing his red velvet Santa hat that his manager from work gave him after his surgery, and it did a good job hiding his still-red scar. He looked so healthy in his beard, his ski jacket, hiking boots, and Levis.

As we walked to him, we saw a cave at the base of his hill, home to a fire ring and broken bottles. Wil wanted to play inside, but we were all business, chopping down the tree. We took turns sawing, calling "Timber!" as it fell. Dragging it back to the truck, we realized it was 16 or 20 feet tall. Trees always look smaller in the forest than they do in our living rooms. My parents picked out a smaller tree that my dad measured for accuracy by holding his arm up over his head, the way we used to measure the proper length of cross-country skis.

After a brief tailgate party with hot chocolate, we tossed the two trees in the truck bed and piled ourselves into the extended cab. "Shall we get some lunch at the fire department?" suggested my mom and we all chimed in "Oh yeah." We were happily hungry.

The long metal building was crowded with rows of tables and tree-cutting families, chattering like a loud village of squirrels. A long line snaked toward the chili at the far end of the room. I had to use the bathroom. Now. So I left a twenty-dollar bill and Wil with Scott, tasking him with getting us something to eat. Needing to go—now—I didn't give him time to argue or define my lunch request any further. After standing in another long line for the ladies room, I came back to find him fuming. He bought two bowls of chili and two glasses of Coke, but Wil wouldn't eat and was whining.

"There would be a good time to leave me alone and a not so good time," Scott whispered angrily as I sat down at the table. "Guess which one this was?"

Why so mad at me all of a sudden? What the heck? I was thinking, wanting to cuss even cruder. *Go ahead,* said the voice in my head, *It's not like you're talking out loud.*

Oh yeah. What the hell? I thought even louder. *How did my bladder screw up our otherwise totally fun day? It wasn't me, it was your damn brain tumor. Back off, buddy, or I'll toss you in the back of the pickup with the Christmas trees and drive downhill really fast around all the curves. Then you can eat my dust, ya big butthead!*

My inner tirade depleted, defeated, I said nothing out loud. It was too much. The fun was over for the rest of the day. We ate lunch in silence, none of us knowing how to extinguish the smoldering anger in Scott. There was no use arguing. I couldn't risk Scott's brain tumor commandeering his voice again.

The conversation came hours later; the realization struck hard. For the first time in the four weeks since surgery, it struck me that Scott had subtle but significant deficits from his tumor. (Deficits, the polite medical term for things you can't do anymore because they cut out that part of your brain which the tumor was eating or would have eaten anyway.) The lighthearted tree-cutting felt so natural that neither my parents nor I realized that Scott needed help. In the quiet of the forest, he was fine. But inside, he could no longer take the clatter of a cafeteria, the decisions of what to buy, how to handle the money and change, and how to keep track of a kid on top of it all. But more than anger at me for deserting him was a deep sadness for himself that he was not the man he had been just a month before. And he might never be again.

We finished eating our chili, but with the fun evaporated, an ingredient was missing to make it taste good. Mom took Wil across the room to look at handmade crafts and Christmas ornaments. Then we drove home, mostly in silence. I left Scott and Wil at home while I drove back to his parent's house to swap the truck for our Honda, and came home to more seething anger that I had left him alone with Wil at the end of a long day. It pushed him over the edge, and we decided to decorate the tree the next day instead. We went to bed exhausted.

The next night, however, an unexpected gift somewhat repaired our tree-cutting debacle. The three of us had just finished decorating the tree and plugged in the lights to shine out the front window when the doorbell rang. It was our shy neighbor, Suzy, bearing bread still warm from her oven. "I saw your lights on, so I thought I'd pop over," she said. "I brought you some bread. I hope you like it."

Scott and I returned to the neurosurgeon's office once more in December. I called to ask for a follow-up appointment because, I told the receptionist, "we have more questions." She sighed and huffed as if it were a terrible inconvenience to make an appointment to merely talk, but squeezed us in at the end of the surgeon's day at five-fifteen. We needed more answers after the radiation oncologist told us Scott's tumor was more aggressive, more infiltrative, than a regular grade-two astrocytoma. We didn't know what that meant. What Scott really wanted to know was whether he was a candidate for another surgery to get more tumor out of his head.

We sat across from the surgeon, he behind his desk, his framed credentials on the wall behind him. I had prepared a page full of questions in my spiral notebook: Could you please explain the second MRI? Is there any value in trying a second surgery, this time with the ICG Wand, in the near or distant future? Are Scott's deficits (cold clammy hands, short-term memory problems, screwed up internal clock, naming and recall, seizure-like shaking in the middle of the night) a result of scarring in the brain? Will it improve? Please explain the pathology of the tumor. How do you see your role now that surgery is over? Are you still the appropriate doctor for Scott's prescriptions? Would a PET scan be useful after radiation?

If you're not dealing with a brain tumor yourself, those questions might mean mumbo jumbo. The only answer that mattered to Scott was the neurosurgeon's assurance that a second surgery was an option after radiation. That's all Scott wanted to know. Despite all our questions, I didn't record many answers, though I know asking mattered as much having answers. When I look at the page of blue ink in my spiral notebook today, I see how I noted that Colorado didn't have a PET scanner in 1998 (positron emission topography, which indicates whether a tumor is actively growing as opposed to scar tissue or to dead tissue, called necrosis). I see how I noted that the frequency of MRIs will vary (depending on Scott's state of mind, so to speak). I see Wil's pretend-cursive squiggles drawn sometime later in black ink as if he could clarify the questions and answers and my memory.

What I do remember about that day is the drive home, me behind the wheel, Scott chattering away with optimism about some future date when he could have a second surgery. *I'm so looking forward to that*, I thought in sarcastic silence. With my body driving on autopilot, I saw my future stretched out into an endless brain tumor battle, except that it wasn't endless. Two to five years, the surgeon reiterated. He put boundaries on a battle he believed we could not win. *Today is the first day I really understand that the odds are against us. I have to prepare myself, just in case. I'm going to need a survival shelf in my head.*

When as newlyweds Scott and I looked at houses to buy in Oak Ridge, Tennessee, we laughed at how so many houses had bomb shelters in the backyard, dug into the oak-covered hills. The town arose to support the Manhattan Project, and most people who lived in the quickly-built wooden houses didn't even know their job was to help build a bomb. But in the decades after the war, they built brick houses. They knew what they had done...and they built bomb shelters...just in case.

I need a survival shelf in my mind. What should I stock it with? To start with, a bottle of tequila, to drown my sorrows if it gets really bad...Hmmm, remember how I got drunk on tequila from too much celebrating on my twenty-second birthday, first at lunch with everyone from work, then with my friends that night? That was the day I met you, Scott. You signed your name on the card that came with the flowers the guys at work bought me. I couldn't read your handwriting. I didn't know who you were. I didn't know then that by Valentine's Day, a month later, we would be inseparable. Oh, too many margaritas on my birthday that year. I even swallowed the worm. I never got that drunk again, but I might need to in two to five years.

As with most of my drive-time reveries, I locked my thoughts in the glove box when I parked in the garage. I couldn't stock anything else on my survival shelf that night. I had to make Wil's birthday cake in the morning. And Christmas would come a week later.

I spent December trying so hard to find the light that I nearly burned out. Scott wanted to make oak candle sticks as Christmas gifts, but he never had the energy. I knew he wouldn't. Most days after radiation he needed a nap. So I shopped online at Amazon.com, then spent much of the month fruitlessly scanning the shopped out malls, coming home empty-handed, emotionally spent.

How could I shop for everyone when all we really wanted was life back to normal. Wil drew a "fold-up computer or calculator" on a page of my journal—very much his father's son, even at five. As it turned out, I spent too much money buying presents for Scott as if trying to fulfill his final requests (not that he made any, the fear was all mine). The theme seemed to be father-son activities to do before you die—such as matching baseball gloves (that they *never* used, not once), a desktop planetarium (that couldn't live up to the actual night sky), a learn-how-to-draw book with watercolor paints and pencils (Scott swore he felt a new urge to create after his brain surgery; he didn't need a book telling him how.)

I felt crushed under the unspoken premise that this very well could be our last Christmas together. But why does it take cancer to realize that we have to value every day as if it could be our last? Nobody knows when their number is up! And *that* made me angry, that almost everyone else in our world was enjoying the holidays, believing not only in Santa and shopping, three wise men and mangers, but also blithely believing in long, infallible lives.

A special delivery one afternoon changed my cynical attitude and melted a bit of my anger. A big box came in the mail, along with a pile of colorful envelopes. The box came from Michigan from the Londry's, friends who moved to Colorado with Scott's family back in 1978—adventurous pioneer buddies whose love was rekindled through emails in the weeks since Scott's surgery. Sitting on the floor of our family room, with the gas fireplace lit, the three of us gathered around the box, excited and curious. I opened the envelope taped to the outside of the package and read a handwritten poem aloud to Scott and Wil. It explained in rhyme how we would receive a package for each of the twelve days of Christmas because they loved us and wanted us to remember so twelve days in a row. (I kept the poem taped to the lid of the box that I opened, but after a few months it finally fell off, so the words have been lost.)

I gasped at their kindness and burst into tears, bewildering Wil. "Mommy, why does it make you sad?"

I pulled him into a hug and said, "These are happy-sad tears. I just can't believe how much everyone loves us. I can't believe how nice they are. Well, I can … but I can't."

"Well, believe it," he said, squeezing me once then jumping over my knees to Scott to be closer to the box. Scott was using scissors to cut the thick tape of the top seam, lifting the lid, pushing his hands into the Styrofoam noodle nest. He pulled out another box covered in Santa paper, which he and Wil ripped off in a flurry, "Oooooh, LEGOs!" they said in unison.

It was the 25th anniversary limited edition. The sturdy plastic box held countless crunchy plastic bags of LEGO bricks, sorted by shape and size. One silver brick came in its own wrapper.

"Chad and I used to play LEGOs for hours on end, days at a time," Scott said. He was touched into silence and just sat there holding the silver brick. Impatient, Wil tugged his arm as if asking the five-year-old Scott to come out and play. Scott responded and the two boys spent the rest of the day opening each small sack, pouring bricks into the box, and building all sorts of LEGO creations until dinner.

As if that wasn't enough, I continued to open the pile of envelopes. In one I found a Christmas letter from my cousin, Terry, with a final sentence that read, "While this holiday season finds us in good health, Terry's cousins Shelly, Scott & Wil are contending with an extended illness, so it would mean a lot to us if you could please remember them in your prayers."

Terry is the middle daughter of my mom's oldest sister and at the time worked for the American Cancer Society. When my mom had cancer and I was an hour away from home at college, Terry came to visit to make sure I was okay. She brought me a copy of *When Bad Things Happen to Good People* and took me out for an afternoon beer at an empty bar. While we talked and I shared how scared I was, I'll never forget how she reached out to me across the table and squeezed me a hand-hug.

Being included in her Christmas card prayer-request felt like another reach-across-a-table hug. It shocked me, but in a good way, like the LEGOs. Along with the emails I knew were being forwarded by our friends to theirs, it seemed we had been wrapped up in the true spirit of Christmas, shipped around the world like a ribbon round a package, and in return, love was arriving daily on our doorstep.

The next day, a second package arrived from the Londry's. In it were three wooden blue birds, ornaments for our tree, in the style of American folk art, hand-painted and tied with raffia. These were the three French hens, and it prompted us to sing the entire song out loud, and then go in search of the alternate irreverent version that someone sent us by email. You know, the one that ends each verse with "and a beer."

On Christmas Eve, completely worn out, I called my parents in tears. My sister back in town yet again for the holidays, cheerily answered the phone and said, "Are you ready for tomorrow? What time do you think you guys will get here?"

The plan was to have Christmas morning at my parent's house to save me the stress of cooking breakfast for a crowd. Earlier in the month, we agreed that would be best. It wasn't. I burst into tears.

"I'm not ready for tomorrow at all. The house is a mess. The presents aren't wrapped. And I can't stand the idea of waking up and having to drive across town." I said this all between sobs.

"Oh," Jenéne said in a long drawn-out word, instantly getting it. "Hang on. We'll be right over."

She and my parents came to my rescue. They cleaned toilets and vacuumed and helped me finish wrapping presents. Then they made dinner while Wil and I sat by the fireplace, reading Little Critter's version of *The*

Night Before Christmas. Scott went up and down the stairs, alternately napping and joining us in the family room.

The next morning we slept in as long as Wil would let us (maybe 8:30) and had Christmas, us three, for an hour. Scott enjoyed opening his presents with Wil. I was happy with the one present Scott's mom drove him to the mall to purchase. It was a soft cotton nightgown, black with three-quarter-length sleeves, like a football jersey. Scott gave me a wink like he thought it was sexy, but we both knew all I wanted for Christmas was a good night's sleep.

As we dismantled the Christmas tree, I thought again about my survival shelf. I pictured it in the back of my mind, through a heavy wooden door with a wrought-iron handle. More than a shelf (but not quite a bomb shelter), I needed a small storm cellar with a series of shelves where, in better times, you might find jars of canned peaches, scrapbooks of photos, shoeboxes of rocks and acorns from childhood mountain picnics, Christmas lights wrapped around newspaper to keep them untangled. In my mind's eye, I added a miniature collection of people, like Christmas ornaments you can't bear to put away. I imagined my people six inches tall, sitting on my survival shelf, legs dangling, milling around, playing with LEGO bricks, waiting to help. I could pick one of my people off the shelf to bring them up to full scale, ready for action. Seeing my people there on my shelf would remind me I'm never alone.

December was dark, but little flames of love sustained us, and, like the season's solstice herself, gave us faith that our days would grow a bit longer and lighter if we could just hold on. Winter wasn't over yet.

All shall be well, and all shall be well,
and all manner of things shall be well.
—Julian of Norwich

12
January in Pleasantville

Subj: Happy New Year from Scott
Date: 1/3/99 8:24:46 PM Mountain Standard Time

Dear Everyone,

Happy New Year and cheers for a good 1999! Scott, Wil and I enjoyed our holidays, beginning with Wil's 5th birthday the week before Christmas and continuing with several celebrations with family and friends. Some days (or hours) were tough emotionally—and still are—as we go up and down this rollercoaster. But we loved seeing everyone during the holidays and, maybe for the first time since Wil was born, purely appreciated the true spirit of the season.

Scott has had 13 of 33 radiation treatments, less than expected by this time due to radiation-equipment breakdowns. It's frustrating to miss a scheduled day, but has also kept Scott from being too tired during the holidays. The breaking equipment is nothing to worry about from a safety standpoint—just means that we won't be done until the end of January or possibly even February. 1:00 p.m. will stay Scott's radiation time.

Along with the fatigue, Scott's hair has started falling out in the target zone of radiation. After a few photos for documentation, Scott's says he'll shave it all off, or at least shape up the edges. Hats help with the winter cold.

Through an acquaintance of my mom, we were given the name of another man with a somewhat similar brain tumor. We spoke on the phone this weekend and hope to meet him and his wife later in January. Just talking on the phone made us feel great (1) to be in contact with someone nearby who is going through something similar and (2) that someone farther along in his treatment, side effects, and tumor stage would take time to help us sort this all out.

Scott had Part 1 of his neuropsychological evaluation last week and will finish with Part 2 on Friday, Jan. 8th. The first part, which lasted a grueling two hours, tested Scott's short-term memory, associative reasoning, writing, and also general knowledge. He was intrigued by the process. We'll tell you about the results when we find out.

Well, that's about it for now. Thanks for the holiday cards, letters and photos. Have a very happy New Year. We'll be in touch.

Love,
Shelly, Scott & Wil Vickroy

When I think of January in Colorado, I think of bright blue skies that follow a day long, feet-deep blizzard, the sun so bright it almost hurts to open your eyes. I think of crisp cold air you breathe in, exhaling in warm wisps. I think of cars so warmed by sunlight that you toss your parka in the back seat and roll down the windows an inch or more. I think of happy geese honking overhead as they steer their V to the nearest city park lake. I think of the subzero weather that almost always comes with the National Western Stock Show and prize-winning steers, dancing horses, and cowboy boots. And coincides with my birthday, which reaps a three-day weekend thanks to Martin Luther King, Jr.'s birthday.

I usually enjoy the freshness of January and my birthday, treating myself to post-holiday clearance sales, a fresh new appointment calendar full of art from Mary Engelbreit or Van Gogh. I spend January thinking of New Year's resolutions, making happy plans for vacations, spring gardening, a new haircut.

That January, though, held a different sense of future plans, as if I should use pencil, not pen, in my weekly planner. The phone numbers I wrote on the inside back cover, an annual habit and quick reference guide, were numbers for too many doctors: neurosurgeon, radiation oncologist, neuropsychologist, physical therapist, primary care doctor—office and pager. The sad thing about that list is that I rarely needed it—I had those numbers memorized.

For me, January 1999 was one steep snow-covered slope dotted with pine trees and unknown, buried obstacles, and I was trapped in a snowball accelerating downhill, collecting fears and facts like pine needles and lost mittens. In Allie McBeal-ish imagery, my head, hands, and feet flailed out from the snowball, mouth screaming out-of-control crazy, wanting to stop and terrified of crashing, shrinking in size as the snowball grew larger.

One day in the first week of January, my mom invited me to a movie. We met at the Continental theatre at I-25 and Hampden, which offers the largest screen in Denver inside and outside a panoramic view of the city and mountains. I was ready for an afternoon escape, and *Pleasantville* sounded like just what I needed. I loved watching as the black-and-white characters turned Technicolor after the modern-day teenager, David, was transported into their world with a magic remote control and took on the role of do-good geek, Bud. Picture Toby Maguire before he was Spiderman, Joan Allen as his prim '50s mother, William H. Macy as Pleasantville's Father Knows Best, and Reese Witherspoon as his slutty sister finding her inner Legally Blond smart girl. At first, Bud tried to keep his sister from changing the townspeople's grayscale approach to life. Eventually, he saw the impact of new ideas, rebellion, and color that comes when you let out what's inside you, and he helped to awaken all of Pleasantville.

Sitting inside the movie theatre, I put myself in Bud's plaid shirt and khaki's, trying to describe the world "out there," which for me was my new cancer-care world set alight by the new awareness I felt about life's fragile luster and the love people were willing to share. Bud called it "Louder, scarier, I guess, more dangerous." At the movie's near-ending, I could see myself as both his mother and girlfriend, having packed him a sack lunch and sweater and saying goodbye when he left them. It felt like saying goodbye, someday, to Scott—hoping to see him again, wondering where he was going, being left behind to go on living in the new version of Pleasantville.

When Bud becomes shaggy-haired David again, back in his own living room, I could see myself as his modern-day mother, mascara smudged face, crying in the dining room. She answers his "What's wrong?" by brushing it off with an honest "Everything's just fucked up...When your father was here, I used to think *this* was it. This was how it was always going to be. I had the right house, the right car, the right life...I'm 40 years old. It's not supposed to be like this."

He replies, "It's not *supposed* to be anything." And I thought to myself, could that be me someday, sad and alone, crying in front of Wil. I didn't want to fall apart like she did.

The final scene struck me. Betty, the Pleasantville mother, sits on the park bench next to her husband and the shy soda-fountain owner turned painter. I felt like it was me on that bench in a pretty pink dress suit, sitting between two versions of Scott, before his brain tumor in his business-dad suit and his after-self in sweatpants, t-shirt and radiation-bald, surgery-scarred head.

Bewildered by change, the husband asks her, "So what's gonna happen now?"

"I don't know...Do you know what's going to happen now?" she replies.

"No, I don't," and he laughs. And they laugh together.

The painter says, "I guess I don't know either."

None of us knew what was happening next. We just had to trust the new palette of our life.

I left the theatre, a hug for my mom for a nice afternoon, and unlocked my car, stunned by the movie. On autopilot, I started the car and drove down the highway, almost rush-hour in the late afternoon. Under winter's brown cloud, Denver was as gray as the movie had been. The movie's last question rolled around in my mind, "What happens now?" I burst into tears, as if my snowballing self had bashed into a tree and exploded.

Alone in the car, anonymous, I let loose and cried, and heard myself scream without thinking. "I am so scared!" Then I yelled, "Please let him be okay." And then, surprising myself at my words, "Please don't leave me." As my sobbing slowed, I hoped something larger than me had eyes on the road and hands on the wheel, and I whispered, "Please, God, get me home safely."

I didn't wait for the right song to come on the radio. I pushed the buttons of my car CD player to jump to the song I needed. I cried while Shawn Mullins reminded me that everything's gonna be all right and to just "rock-a-bye." I pushed the skip-back button to play the song again and this time I just breathed while he sang. The third time, I sang along. After that I tuned to KBCO for a traffic report.

The clouds over the mountains turned crimson. I gripped the steering wheel, continuing home. I knew that at least for today Scott was still safe and alive, even if I didn't know yet whether his radiation treatments were doing any good. I'd been trying so hard to be brave and strong all these months, and only that day did I realize how much I needed to voice my fears out loud, if only to myself.

After a week of constantly being on the verge of tears, I told Scott what happened. We were lying in bed one night and I just finished reading, *The Education of Little Tree*. In parts I laughed out loud, but at the end I cried when the grandfather dies. The Cherokee have a death ritual to say good-bye, saying, "This time has been pretty good. Next time will be better. I will wait for you."

Scott held me while I cried, waiting until I could talk, not needing specifics. We talked a long time, about radiation, his feeling physically worse, how Wil was coping and missing his friends, how the movie had made me react, not knowing what's next. We didn't come up with a plan, no solutions. It was almost as if screaming out loud in the car, "I am so scared," were such powerful words that I stayed stuck being scared for a week.

When I woke up the morning after our talk, my energy had shifted and I felt able to breathe. I was ready to send another email to our faithful friends and speak more truths out loud. I was ready to offer honesty in my messages, not just sugarcoat our crazy existence. Next to my computer, as I began to type, I noticed a quote in my Mary Engelbreit planner. Abraham Lincoln's voice lifted off the page with these words, "The best thing about the future is that it comes only one day at a time."

Subj: Latest on Scott - 1/14
Date: 1/14/99 9:53:31 AM Mountain Standard Time

Dear Everyone,

I haven't written lately because not much is new. Scott has been getting through the daily radiation with no health problems and the equipment has been working just fine. Scott has been going to physical therapy about once a week for strengthening exercises, working out at the rec center almost daily, and is having weekly Healing Touch sessions. All that seems to be helping a lot with his side effects.

Scott will have his last radiation treatment on Tuesday, January 26th (assuming no further equipment breakdowns). Then we will play the waiting game for 4-8 weeks until the doctor decides we can have the next MRI, which hopefully will show how much the tumor shrank from radiation. (The long wait is because radiation causes brain swelling, which needs to recede, and the tumor continues to shrink for awhile.) Depending on the MRI results, we'll proceed to whatever is next.

Scott attended a men's cancer support group on Tuesday this week, which is sponsored by a great organization in Denver known as Qualife. Scott was by far the youngest of the 16 men there and most had prostate cancer, but two others had brain tumors (one man even had the same surgeon as Scott). Scott said it was an upbeat group with a lot to talk about, and despite the differences in cancer, their experiences are very similar. He enjoyed it and plans to continue going to this twice monthly group. Family members are invited to the second meeting every month.

Even though the physical stuff seems to be improving or stabilizing, I must admit that mentally it seems to be getting tougher. The Great Unknowns are waiting for us after the radiation is over. We're trying to figure out how to get on with Living, preparing for what may be next and researching treatment options, trying not to be scared all the time (that's me more than Scott), and making every day count. Some days it seems that the week of surgery was a piece of cake compared to the longer-term wondering, waiting, and wondering some more. So, bear with us as the ups and downs get steeper. And please keep in touch.

On a lighter note, Wil is glad to be back in preschool after the holidays (I can't be-lieve that in two weeks I'll be registering him for kindergarten!) Wil had to bring a "W" word to school this week and after thinking for a minute said "I could bring myself." :)

Love,
Shelly

They're changing guard at Buckingham Palace.
Christopher Robin went down with Alice.
Alice is marrying one of the guard. "
A soldier's life is terrible hard,"
Says Alice.
—Alan Alexander Milne

13

Changing of the Guard

That tune hints at something both jaunty and haunting. I picture Christopher Robin holding hands with Winnie the Pooh and Alice in Wonderland, watching as the guards click-clacked away behind the palace fence. (I have no idea whether the lyrics meant that Alice, but that's how my brain sees the song.)

As we began to anticipate the long wait after radiation, we had time for more research to determine the next steps in our march, which led to an itchy sensation. It seemed as if the universe were suggesting it was time to change the guard.

Seeking more facts about brain tumors in general and possible treatment plans was one aspect. We owed it to ourselves to discover what else was out there that might help Scott survive not only his malignant tumor but the side effects of treatment.

For instance, we found a new physical therapist who specialized in neurological rehabilitation, showing Scott exercises like standing on one leg on a foam cushion to improve his balance. She reminded him to use his right hand as much as possible so that his left brain didn't give up on the motor functions just because they were harder to coordinate.

Then I learned of a workshop the first weekend in March for brain tumor patients and families hosted by the National Brain Tumor Foundation and M. D. Anderson Cancer Center. This conference seemed kind of creepy to me, being surrounded by a hotel full of brain tumor patients—maybe much more desperate with higher-grade tumors. I was both intrigued and scared to dive deeply into workshops that would explain the way brain tumors grew, how surgery was performed, whether new treatments were available, how to cope with side effects and rehabilitation. The workshop flyer promised a lot of answers, as well as an offer to get consultations with the brain tumor experts at M. D. Anderson Cancer Center. And the cost of it was only a few hundred dollars, plus airfare. It seemed feasible. The timing would be right for seeking second opinions because by then we would have Scott's post-radiation MRI and be ready to decide on the next steps of his treatment.

Scott continued getting Healing Touch treatments from Pam, who always brought her massage table to our house and set up shop at the foot of our bed where there was space to walk around the table and move, add, or clear energy wherever Scott seemed to need it most. Wil often helped her set up the table, pulling a narrow fitted sheet over the padded tabletop, placing a pillow at one end, putting a relaxing CD in the player.

One afternoon, after Pam gave Scott a Healing Touch treatment, Scott found himself in a conversation with Wil about death while otherwise creating houses with LEGOs.

"Are you going to die, Daddy?" Wil asked.

"Well, we're all going to die someday, Wil," he answered, always wanting to tell his son the truth. "But we never know when. I'm not planning on dying anytime soon. I guess it makes me sad to think about it, though. I would really miss you and Mom."

Wil was quiet for a minute, processing, and then patted Scott on the arm. "It's okay, Dad. If you died, I could climb on Pam's table and she would help me talk to you. And I would still draw you pictures."

Scott couldn't answer, except to smile. Wil didn't need a reply. Scott told me about their conversation later that night, "I have no idea where he got that idea. Do you think it's okay he believes that?"

"I don't know. Maybe he knows something we don't. I don't think it could hurt."

Later in January, an email arrived from our Healing Touch friend, Joan, who wrote that she knew a woman named Janna who recently moved to Denver after some years in Australia. She considered this woman gifted at Healing Touch and a medical intuitive (admitting that Janna wouldn't use that term herself). Because of her years of experience, her depth and breadth of training, her certification not only as a Healing Touch practitioner but also a certified instructor, perhaps Janna might provide a deeper level of healing than Scott was getting now, Joan suggested. Joan gave me her full name and phone number. Joan's endorsement seemed too full of promise to ignore.

I called Janna and told her about Joan's referral and that Scott had a brain tumor. "So are you available for a session anytime soon?"

"Of course," she replied. "I can come to your house, if that would be easier. What day works best for you?"

The first time I met Janna was at the curb outside our house as I helped her pull her massage table from the back of her SUV. Shorter than me, with a short blond bob, and quick to laugh, it was Janna's brilliant blue eyes that impressed me first. I thought I saw an old soul behind those eyes, or at least someone full of compassion, humor, and possibility. *I wouldn't mind having some Healing Touch sessions with Janna myself,* I thought right away. *I hope Scott likes her.*

He did like Janna. As much as he also liked Pam, who was much younger, Scott sensed a different energy with Janna during their sessions. She also got Scott talking—about his fears, his attitude, his motivation to undergo treatment. I never knew the details of their sessions, only what he was willing to share, but I could see a shift in Scott. It seemed his inner samurai was waking up and getting stronger.

Soon we told Pam that we'd found someone else. It was hard, letting her go, because we didn't want to hurt her feelings. But Scott's health came first, and that meant making sure his entire team was tip-top. In a way I think Pam was relieved. I wonder if her inner novice-healer was able to work with Scott's samurai energy.

I know Pam was the perfect person for Scott to begin with, but as his journey progressed, I believe he needed someone like Janna to help him go further. I also believe the saying is true that when the student is ready, the teacher appears.

Most people begin to feel tired after a few weeks of radiation therapy.
Feelings of weakness or weariness will go away gradually
after your treatment is finished.
— "Radiation Therapy and You,"
a National Institutes of Health publication

14

Radiation Fatigue

Midway through January, Scott and I went to see a screening of a movie we had invested in, called *Picture of Priority*, about teen suicide prevention. A couple of years before that, a man Scott worked with asked him to help fund it. I wasn't thrilled at the amount we spent at the time, but I believed in the movie's goal to create a film that would raise awareness about the warning signs of suicide and how to get help. It would be filmed at Lakewood High School, where my parents both went, so I figured that was a synchronistic sign to say yes. I've wondered since if maybe the movie kept me from slipping into despair.

We went to Bruce's house to watch the movie with some other investors (family, friends, coworkers), sitting in his darkened living room on kitchen chairs. Less than halfway through the riveting movie, Scott got up and went to the kitchen for a glass of water. A few minutes later, he whispered to me that he needed to sit further back in the room, away from the screen. He dragged the ladder-back chair to the furthest edge of the room where he could still, barely, see the movie.

When it was over, the teen's suicide averted, and the suicide warning signs scrolling before the movie credits, Scott motioned to me with his fingers and a jerk of his head that he needed to leave.

Once we were in the car, Scott said. "I'm pretty sure I had a seizure. I'm feeling dizzy."

His face was flushed and hot. Although it was Saturday evening, I thought our walk-in clinic would be open. We drove straight there, only to find it closed. I called our family physician from my cell phone and she said, "Don't sweat it. Just come in tomorrow if Scott's still feeling bad."

I looked for warning signs from the previous week. On Friday he spent the day in the basement with the electrician who Scott's dad hired to help us finish our basement. By nighttime, Scott could barely walk up and down the stairs. I overheard Scott on the phone to a friend, "It's been a damn hard week. It's getting harder and harder to function."

Scott rarely wrote emails during his treatment, as the ability to write anything, whether by hand or by keyboard, had turned off in his brain. Clinically, that's called dysgraphia, a symptom common to tumors of the parietal lobe. One email Scott did write was in reply to his friend, Kevin, who was wishing Scott could go downhill skiing with him in Japan. Here's what Scott wrote:

Hi

Still breathing. I think... Been a hard week. Every day is a blind date. I think you can understand how tiring that can be. I want my life back. Hell. Any life. I suppose I would complain even more if it was boring

Remember I used to say "If it was easy it wouldn't be any fun'... I could do with a little less fun right now. Or maybe, just for a few minutes.

Thanks for thinking of me. Sure do miss you. Don't hit any trees.

And Kevin... Just in case I haven't told you... I love you, too.

Around the same time, Scott's cousin-in-law's father was diagnosed with a suspected brain tumor. Scott made the effort—which took him a long, long time—to type a personal email with advice.

Hi Doug and Julie

I think I know a (very) little of the frantic panic oh my God how can this be happening what am I going to do...that you may or may not be going through (I hope not going through).

Remembering back 3 months ago to when all this was/is happening to me, the thing I wished I would have done would be to slow down. Think. Make things makes sense to you. This is your life. Your body. It's your choice. Some choices you can't unchoose. Most you can.

Make your doctors a pin/label that says: I DO NOT KNOW

Make them wear it all the time they are around you. If they don't, wear some for them. If they do (somehow) think they know something, then rephrase the question. The doctor who leaves plenty of room for something unexpected — that's a good doctor.

Now for some brain jokes/sayings (all original of course)...

1) I know some brain jokes. Now let me see...

2) You just need to take it one day at a time. By the way, what day is it?

3) Just imagine all those brain cells I lost drinking. Well, now they're trying to come back.

One Sunday in January we went to church with Scott's parents, unusual for us since the annual Christmas Eve service was almost the only time we went to church together before the tumor. I sat in the pew thinking about how changed our family already was by Scott's brain tumor. That day, instead of fuming over the recurrent misspellings of hymns in the Christmas program, I could enjoy the regular January sermon about appreciating God's beauty in Colorado and finding your special calling in life. And like frosting on a cake, instead of the usual organ, a casual group played guitar music. I sang along to the music, my hippie-Catholic-flower-child surging out of my heart at the sound of the John-Denver-like tunes. *Now* this *is church music,* I thought, and I felt like crying.

Scott whispered with a laugh, "I'm fighting an urge to walk up to the altar. Like I should stand up there and tell everyone how blessed I've been by so many people helping me. How it's restored my faith in humanity."

"Go for it," I challenged him in a whisper.

"Nah, never mind." Scott's inner introvert vetoed his urge to testify. I wish I could have seen him do it. Another strand of the protective band around my heart unsnapped, awed that Scott felt the urge at all. *What is it about church?* I thought. *How it breaks down our defenses.* It made me want to cry. After the service, while standing outside the coat room, Wil handed me a crayon-covered paper from Sunday School on the topic of Jesus healing the sick. *How ironic,* I thought. I almost started to cry.

I was overwhelmed by every bit of the morning at church. And then Reverend Jane walked up to our family to say hello, the same Reverend Jane who had prayed with us moments before Scott's surgery.

I burst into tears at the sight of her, hugged her, and cried even more. Scott and his parents stood there looking embarrassed, as was I. Reverend Jane looked at me funny when I finally relinquished the hug with a soft, "Sorry about that."

She commented with characteristic grace, "Sometimes we feel closer to someone we've prayed with."

I don't know if that was it or if I was just so tired of holding back tears. I couldn't wait to get out of that church. It was as if I tried to leave my tears, fears, and panic on a pew in the back of the sanctuary for a priest to find like a lost baby and send out for foster care. Do you think our tidal wave of tears in church is a reason why some of us leave and never go back?

Over the next week, Scott went downhill physically, which we attributed to fatigue and possibly swelling from radiation. He felt terrible—shaky, dizzy, nauseas, unable to focus his thoughts. We saw the on-call radiation oncologist, who chalked it up to fatigue from radiation. He said that while Decadron could help if the problems were caused by brain swelling due to the radiation, it would take a few days to take effect and rest was the best remedy. Tired of so many pills, Scott opted against the Decadron.

One morning, as we were waking, Scott told me his dream. I thought it so vivid that I jumped out of bed to transcribe it into his journal, which otherwise was still blank.

"In my dream I was in a speed boat with another man driving, who was younger than me. It was a fast-moving river and he was driving the boat upstream. I remember thinking it was strange that the boat's steering wheel was on the left; usually boats are steered from the right. I got the feeling that the other man didn't like me, but he knew he had to be partners with me. So we're heading upstream and we come to an island and we land on the beach. We see an old man fishing offshore, standing knee deep in the water. Then he was getting sucked downstream, like he was so tired from fishing for so long and battling the current. So the young guy and I jumped out of our boat and helped pull the old guy onshore. And I think there was a young woman there on the island, or maybe she'd been in the boat, I don't know."

"Wow," was all I said at first, still writing in his journal to capture the details, but recognizing the possible symbolism. Almost every day we would ask each other, *Did you have any dreams?* so we were practiced. "It's like the island represented 'Rest' and your brain is the old man battling the current of radiation, being so tired and all. And you're in the boat, but you don't get to drive. I guess that babe on the island was me." And I grinned at him, but he wasn't smiling. We both just wanted to lay there awhile and ponder the dream.

How can you feel so tired when you just woke up? Thank goodness radiation was almost over. But then the waiting would begin.

Subj: Update on Scott - 1/25
Date: 1/25/99

Hi Everyone,

Scott is feeling a bit better, having rested over the weekend and just knowing the end of radiation is almost here. Tomorrow (Tuesday) is his last radiation treatment. YAY! Then he'll need 4-6 weeks to recover (the fatigue will continue for awhile as his brain recovers). The doctor said Scott's problems last week were likely due to fatigue, as well as some swelling—but that it was impressive that he made it through all the radiation without needing any anti-swelling medication (steroids). She said most brain tumor patients need the steroids, so it was "a testament to Scott's fortitude" that he didn't. Scott attributes it to the 5-day break he got at Xmas and New Years, and I think the Healing Touch made a big difference.

We did make reservations for the brain tumor conference in Houston, March 5-6. We plan to go a few days earlier in case we can meet with a specialist from MD Anderson Cancer Center. Just to clarify my earlier message—we're seeking 2nd opinions from specialists in Houston because it's a good opportunity to do so since we'll already be there. But we do have confidence in our doctors here in Denver. We'll just need to broaden our research now.

I have subscribed to an email list for brain tumor patients (which includes doctors, too) and in one day already received some information on specialists around the country. It will be an interesting and valuable resource to be on that list.

Several people have told us about seeing Dr. Keith Black on CBS Sunday Morning last weekend and I have found some contact information for this doctor (he is us- ing "vaccines" for brain tumors, as well as neurosurgery advances). It's always good to have more information, so thanks for that.

I registered Wil for kindergarten this morning, and now he wonders why he has to go to preschool today. :)

We'll keep you posted during the next 4 weeks until Scott's next MRI. Pray for quick recovery and lots of good rest for us. THANKS

Love,
Shelly, Scott & Wil

Subj: Update on Scott 1/29
Date: 1/29/99 10:47:08 AM Mountain Standard Time

Dear Everyone,

Thank goodness that radiation is all over for Scott. On Monday this week, he said the treatment "damn near killed me." The last two days the beam is focused on a smaller area for a "boost" of higher radiation, and Scott really could tell the difference. He felt awful during and after the treatment, like his brain had been

"fried." He didn't know if he would go through the last and final treatment on Tuesday—he wasn't sure until he actually walked down to the radiation room and lay
down on the table. But he did, and he's glad to have finished the process so that
nobody could say he should have had the final dose—not that he's convinced one
day would make the difference. Anyway, he has been increasingly tired this week,
which we hear is pretty common. This could go on 3-6 weeks before he feels recovered from all of the radiation.

The next MRI is scheduled for 4 weeks out. We will meet with both the surgeon and
medical oncologist two days later to hear the results and see what, if anything, we
should do next. The following Wednesday we leave for Houston and will have an
all-day consultation at MD Anderson Cancer Center on Thursday, March 4th. The
conference/workshop for brain tumor patients will be that Friday and Saturday.
We're looking forward to Houston, as we've heard great things about the quality of
these conferences.

We met with the neuropsychologist this week and received a 10-page report on
Scott's neuropsych evaluation. It was interesting, but not surprising to us, to hear
that Scott scored very high on many areas (he remains "exceptionally" intelligent),
but his brain is processing information slower. [That's the extremely simplified version of his test results, of course.] For any of you out there who ever saw the movie "Blade Runner," that would explain a lot about the testing process and Scott's
enjoyment at having been through it himself now. If you haven't seen the movie,
go rent it (says Scott). :) Scott also said Wil's kindergarten assessment test was
surprisingly similar.

Because Scott is continuing to have mild seizures (not fall-down flopping around,
but more like unexpected, intermittent "brain static"), we are going to see a neurologist who can be in charge of the anti-seizure medicine and follow Scott's progress from that standpoint (it has been the surgeon up to now). So, our doctor
team is growing. I know you're curious, so to give you an idea of how unexpected
a seizure can be, Scott was reading an item on Wil's kindergarten-readiness test on
recognizing patterns such as red-blue-green-red-blue-green—his brain did NOT like
that thought process (and remembered the similar test from the neuropsych), and
Scott felt physically ill—i.e., focal seizure.

Last night, he was talking to a friend about computer keyboards (that's all he could
tell me without feeling worse) and BZZZZ, focal seizure, gotta lay down and not
think about anything! WIERD, huh? As if those types of thoughts use the brain cells
that are in the tumor area. ??? It's hard for him to feel fine one minute, and very
much NOT good the next—with no warning or recognizable reasons. Maybe different seizure medicine will help. Surely the recovery from radiation will help, too.
"For those of you thinking I had a fat head, well, now it's for sure." (That's from
Scott).

On top of Scott's stuff this week, I had two big extra worries. My sister, Jenéne,
who has been sick with excruciating headaches for two weeks, had an MRI this

week (which luckily, thankfully, showed nothing) and she is starting to feel better. BIG WHEW! And my grandmother (dad's mom) went through surgery this week to rebuild her bionic knee. And thank goodness, she pulled through the surgery, too.

So, that's been our week. More rollercoasters with unexpected tunnels and turns. We scream, we laugh, we want to throw up. But we're not getting off yet. :)

Have a good weekend. Will keep you posted.

Love,
Shelly & Scott

Sure, people need Jesus, but most of the time,
what they really need is for someone to be Jesus to them.
—*Reuben Welch*

15
Parallel Lives (Meeting the McDowells)

Long before Scott told me he loved me, he gave me a clue that he thought I was the one. Only a few weeks after we started dating, Scott brought me a thick hardback book to read by Richard Bach, *The Bridge Across Forever: A Love Story,* about soul mates and how Richard found his in Leslie Parrish, who we both remembered as the blond bombshell who falls for the god Apollo in an episode of *Star Trek.* As much as I liked the book's message, I liked it even better that Scott retrieved it from his previous girlfriend so that he could give it to me. Two years after that, we rushed out to buy Bach's next book, *One.* In this book, Richard and Leslie meet many of their alternate selves through a strange twist of quantum physics in an airplane. If you've ever met someone with a similar life and said, "That could've been me," well, Scott and I say, "There went another Richard and Leslie."

One of the hardest things about Scott's brain tumor diagnosis was the sense of being the only one, ever, anywhere, with a brain tumor. Sure we heard stories through friends of others who had survived, but we didn't know any in person. Meeting the McDowells was like finding Richard and Leslie.

It was my mother's friend, who she knew through teaching, who first emailed us about Reverend Clyde McDowell. She had been in his congregation when he served as senior pastor at Mission Hills Church, which happened to be where my stay-at-home-mom's group, FEMALE, had been meeting for almost two years. That was my first clue that synchronicity was at work. Feeling shy about intruding into the life of a stranger, we hesitated to make the call. Then one of my neighbors down the street sent us his name, too, because she also went to church at Mission Hills and had heard about his brain tumor. So I figured it might be preordained for us to meet.

Dr. McDowell had recently been appointed president of Denver Seminary, not only a man of God but one of God's top dogs. His wife's name was

Lee. She answered the phone when Scott called their home. "May I speak to Clyde McDowell," he asked.

Scott heard a protective hesitation on the other end saying "May I ask who is calling?"

Scott realized he needed to clarify his reason for the call. His words came out in a pile at her feet, "I have a brain tumor, too. We were wondering if we could talk to you sometime."

The voice on the other end warmed as she said, "Yes, of course. What can we do for you?"

Her husband, she explained, was in the midst of chemotherapy treatment, so it was a few weeks before we could meet in person. It was the end of January when they came to our home, in the early afternoon while Wil was at preschool. Wanting to be a good hostess and show my gratitude for their visit, I baked two pies, pumpkin and apple, because you never know what kind of pie a person will prefer. Scott and I were both nervous because we had never invited a priest or a reverend to our home before, much less a seminary president. I must admit I was feeling like a heathen.

The doorbell rang. I opened the front door to find a tall, athletic yet tired looking man in a business suit and his beautiful wife, with long blond hair, who wore a dress suit. Scott and I were in jeans. I guessed they were a decade older than us, maybe more. We shook hands and I showed them to our family room where they sat on the couch, and I offered them pie with hot tea or coffee. Lee had the pumpkin pie and Clyde, the apple.

While we all nibbled pie, I summarized Scott's story of diagnosis, surgery, and now radiation, and then Lee explained Clyde's story, briefly. His tumor had been diagnosed the previous summer as a grade-three astrocytoma. Two surgeries had failed to remove the tumor, so it was deemed inoperable. After two different chemotherapy protocols, his tumor had the opposite reaction than expected. In a few days they would be returning to San Francisco to be assessed by the doctors there, where his clinical trial was based. Clyde's tumor was in his left frontal lobe, the communication center, which affects speech, an obvious irony for someone in his profession.

Finally I asked what sounded like a stupid question to ask a man of God, "How do you deal with all this?" I figured "my faith" would be his short answer but I was hoping for more insight.

He smiled and handed me a narrow, thick pamphlet on white paper. It was titled "Reflections on an Unexpected Journey." He wrote it, he said, during his radiation treatments in San Francisco, with help from his wife. Perhaps his writing would explain better than he could now.

They left soon after, with an invitation to stay in touch. They walked down our sidewalk holding hands. As soon as Scott shut the door, he saw the pamphlet's back cover where the McDowells were pictured in a black and white photo. Scott held it out to me, "Look at this. This is exactly how I pictured Clyde in my mind before he arrived. Not the tired brain tumor patient he was today, but this man, healthy and strong. I pictured his face exactly. Isn't that strange?"

Scott had a soul connection with Clyde, having met the man, hearty and whole, in his mind before he ever arrived on our doorstep. On the surface, I saw a lovely couple with nearly grown children whose life had been derailed, whose new career must be set aside, who were struggling to reconcile their theology with suffering, yet still could trust in God's greater purpose. I wondered how different it would be if Scott's tumor had arrived when he was 48 instead of 33. Meeting the McDowells was, in the slimmest but truest of senses, like meeting an alternate version of us, older and wiser, but maybe just as scared and confused, and yet, still as hopeful.

I was relieved beyond belief that our meeting had not become an effort to evangelize or convert our religious thinking. Our meeting was not between a reverend, his wife, and two souls needing saved. It felt like a meeting of equals, two couples dealing with brain tumors. Perhaps from their view, the visit to our home was an obvious extension of pastoral care—we called and they came.

I cannot speak for the McDowells about what our meeting meant to them or even begin to transcribe Clyde's thirty-one pages of personal reflections. Yet one part from his pamphlet speaks to me now in how I see parallels between Clyde's life and Scott's, in how they grappled to interpret the new version of their reality, seeking answers to the question of "why me, God, why now, when I had other plans?"

"Surely, all of my life has been the intelligent pursuit of excellence in my profession. The Master's degree and Doctoral program were all human efforts to raise my competence and impact. Yes, God has put in my heart, like in many others, a desire to make a difference in this world. I want to leave a legacy of impact on the world...I am reminded that God did not come to save the world so that He would produce many highly efficient and competent leaders, but rather He would bring about changed leaders with changed hearts and changed motives because they had experienced that One who is the "Lover of our Souls" and the "Friends of all Friends."

As I read his words, I thought about the legacy we all hope to leave, how it's not always granted to us to know what impact we leave on the world. Perhaps if we ever leave a legacy, like the Indigos Girls sing, it's that we loved each other well. Perhaps part of Clyde's legacy was to inspire us to pay it forward.

As we cleaned up the dishes and put plastic wrap on the leftover pies, Scott and I talked about how impressed we were by the McDowell's calm grace and their willingness to interrupt their own treacherous, hectic journey to spend an hour with us. They didn't come to solve our problems, but to share a slice of pie and their compassion.

"I hope we can do the same thing for other patients some day," I said.

"Me, too," he agreed.

You can meet someone with another type of cancer and feel some sense of connection. But until you meet someone with the same diagnosis, in the same boat, the same situation, you can't help but feel alone, as if nobody has walked in your shoes. Simply put, meeting the McDowells was a moment that mattered. After that, we felt the presence of more footprints on our path. Our paths would cross again.

We can't solve problems by using the same kind of
thinking we used when we created them.
—Albert Einstein

16
Seeking Second and Third Opinions

Winter inched us closer to the welcome completion of Scott's treatment, phase one. While Scott's brain was accumulating a lifetime dose of radiation, our hearts accumulated worry and our minds accumulated facts for decision-making. We were inching closer to the edge of a cliff and must soon decide how to proceed. Would we close our eyes and jump? Would we get to the edge and find a way to continue on a well-paved road, or at least a footpath? Thank goodness for the people you meet on the road who point you toward hope.

In the waiting room on one of the last days of radiation, Scott met someone who pointed the way. When he met her, he stood watching the tropical fish, which he did every day like meditation to prepare himself for the next blast. It was a day out of radiation's forty that my mom had driven Scott to his appointment, so he told me afterward.

"I met another brain tumor patient today, a woman with a glioblastoma, the grade four. She's having radiation and chemo at the same time. I wonder why I wasn't offered that?"

"We *did* ask about radiosensitizer drugs, but she told us no." I reminded him of our original conversation with the radiation oncologist. *Hmmm… wonder why*, I thought to myself. *Too late now.*

"Her name is Allie," Scott told me. "She has an entire team of doctors with a new brain tumor program, and they're right there at Swedish, same as the radiation department."

That's all he could tell me, so the next day at radiation, I met Allie myself to find out more. Scott introduced us just before he walked through the heavy double doors into the radiation room. I liked this round-faced, bald, black woman who wore a floppy, purple velvet hat with a yellow silk flower. She exuded a flair for living. Allie told me her story, which started less than two months before.

"I was walking down my stairs at home, and the next thing I knew I woke up in ICU hearing I had a brain tumor."

"Wow," was all I could say, as my head blessed our luck at having some days to get used to Scott's diagnosis, meet the surgeon, have a party, to be somewhat prepared. Allie continued.

"Turns out I had a grand mal seizure. It threw me down the stairs. It was pure luck, or God taking care of me, that my sister came by my house that morning. We were going to go shopping. She found me lying there, unconscious, and called 911 and then called John, my husband, at work. The ambulance brought me to Swedish and I had emergency surgery. When I woke up, I was introduced to a doctor who told me I had a brain tumor, the worst kind."

"I was lucky they brought me to Swedish. The doctor, Dr. Arenson, has just started a brain tumor program here. He is a pediatric cancer specialist but now he also treats adult brain tumor patients. He has a whole team of doctors who work together. We all sat down in this conference room, and, at one time, they all gave us their opinions. So that's why I'm having chemo with my radiation. They say it's a better combination than just radiation alone, at least for my kind of tumor. If Scott needs more treatment after radiation, you should call him."

Scott came out and the radiation technician came over to get Allie, so our conversation ended. But the seeds of hope had been planted. I went to the check-in desk and asked for Dr. Arenson's phone number and how to spell his name. I was excited to know a team of brain tumor specialists existed in Denver besides the teaching hospital. For some reason, and perhaps I misunderstood at the time, University of Colorado Health Sciences Center (which everyone calls University Hospital), wasn't covered in our insurance network. Also, I was miffed at the same time to hear our radiation oncologist was part of this new team but had not told us about it.

I suppose the team is *brand new,* I thought. *Maybe that's why. Thank goodness we met Allie.*

In early February, after radiation ended, we met Allie's neuro-oncologist. Dr. Arenson was part of a childhood oncology practice near the downtown triangle of hospitals: Presbyterian-St. Luke's down the block, St. Joseph's (where I had been a candy striper in junior high), and The Children's Hospital. It was also within walking distance of the Qualife house (where Scott attended a men's cancer support group), City Park Zoo (where I worked after college in the concession stands feeding Popsicles and snow cones to happy children), and Sushi Heights Restaurant, where they made the best ginger salad dressing and a decent tempura-teriyaki platter.

It was a little weird to stay on the elevator when other adults in the elevator got off on the second floor, at the Rocky Mountain Cancer Center. One person asked to make sure we knew where we were going. We must have looked scared, not to mention kid-less.

The office was a welcome relief after months of boring adult doctor offices. Colorful little tables and chairs offered crayons, games, and books. A 100-gallon saltwater tank of neon colored fish burbled in the corner. The walls were an art gallery of the most gorgeous black-and-white photography of cancer-bald children. Katy Tartakoff knew how to capture the cancer-free beauty of those souls peeking out from their light-and-shadow faces. I recognized her work because Scott's mom arranged a surprise portrait for Wil the Christmas he was two. In the resulting picture, Wil's face was solemn above his top-buttoned plaid shirt and Oshkosh overalls.

A smiling nurse escorted us to Dr. Arenson's office, which was down a bright hallway beyond the circle of treatment rooms where silly nurses joked with jolly doctors and made the children giggle. When we arrived, Dr. Arenson stood and walked from behind his large desk to shake our hands. Dr. Arenson is shorter than me, with brownish-gray hair in a shaggy style over a short beard, and he has a runner's build. His stethoscope is always around his neck, above a necktie, and he rarely wears his suit coat. His hazel eyes are kind and sad, as if he's seen so much cancer that compassion overflows onto his cheeks. I saw a fighting spirit in him, too, combined with a confidence in his treatment plan.

I don't remember the specifics of his presentation that day, telling us about the new team at the Colorado Neurological Institute. He said something about how he'd had good luck with a chemotherapy regimen for children, one with a different combination of drugs than the standard regimen used for adults, and he listed the names of the drugs. Out of the haze of details, I remember hearing him say, "We believe cure is possible, if treated early enough and aggressively."

Cure is possible? I thought. *What a contrast to the doctors and statistics who say no cure exists for brain cancer.*

I asked him about alternative medicine, like high doses of vitamins or certain herbs, if he ever supported supplementing his treatments. "Most are unproven," he said, "And I'd rather see research that proves the effectiveness. Some herbs interfere with chemotherapy drugs. I think multi-vitamins are fine. But if you ever see something on the Internet or hear about a certain treatment, you can bring it to me and I'd be happy to make phone calls to check it out further."

At a certain point in the conversation, he reached over to his bulletin board and took down an old piece of paper that was once torn from a yellow legal-size pad. On it, handwritten, was a numbered list of names and the dates of diagnosis. There must have been at least thirty names, and only a few were crossed out.

"These are my patients," he said, pointing. "This many are more than two years out from their diagnosis; they're ahead of the statistics."

More than anything else in that room that day, I remembered his list. This man clearly cared about his patients as individual children with names and he intended to give them a chance to grow up.

Honestly, he scared me. I was afraid of his notion that chemotherapy should be even more aggressive than normal. I think it even scared me to hear his assertion that cure was possible, if treated early and aggressively enough. Maybe because I hoped we were early enough and because it wasn't a promise of an easy, quick fix. It meant taking a risk for an uncertain outcome. His "let's be frank" talk said there are no magic bullets, but trust me, this has worked and here are the names to prove it.

Before we left, Dr. Arenson said one more thing that surprised me (which I learned later he says to all patients). "I believe part of the strategy toward healing is spiritual. I hope you will spend some time connecting with your higher power, if you have one."

I didn't know what to make of that, except I agreed, and at the same time was amazed that this doctor was somehow an interfaith advocate. It was refreshing, encouraging, and mysterious.

We left his office with a deal to have a team consultation at CNI after Scott's next MRI, which was already scheduled for the following week.

The day of the conference began early. Check-in at six, MRI at 6:30, conference at 8:00. This MRI included something called SPECT, or spectroscopy, which no other doctor had ordered before. As we'd learn soon, the SPECT showed a chemical spike to indicate tumor activity and differentiate tumor from healthy brain tissue.

We waited outside the conference room, in the hallway near the Swedish Hospital cafeteria. A not very pleasant smell waited with us: coffee, eggs, and Clorox from the steaming dishwasher room. Finally the door opened and we were invited inside to sit at a square of tables. Occupying chairs on three sides were the CNI Brain Tumor Team: our neuro-psychologist who gave us a wink and a smile, saying, "Hi, friends." Our radiation oncologist said hello, too. Next at the table were two neurosurgeons, a pathologist (who determines the type of tumor you have), a neurologist (who helps control seizures), a radiologist who would officially read Scott's MRI of that morning, a social worker (who is also called a patient care coordinator), a woman from the hospital's tumor registrar (who keeps statistics), and Dr. Arenson, neuro-oncologist, and one other medical oncologist.

Scott set our video camera on the table, pointed away from any faces, and said, "We don't have a tape recorder but we brought this so we can listen to it again later…so we don't miss anything."

No one disagreed, and the conference began.

The neuro-radiologist put the new MRI films on an overhead projection screen and we saw the status of Scott's tumor. Without the fluid-filled cyst that was drained in November's surgery, the tumor looked smaller to me. I was still figuring out how to read an MRI, how to look for the areas of bright whiteness that signify tumor. Scott's previous films were not there for comparison. They'd accidentally been left at Dr. Arenson's office, clear across town. The pathologist confirmed from having seen the original biopsy slides that the tumor was still a grade-two gemistocytic astrocytoma. But as Dr. Arenson said, because of "significant" areas of bright white enhancement on the MRI, the tumor didn't have the typical appearance of a low-grade tumor, "We all feel queasy when we look at it. If it's not eradicated, it will become more aggressive."

I took notes as a neurosurgeon described how he'd highly recommend a second resection, how it was possible to remove tumor without losing function due to the tumor's location. "We would use stealth," said the surgeon. He wasn't talking metaphorically. He was referring to a surgical technology called frameless stereotactic radiosurgery, nicknamed stealth. "Did you have stereotactic the first time? No? Well, you would have an MRI in the early morning before your surgery. Then in the O.R. we would have a probe and could point to a place in your brain, then look up on a screen to confirm whether the tissue was tumor or not. We don't want to cause you problems neurologically. Stealth allows us to be more comfortable and more aggressive in the resection. Your tumor is posterior to the motor cortex, so …"

The neurosurgeon was getting into "blah blah blah, Ginger" territory and I wasn't following all his jargon, but Dr. Arenson translated by saying, "Surgery is the most important initial thing to be accomplished. Radiation might have helped demarcate the edges of the tumor. We recommend surgery as long as it is a risk you would accept. Then we would discuss additional treatment based on what we find in there, if it's a higher grade tumor. Either way, we would consider chemotherapy, which will be most effective if surgery happens first. Chemo has a much better chance if it only has to deal with the least amount of disease possible.

"The single most important determinant of outcome is the amount of tumor removed at the beginning," Dr. Arenson reiterated. Then he and the neurosurgeon talked back and forth about a study they knew of that showed how the gamma knife could be used as a follow-up treatment on a small amount of residual tumor and that such treatment could improve a patient's outcome even further.

With more brevity than I ever managed, Scott asked, "What are the risks?"

Several doctors spoke at once, then allowed the neurosurgeon to continue. What I jotted in my notes were "visual/spatial/association, weakness on right side, eyesight, second surgeries = more risk of swelling, bleeding, infection." He added that before the actual surgery, we would sit down and talk about the risks in more detail.

I asked, "Can't you call our first neurosurgeon to find out why he didn't remove more in the first place, or maybe what it looked like to him?"

The team neurosurgeon refrained from scoffing, allowing that it might be useful to review the original "op report," and maybe he could make a call. I realized we were dealing with rivals, competitors, not call-em-up friends.

"It wouldn't matter," he replied. "We need to go back in and remove as much as we can."

When it seemed we were done, Scott said in a long, drawn-out breath, "Ohhhhh-kay."

Dr. Arenson understood the ambivalence, "That may not be what you were hoping to hear. What we're here for is to try to help you and be as objective as we can. Each of us is available to you afterward, anytime, if you have any more questions. We'll keep the dialog going."

And then he defined the types of treatment approaches in a way that I've never heard clarified.

"There are two different philosophies for treating brain tumors; they're not right or wrong, just different. The first approach is to do the least harm, not being overly aggressive. Our approach, very clearly, is to be on the aggressive side of the fence, more so than most other places would be. That's our focus. You're otherwise young and strong, and so we think you are a good candidate for this approach."

We told the team thanks, we'll think about your offer, but first we're going to hear our first neurosurgeon's advice and also we're going to Houston to consult with the experts at M. D. Anderson. We'll be in touch. So we left the conference feeling okay—okay about the post-radiation tumor because we had just found a team willing to work at a shot for survival.

Had I looked back at the conference room before leaving, I believe I might have seen a shimmer of atmosphere suggesting Camelot and the Knights of the Round Table, and I might have heard the clinks and clanks of shining armor. I felt the subtlest hint of having just met our foresworn heroes who had pledged to seek the Holy Grail, the cure for malignant brain tumors, and fight for Scott along the way. Did I hear trumpets?

We didn't meet with our first neurosurgeon until the following Thursday. It was a long, naïve wait. There is something to be said for ignorant bliss.

At our appointment that day, we looked again at the films in his office. By then he had seen them and the radiologist's written report that compared them to the scan taken December 6, just before radiation.

"The tumor has doubled," he said without warning.

"What? Say that again. How could it double *during* radiation? I thought the radiation was supposed to be shrinking it." It was as if Scott and I were speaking with one voice.

"Sometimes it happens."

Yeah, shit happens, I thought. And he went on to say, clinically cold, how he felt it was too dangerous to attempt another surgery, given the location of the tumor and the neurological deficits it could cause for Scott, ruining the quality of whatever time he had left.

Scott was stunned and disgusted. This man was giving up? Unbelievable, especially when less than a week ago we had sat with an entire team who believed cure was possible and agreed second surgery was feasible — not too risky at all.

Whatever the surgeon said next came out sounding to me like, "You're basically screwed. Better go home and get your affairs in order."

We never saw him again after that.

It's a good thing we met with the team at CNI first. What would we have done if we hadn't thought to get a second opinion…and a third? Our original neurosurgeon's view epitomized the "other side of the fence" that Dr. Arenson had spoken of, the "Do no harm" camp. But to me, believing that *was* doing harm. It was denying that other options existed, denying Scott the chance to fight, and denying us hope.

In contrast to the doctors at CNI who sought the Holy Grail with courage of conviction, I had a wicked vision of this surgeon acting in Monty Python's version. In my mind, he had already flung Scott over his shoulder and was heading—without mercy or emotion—toward some gurney-pushing guy who was shouting, "Bring out your dead."

"I'm not dead yet!" Scott would say. This doctor would argue with the gurney pusher, saying, "Well, he will be soon. He's very ill."

"I'm getting better," Scott would say, to which the surgeon would insist, "No, you're not. You'll be stone dead in a moment."

Unlike the poor bloke who was thrown, dead, on the cart after a quick whop to the head, Scott would jump down and run. "Run away!"

The next thing I remember is sitting behind the wheel, stopped at a red light at 8th and Josephine, right there across from Congress Park where I had my First Communion as a lace-clad first grader, back when our hippie Catholic congregation had rebelled, split off, and held church outdoors all summer. It was no different to me than pulling up in front of a church, within arm's reach of grace. Still stunned, I was saying to Scott, "I can't believe it. How could this happen?"

And straight from the heavens and KBCO I heard these words sung into my heart, "In the arms of an angel, may you fi---i-yi-yind some comforting."

My heart melted and my grip on the steering wheel relaxed, as I said to Scott and the gods, "Oh, how nice of the universe to send us that song."

I started to cry but I stopped right away. The light turned green, and I had to drive home.

"It's okay," Scott said. His anger at the surgeon's write-off had fueled some samurai fire to keep fighting. "We have other options. We still have to see the other oncologist this afternoon. We'll go to Houston and see what they say. And we have CNI. We do have options."

That moment and song are etched in my mind. It suggested something bigger was watching out for us. The song didn't promise an easy fix or a certain outcome, it merely offered the arms of an angel for comfort along the way. And comfort me it did.

Later that day we met with yet another doctor, the medical oncologist who the surgeon recommended, who our primary care physician had interned with, and who the radiation oncologist said we would like. It was good to have yet another opinion in Denver, and we liked what he had to say.

Having seen the MRI-doubling report and heard our take on the surgeon's opinion, he said, refreshingly, "I'm not a brain tumor specialist, I maybe see one or three brain tumor patients a year. I think you're smart to consult with doctors who treat brain tumors every day."

He suggested that while we were at M. D. Anderson, we ask them about a treatment using Gliadel wafers (where during surgery these chemo-filled wafers are left to dissolve in the brain), or gene therapy, or vaccines, or anything else they could offer, plus their opinion on the treatments offered so far.

He said, "Ask them, if not this, then why not? Don't just ask them their reasoning *for* a certain treatment, but also why they are opposed to a certain treatment."

The doctor also suggested that we ask to meet with one of the M. D. Anderson neuropsychologists and find out whether they would be involved before or after surgery.

We respected his ideas and his honesty to admit he wasn't our best bet. He said he could offer a basic regimen of chemotherapy, but we liked that he was thinking outside the box, beyond his ego or bottom line.

The visit with him was a reprieve in the day, like stopping at the castle of a kind old knight who gave us bread and wine for sustenance and sent us on our way with a kind wave, "Farewell."

*It's never too late—in fiction
or in life—to revise.*
—Nancy Thayer

17

Fourth Opinion in Houston

Subj: Scott - off to Houston - 3/2/99
Date: 3/2/99 7:59:44 PM Mountain Standard Time

Dear Everyone,

A quick note to say that we're off to Houston tomorrow, Wednesday morning. Just in case, and unless we hear anything significantly different in Houston, we have tentatively scheduled surgery for the Friday we return, March 12, at 8:30 a.m. at Swedish Hospital. All that may change, but we didn't want to lose time by not scheduling it. SO, thanks for all your support and prayers. We'll keep you posted.

Love,
Shelly & Scott & Wil (who is staying with grandparents this week)

In planning to get second opinions (actually, fourth) from the brain tumor specialists at M. D. Anderson, we had to send Scott's medical records in advance. Standard procedure, this included copies of all his MRIs and the biopsy slides from the November surgery so the pathologists could look for themselves to determine Scott's type and grade of tumor. Dr. Arenson also offered to send a summary of the CNI team consultation so that M.D. Anderson experts could comment on CNI's chemotherapy protocol and plans for a second surgery. I appreciated his willingness to let The Experts compare apples and oranges.

When I made Scott's appointment at M. D. Anderson, I was told it was likely that the doctors would offer immediate surgery and to plan for that possibility. I couldn't imagine sitting all by myself in a Houston hospital while Scott underwent surgery or asking our parents to buy plane tickets, too. Neither could I imagine jumping on an airplane every few weeks for chemotherapy appointments. It sounded costly in more ways than one, but I tried to keep an open mind in case The Expert's opinion sounded like a much better offer. I could find ways to make it work if I had to.

While I was confirming hotel and airline reservations for the conference, pulling together our medical records and compiling a long list of questions to ask the specialists in Houston, Scott made his own preparations. He spent an afternoon behind the locked door of our bedroom sitting in our glider-rocking chair. He sat a few feet away from a tripod topped with our video camera, the one he bought the day after Wil was born but hadn't used much in recent years. Before he closed the door, he told me he was taping messages to me and Wil, his family and friends, in case he didn't come back—either from a surgery in Houston or surgery at CNI. I resisted the urge to stand at the door, listening, and to this day I have never watched his tapes.

A few nights before going to Houston, I had a weird dream. *I am walking though the dim hallways of Steele Elementary School, which morphs into South High. I am coming to school to pack my things and say goodbye to my friends, because I am moving. I haven't been to school since November and now it is March, just before spring break. I wonder if I have enough credits to graduate or if I will have to repeat the school year. In one room I meet my childhood girlfriends, who are having a slumber party in a high-ceilinged room with tables topped by sewing machines. I can't stop wondering how well those machines stitch and if I could borrow one long enough to sew curtains for Janna. Then my grown-up friend, Kathy Matsey, gives me a going-away present, a pair of white baby boots tied together by their laces and a clump of baby's breath tucked in. On the soles of the shoes she has written, "Trust" and "Have Faith in the Every Day."*

When I woke up, I wrote the dream in my journal, aware of so many mixed metaphors. I decided to take a literal hint from the dream. A few days later, Wil and I ditched preschool and traded in my old Singer for a new Elna. We were both excited to go home and sew new clothes for his bunnies and tiny Rugrat dolls. I wondered if I would ever have time to take the Elna training class offered by the store, not that I needed it, except maybe for button holes. Perhaps I needed my new sewing machine as a commitment to keep on living and doing what I loved, no matter what happened in Houston.

Later that afternoon, we took Scott to Janna's for a Healing Touch treatment to boost his energy for the trip. Afterward we took Scott to the driving range. Wil and I sat in the car, chatting about what to sew first, watching Scott alone in the spring wind. He looked good swinging his golf clubs. I wondered when (or if) he would be able to do that after his next surgery. The day had been a pleasant diversion, almost hopeful, letting us ignore the tumor for a stretch. That night, as if guilty for playing hooky, I spent an

hour reading messages on the BRAINTMR loop, researching more treatment options as if cramming for a test. My sad fear crept back in. I vowed to
never go online for brain tumor research at bedtime.

The airplane ride to Houston was uneventful. I read printouts of research and Scott slept. We managed to get our luggage and a rental car and
navigate the city's traffic from the airport to Homegate Studio & Suites
(available to cancer patients at a reduced rate). We stayed in a suite with a
kitchen and living room, but couldn't see any restaurants in walking distance. Surrounded by palm trees and green grass, the retro décor, and bro-
chures suggesting a visit to the NASA Space Center, I felt like one of the
astronaut wives in *Apollo 13*. (They never seemed very happy, always being
left below while their husbands ventured off-planet.)

On Friday morning, we drove a few blocks and around the corner to M.
D. Anderson and let a valet park the car. It was there we met our third waiting-room angel. It happened just before our chemo consultation with a
neuro-oncologist. The large, clinical waiting room on the umpteenth floor of
the M. D. Anderson Cancer Center Tower was an expanse of tile floors, row
upon row of chairs, and windows that looked south over Houston. Our "patient escort" tour guide handed Scott's chart to a nurse at the counter and
showed us chairs on which to wait for our consultation. Across the room we
made eye contact with a man wearing a suit with a bolo tie and cowboy
boots, sporting long gray hair tied behind his neck. He smiled then sauntered over to us, holding out a brochure. "Why our pastor wears a ponytail"
was printed on the front.

"Hello, my name is Reverend Tim Herron," he said, shaking Scott's
hand. "I'm guessing you're here as a brain tumor patient."

"Yes, we flew in from Denver for a consultation," I answered, "and also
to attend a conference for patients and families put on by the National Brain
Tumor Foundation."

"I'm a brain tumor survivor, myself," he said. "M. D. Anderson lets me
hang out here in the waiting room so I can share my story with others. I became a reverend so I would have a hall pass into hospitals."

From this reverend I braced myself for a sermon, but that's not what we
got.

"When were you diagnosed?" I asked.

"Ten years ago," he said. "They don't even use the same kind of treatment anymore," he added, predicting the same question new patients al-

ways ask him, begging the recipe for his magic cure. "It wasn't the treatment that saved me. It was my five children. I wanted my kids to grow up with a father, and I figured the best person for the job was me."

A nurse called Scott's name, so we couldn't talk longer but just waved goodbye.

The consultation lasted several hours. First Scott offered up his arm to let a nurse draw a tube of blood which, she explained, would be used for a research project titled "Brain Tumors: Biologic, Molecular and Genetic Studies." We would never know the results specific to Scott but could be proud knowing we had contributed to their research, she said. And we would be added to the cancer center's mailing list to receive a patient newsletter.

Next, Scott was evaluated by a tall, red-haired woman doctor, a resident I think, who asked a ton of questions and answered "Fair enough" to almost everything Scott had to say. We were getting good at summarizing Scott's initial symptoms and his treatment so far. Then we met the neuro-oncologist, who struck me as warm and likeable. The first thing he said was that the pathologist had reviewed Scott's biopsy slides and classified it as a grade three, not a grade two, using the term anaplastic astrocytoma even though the tumor clearly included gemistocytic cells. As I understood it, some cancer centers use a three-tier grading system where some of the middle grades are lumped together. The basic treatment regimen is the same, he said, so it really doesn't matter. In fact, calling the tumor a grade three actually defines more treatment options. We have more clinical trials for higher-grade tumors, he told us. It was like hearing, "In our high school you would be a ninth grader, but we call them freshmen, and we let you take extra-hard AP classes."

We left the consultation feeling great because The Experts had spoken and answered our long list of questions. First, they concurred with the need for and safety of a second surgery, and said if photodynamic therapy was available with surgery in Denver to seriously consider it, having heard good things about the results. Happy to hear a thumbs-up for surgery at home, I could listen when he said various clinical trials were available if we wanted to come back for treatment. He recommended a new wonder-drug called Temodar that was nearing FDA approval, a drug with promising results and tolerable side-effects. He also said he would offer us the standard PCV regimen.

Then he said he believed Dr. Arenson's chemotherapy regimen was much more toxic than necessary. "Overkill" is what I wrote in my notes.

This felt like vindication of our fears. And he gave Scott a prescription to fill right away for Decadron, to decrease the brain swelling that he said was causing Scott to feel dizzy.

After we left, I drove straight to Walgreen's to fill Scott's prescription, to a grocery store for granola bars and apples, and then to another hotel to check in for the conference.

When we got to our room, we were so tired and hungry that we ate all our snacks and didn't bother going downstairs to dinner. My inner introvert and I didn't have the energy yet for brain tumor small talk with other conference attendees.

On Saturday morning, we awoke somewhat refreshed and ready to dive into the details of brain tumor treatment at the "Hope" conference. In the darkened hotel conference room, about 200 patients and caregivers were holding hands, some taking notes. Others just listened to speakers or watched the slide shows with motionless exhaustion, moving only to shake their heads or nod as if to say, *I know, I know. Been there. Done that.* I was one of the avid note-takers. Every few pages I had to skip ahead in my spiral notebook, having found blue-ink drawings from Wil that felt like long-distance kisses.

At the session on neurosurgery—"Is My Tumor Operable?"—the accompanying full-color slide show was dramatic and gross, yet fascinating. The magic-marker on a shaven scalp showed where the incision would go. We saw clamps on the scalp, a glimpse of bone, power tools, then brain and tumor mass. I shut my eyes a few times, but then I peeked.

The session on tumor pathology— "Is My Tumor Malignant?" —was the most educational for me. We were viewing what a pathologist sees on a biopsy slide, tumor cells stained purple mixed with normal gray brain cells, at the microscopic level. First, an encapsulated benign brain tumor. "See how there is a distinct margin to the tumor? We can excise this during surgery and be fairly certain that no tumor cells are left behind."

Next slide: a glioblastoma multiforme, the deadliest grade-four GBM. "See how the majority of tumor cells are here...and here." It looked like shadowy fingers reaching into the brain, unevenly heading in different directions. "But look to this area over here, away from the primary tumor site. These sparse cells are also malignant and can grow at an alarming rate."

Seeing evidence on those slides of the aggressive and diffuse nature of these malignant cells gave us vivid information that made all the difference in our decisions that week, and also down the road.

"New Treatments for Brain Tumors" gave us insight into research in the works, but left me with the impression that there really was no cure now but might be in a decade. The doctor we'd consulted with gave a sobering talk on the physical effects and toxicity of therapy. I was especially alert to the long-term effects of radiation and the likelihood of birth defects or sterility from chemo.

I was relieved and rejuvenated in the session, "How to be a Parent During Brain Tumor Treatment"—thankful to hear new ideas and meet other parents with similar issues, like sleep changes and school phobias. Play therapy and drawings can help children work through their fears, we heard, and it's important to add security to their world by maintaining boundaries and limits of discipline. "Honesty is important, even if it hurts," said the child psychologist to the crowd of mostly-nodding mothers. "Their imaginations could make it even worse."

After lunch we attended even more sessions on complementary medicine, where we heard about shark cartilage and potential herb-interactions with chemotherapy. We were starting to fade by the time we sat through the session on putting research advances in perspective, and then another on chemotherapy. By the end of "Managing Medication Side Effects," we were worn out.

Most heartening of all, and worth the whole trip, was meeting the veterans of brain tumor survival, people who had endured the treatments and outlived the statistics. We listened to david m. bailey (who officially uses all lowercase), wearing a tie-dyed T and bandana, singing original lyrics as he played guitar. *Love the Time* renewed our spirits. We cheered—and cried—with the other attendees. I bought his CD.

At some point in the afternoon, we had a stand-by-a-table consultation with the neurosurgeon whose presentation had enlightened us that morning and who also chaired the conference. He looked at Scott's MRI films, which I had retrieved from our hotel room upstairs during a break.

"I would be able to remove seventy to eighty percent of your tumor, based on its location, but not likely more," he said "Ideally, though, you'd want to remove ninety to ninety-five percent for the best chance of long-term survival."

It was hard to believe as we stood there that we were talking to the lead neurosurgeon at M. D. Anderson, hearing him say he'd gladly perform Scott's surgery, the very next week in fact, if we wanted to stay in Houston. We realized that the opinion we wanted to hear was one that concurred with CNI's plan. It was enough to know that our hometown team of brain tumor specialists would perform surgery in the same way with the same tools as this renowned specialist. But in Denver, we'd be with our son, our friends and family for support. We were ready to go home.

Scott and I talked a long while before falling asleep that night, even though we both felt so drained by the day. Maybe because we were so drained, we had nothing but the barest truths to speak.

"God, I'm tired. These two days feel like a week. It's hard to believe I'll be out of surgery by this time next week. The way I feel right now, I don't know how I can make it one more week. I feel like shit. It's getting worse, like the tumor is growing faster now."

"We don't know that it's growing. You could be feeling bad because of the radiation swelling. The Decadron should start helping pretty soon, I would think." But Scott didn't want a cheerleader.

"I feel like I'm shrinking away, inch by inch, day by day," Scott said. "I'm worried that it's only going to get worse for all of us."

I whispered, "Oh honey," thinking *me, too*. I was too tired to wake up my inner Pollyanna for more chipper words, so I tucked myself tighter into his arms where we lay on the bed, and I let him keep talking.

"I feel like I've given God an ultimatum," Scott said, "Either take me on the operating table or make me all better."

That made me sit up again, pushing off his shoulder to look in his eyes. "Really?" I asked. "That's pretty black and white."

"I know."

On Monday, we debated whether to catch an earlier flight or enjoy a day as tourists pretending it was spring break after all. We opted for tourism and drove twenty-five miles south to the Space Center. The sky turned darker through the day and after an hour in the visitor's center, most of that time in the gift shop buying freeze-dried ice cream for Wil and a videotape of NASA history for Scott, we left, afraid of missing our flight.

I drove us to the airport, chased by thunderstorms that seemed to echo the lightning storm in Scott's tumor-swollen brain. Murphy's Law went into effect and we sat for hours at the airport, delayed by bad weather, not getting home until ten o'clock that night.

From our single hour as tourists of Houston's Space Center, I couldn't help feeling that we had been given a good-luck send-off from the spirits of courageous explorers, as if we had touched the moon-dusted sleeves of the bravest of the brave, men who had stood on the surface of our lucky moon. I can't decide which quote I like best to sum up our fact-finding, fourth-opinion-seeking mission to Houston, and our decision to have Scott's second surgery in Denver.

There's this one from Gene Roddenberry, who created *Star Trek*, and inspired *Star Trek: The Next Generation*, which gave Scott his nickname of Data: "Our prime obligation to ourselves is to make the unknown known. We are on a journey to keep an appointment with whatever we are."

Or this quote by Jim Lovell, commander of the Apollo 13, which was doomed to explode but landed back on earth thanks to ingenuity, duct tape, and not losing hope. "From now on we'll live in a world where man has walked on the moon. It's not a miracle, we just decided to go."

Perhaps even more apropos to the process of seeking second, third, and fourth opinions is a quote from my Mom, who heard it from another cancer survivor at a talk about choosing your treatment steps. Mom said "It's a known fact that even the astronauts make hundreds and thousands of course corrections on their way to the moon. Like them, it's okay not to know exactly how you're going to get there, but to trust in the process."

Having decided upon our next steps, we spent the week preparing for Scott's second surgery.

Subj: Update on Scott - 3/9/99
Date: 3/9/99 10:15:46 PM Mountain Standard Time

After 3 appointments today, we have decided to go ahead with surgery this Friday in Denver. For most of the surgery, Scott will be asleep under general anesthesia, but will then be awakened to give the surgical team feedback on his capabilities. They are concerned that the tumor may have grown into the motor cortex -- they won't be able to remove it all, but with him awake they can push the boundaries as far as safely possible. (80% is likely the maximum, but ideally they'd want out 90-95% for this type of tumor.) It freaks me out to think of Scott awake, but he's looking at it as a great scientific experiment. The neuropsychologist we've been working with since December will be in the operating room, asking Scott questions. We couldn't be happier that this great guy is on our team and will literally be holding Scott's hand during the operation.

One new development with surgery is that Scott has opted for a clinical trial called photodynamic therapy (PDT). Swedish Hospital has been involved with this for about 16 years (one of the surgeons on our team helped pioneer this treatment). On Thursday morning, Scott will be injected with a light-sensitive drug (Photofrin). On Friday at the end of surgery, they flood the empty tumor space in the brain with some solution and then put a fiber optic/laser light inside, basically giving the bordering tumor cells such a bad sunburn they die. The drug is absorbed by fast-growing cells, such as skin cells and tumor cells. Those are the cells that then die when exposed to sunlight (it's the red light of the spectrum).

The one side effect of treatment is that for the next 4-6 weeks, Scott will have to avoid all exposure to direct sunlight, as well as incandescent light (regular light bulbs). We'll have to replace our light bulbs with fluorescent light, keep our windows shaded, and if Scott leaves the house, he'll have to be covered head to toe, every inch, with cloth and sunglasses (like The Invisible Man). That will be REALLY hard, but worth the results.

I'm feeling less frightened this time (or I'm doing a better job not thinking about that at least for today). Scott is sure that the surgery is the best next step and confident in the team here. He'll definitely wake up with less peripheral vision, but we hope and pray that he will not suffer any paralysis (yes, it's a risk) and that he'll still be the same old Scott we know and love.

Thank you for sticking by us on this long, so-far four-month journey.
We have a long road ahead to recovery, but every day is a blessing.
The longer the road, the better. Please say a little prayer for us. :)

All our love,
Shelly, Scott & Wil

You don't get to control any outcome,
only every choice you make along the way.
—Stephen C. Paul

18
Haircut Before Surgery

I knew it was nearly midnight, almost Friday, because the hospital seemed a bit darker and quieter and the nurses from the night shift had settled in. I could tell when I went to the desk to ask for a pair of scissors. We decided to cut Scott's hair and shave it as close as possible, rather than waste time in the morning doing it—or settle for a partially shaved head and have to trim around the stitches later.

Scott sat in a chair by his room's sink. He sat on the well worn visitor's chair, and it was too short for a barber's chair. *If the nurse comes in,* I thought, *she's going to run into us with the heavy door.* A white towel hung around Scott's shoulders, and under that was a blue hospital gown with paisley-like squiggles. He wore his gray sweatpants, not fully succumbing to hospital attire. I stood behind him, scissors poised, electric razor on the sink counter, charging up. The IV in his right arm was hooked up to a chrome pole on wheels, and I maneuvered around that, not wanting to become entangled. I wet his hair, running a comb through his wiry brown and gray hair, which was already thinned quite a bit in the back thanks to radiation and male-pattern baldness that his thirty-three years were forcing on him anyway. The fluorescent light over the sink seemed too bright, compared to the dimness of our private room and Denver's night sky beyond the heavily curtained window.

"Are you ready," I asked, and the question seemed a lot bigger than words.

"Cut away," he said with mock courage, and that seemed braver than words. I started to trim, taking his hair as short as possible with the scissors first. Clip, clip, snip. His hair floated to the linoleum. I kept trimming, combing as I went. We were both thinking but not saying, *Is this the last haircut?*

The next morning, about 5:30, Scott would be whisked from the ninth floor of Denver's Swedish Hospital to the third floor where his surgery would take place. Scott would be awake for part of this craniotomy so that the surgical team could monitor his cognitive and motor functions while they tried to remove as much as possible of the malignant brain tumor.

Scott had been admitted a day early to receive a drug called Photofrin, a light-sensitive drug that was key to the stage-three clinical trial called photodynamic therapy. I was allowed to stay the night.

Scott's hair was as short as I could get it with scissors. "Can you hand me the razor now?" I asked, setting the scissors on the counter and brushing off hair from his neck and the front of my t-shirt. *He looks good with hair this short,* I thought. Short hair made his blue eyes stand out even more, though his face was a bit rounder than normal from the Decadron, a steroid to control brain swelling but seems to swell everything else.

I started in with the razor, creating a new kind of fashion statement. It was a hard to shave around the existing curved scar on his skull, because it wasn't smooth but caved in, a groove. I handed him the razor so he could shave off his mustache and beard, a typical springtime tradition anyway. Every spring it always shocks me to see his chin and lips without hair. It was like shaving a decade off his face.

Neither of us had much to say that night, but we weren't ready for sleep either. It was nice to have a grace period of quiet time to gear up for tomorrow's surgery. The whole day had been kind of nice—if you can call it that when you're checked into a hospital awaiting surgery. At that moment, I wasn't thinking about tomorrow, but recalling our afternoon.

Wil came to the hospital in the afternoon with Aunt Amie and Lance. Wil was going to stay fifteen minutes, but it turned into three hours. While Scott was having the Photofrin injected into his IV and glibly entertaining guests, Wil and I became hospital tourists.

"Here's the waiting room where I'll be sitting for the next few days," I told Wil as we walked around the corner into the expansive Intensive Care waiting room.

"Oh, look at the fish!" he said, running over to the aquarium and standing on tiptoe to see the clownfish hiding behind the live saltwater plants. I looked around the room, checking whether the chairs were wide enough to sleep on. A few people were there, staring at TV or reading magazines. Windows overlooked the south hospital entrance and I could see the bare crab apple trees below. It was a blue-sky Colorado day. I didn't know yet that tomorrow the trees would be dripping with a wet, spring snow.

Wil and I left the ICU waiting room and sauntered back down the hall. To help people find their way to Radiology for MRIs, CT scans, and x-rays, the hospital had installed black diamond tiles on the floor. We followed the trail as if on treasure hunt. Wil wanted to play hop-scotch. "Watch out!" I said, pulling him mid-jump as orderlies pushed an empty gurney past us. We retraced our steps to the operating room. On the right, I pointed out the double door to the operating rooms, "where Dad will be tomorrow." On the left, I pointed, "Here's the other waiting room." We peeked into the narrow and crowded surgery waiting room painted a listless yellow. It was full of anxious and tired families who didn't need to be part of a curious pre-schooler's tour. I saw the back of a surgeon in blue scrubs through the window of a private "get the bad news" room, speaking to a young woman who was twisting a tissue in her hands, not wiping the tears in her eyes. *Would that be me tomorrow?* I wondered.

"Let's go," I said, not wanting to stop and ponder that question. "Should we go get Aunt Amie, now, and give her the tour?"

Wil was happy to retrieve Amie from Scott's room and, with authority, began the tour anew. He was in charge now, showing her all the places he just learned about. "You really know your way around," Amie teased. "Are you sure you haven't been here before?"

We ended our second tour in the cafeteria ("It stinks in here!" Wil noted), then rode the elevator back upstairs to the ninth floor. Holding my hand and Amie's, he chirped about the tropical fish, the cool automatic doors he had seen, asking if children can stay in this hospital. I reminded him that our neighbor's son, Noah, had been born here at Swedish. It was typical Wil, non-stop talking, not quiet and scared like the night he visited Rose Hospital after Scott's first surgery.

"I like *this* hospital," he said to Scott, bouncing into his bright room at Swedish. "It's a lot nicer than the other one. They have clownfish!" he announced. "Can I draw you a picture?" Wil stopped at the dry-erase board where nurses leave notes about fluid intake or chemo protocol. Today the board was empty, until Wil drew a happy family threesome, standard stick-figure style. "This is to keep you company, Dad."

It was significant to Scott that Wil, who draws daily like prayer, had sketched him into the picture. "He hasn't drawn me in a picture for over a week," Scott said to me later. "Today was the first time he put me back in the family." I hadn't noticed and felt instant guilt, as if I should be much more aware of Wil's fragile psyche. I didn't disagree with Scott about Wil's artwork omissions. It seemed Scott was taking Wil's freshly-drawn picture as a good omen that he was here to stay.

Kevin and Paul, Scott's college roommates, were also in the room with Amie and Lance, hanging out with Scott, sharing standard small talk, interspersed with polite questions about the technical details of tomorrow's surgery and today's preparation.

"They already injected the drug," he was explaining. "By tomorrow, all my cells will have soaked it in and be sensitive to light. It gets absorbed by the fastest growing cells, like skin, and the fast-growing tumor cells. So tomorrow, at the end of the surgery, they'll shine a laser into the tumor cavity and theoretically kill off an additional margin of tumor cells—the invisible ones too small to get with the knife. The rest of my body will be light sensitive for six more weeks. I won't be able to go outside in the daylight or I'll get an instant nasty sunburn."

"Did you cover up all the windows in your house yet, or change the light bulbs," asked Kevin, who knew some of the protocol we'd have to follow. For the next six weeks, Scott could only be under fluorescent light bulbs when indoors, and could only go outdoors before dawn or after sunset. It would take that long for the Photofrin to leave his system. We figured it was worth the hassle for the promising benefits of PDT, as photodynamic therapy was called. In 1999, PDT was approved for several diseases, including esophageal cancer, early-stage lung cancer, age-related macular degeneration, and some gynecological cancers.

"No, we'll have a few days to do that before Scott comes home. Dad's going to Home Depot to buy a whole box of light bulbs this week. One of our friends from Fort Collins offered to come down and install the light bulbs for us. Besides that, I think our curtains and wood blinds will be enough protection. I might have to tape sheets on the windows here and there. I did find some great new hats and gloves for Scott to wear, though. He's going to look like Lawrence of Arabia!"

When I informed our friends via our still-growing email list about our decision to have the second surgery in Denver with photodynamic therapy, I sent out a lighthearted challenge to complete this riddle: "How many brain tumor patients does it take to screw in a light bulb?" My private, grim thought was *It doesn't matter, the light bulb outlasts the brain tumor patient.* I needed a better answer.

Thankfully, we received this cheery email reply, "None, their friends will do it for them" from a long-time friend and coworker programmer with

Scott in his first post-college job. Mike sent a reply-all to our latest email, suggesting donations to cover the $19.95 cost per bulb. He was blown away (as we were) by the generous response of our friends.

"Well, kiddo, we'd better get going. Kiss your mom and dad goodbye," Amie said to Wil, wiping some of the black marker off his fingertips with a wet paper towel. As the discussion was heading toward medical side effects, Amie didn't want to hear anymore or expose Wil to any gory details. What Wil understood was that Dad was having "sunshine medicine" with his surgery to help the tumor go away. Kevin and Paul saw the chance to leave, too, so they waited until Wil was out the door then hugged Scott and said goodbye, too.

I walked them all to the elevator, with a final kiss and hug for Wil. "I'll call you at bedtime, honey bunny." Wil was off to our next-door neighbor's house again. It was a blessing to have family in town and friends next door who felt like family. Years later, Wil still recalled that after the first surgery while playing Barbies with Andrea (almost two years older), that he started crying because he was so sad and scared about his dad—and how she put her arms around him to comfort him. As I headed back to Scott's room, I thought to myself that every child should have someone safe to cry with and not always have to be brave.

"Me, too," I add out loud, grateful to have cried more than once on the couches and kitchen chairs of my parents and neighbors.

On the car-ride home, Amie and Lance asked Wil if he had visited Scott at the first hospital last winter. With preschool logic, Wil answered "Yeah, but I'm not afraid of Dad in this hospital. Did you know that kids can get brain tumors? They can even have a bald head if they want to. ... If I ever got sick, this is the hospital I would want to be in." Apparently, tropical fish make all the difference.

Back in the room, with visitors gone, Scott was sitting on the bed fussing with the IV tube and the sheets. No longer a party host, he looked like a patient. Tired. Plugged into machines.

"Whew," he said, looking up. "Saying goodbye to Wil was harder than I thought."

"Why?" I asked, surprised because Scott seemed nonchalant as I watched him hug Wil, then pat his little back when he turned away.

"Because...that might be the last time I ever really see my son," Scott replied.

"Do you feel like you might not make it through the surgery tomorrow," I asked, even more surprised. *Whoa, wait a minute,* I was thinking, *what happened to our pact for joint optimism regarding this event! I can't do it if he's not up for the game, too.* I sat down on the hospital bed next to him.

Scott was choked up when he answered, but then swallowed and became a bit defiant, as if I should have remembered the risks he was willing to face. "The doctors said that I could lose my vision with the surgery. I probably won't see Wil the same way anymore, or anything else for that matter."

I didn't catch his deeper meaning. "No, Scott, they were talking about your peripheral vision possibly becoming more narrow, not going blind," I said, holding out my hands then drawing them together. I meant to demonstrate, but it came out feeling more like a helpless shrug. I leaned against him and gave a heavy sigh.

Pressing my point didn't matter—the risks of surgery were huge and subjective, and there was no way of knowing what would happen tomorrow for sure. I knew that each brain tumor patient's risk and prognosis is different—different tumor type, tumor size, tumor location, patient's age and overall health, not to mention attitude toward the process.

Twice that day we continued The Talk we'd been dipping our toes in for months: What to do if Scott died. Funeral or party. Cremation or coffin. Where to be sprinkled or buried. Scott's insistence that I someday remarry. I know it sounds heartless, as if by discussing Death we were giving in to Doubt. For us, though, it diminished some fear. I must admit frustration when Scott said the decision on his burial or cremation was up to me, he didn't care. I didn't press him further, because I needed to believe that it wouldn't be an urgent issue tomorrow.

"Hi there, you two," said a cheery voice and a welcome diversion. Our neuropsychologist strode into the room, holding Scott's chart and what looked like an oversized deck of cards. He had drawn up some flash cards with simple math equations, pictures, and word-recall tests. He was testing Scott before surgery as a benchmark for how his brain was processing information. Answering twelve minus five took Scott almost ten seconds.

This doctor was one of our reasons for electing to have Scott's second surgery at Swedish. He would be talking to Scott as the two neurosurgeons chipped away at the tumor. A neurologist would also be on hand, monitoring a real-time three-dimensional MRI of Scott's brain so that the team could map precisely which regions the knife was nearing. The team had state-of-the-art tools that allowed them to be as aggressive as possible in removing Scott's tumor, stopping just short of leaving him with deficits that would interfere with his quality of life. Scott had his own opinion about that.

"Who are they to say what deficits are acceptable for my quality of life," Scott said more than once during the recent weeks as we researched our treatment options. Scott was willing to have deficits, like less eyesight or impaired mobility or less use of his right arm, if it meant enough tumor were removed to give him a shot at long-term survival. Since his diagnosis, he'd already given up the independence of driving and the deep satisfaction in his career. Through our research and in getting second, third, and fourth opinions, we had learned that everywhere you went, everyone you asked had a different opinion on what risks were worth taking. I was relieved that we had armed ourselves with enough knowledge to be able to make that risk assessment ourselves.

And that brought us to Scott's haircut and a clean-shaven head for surgery the next morning, the final touch on doing as much as possible to prepare for the day. (I've since heard you shouldn't shave before surgery to prevent the risk of infection. Oh, well.) Now, there was nothing left but to trust in our guts and our God that this second surgery was Scott's best bet for survival.

I pulled the towel from his shoulders, careful not to let any itchy hairs down his back. He stood up and grabbed the IV pole, then wheeled it over to the bed, saying "I'm ready to sleep."

I carried the chair back near the window then threw the towel onto the floor by the sink and began to wipe the floor. *Good enough,* I thought, *they can clean the room tomorrow while we're out.* Scott was already under the sheets. A nurse came in to check his stats and was startled at Scott's transformation. "Oh! You look pretty good for a bald guy. Here's an extra blanket for you," she added, handing it to me as I settled into the narrow recliner chair next to Scott's bed.

The night passed quickly, our sleep interrupted several times by nurses.

"Time to get up," Scott said, reaching from the bed to touch my shoulder. It was 5:15 a.m. He was alert, his day had arrived. "Get ready."

"I'm ready."

Let all these be possible:
peace of mind, strength of spirit,
joy at light of day, laughter abundant.
—*CNI Healing Service*

19
Awake Craniotomy

Having slept in my jeans and fleece sweater, as well as my shoes, I was ready to leave when the wheelchair arrived. I threw my backpack over my shoulder and put my hand on Scott's as he rolled down the hall. We took the private, staff-and-patient elevator to the surgical floor.

In my mind, I kept repeating my new mantra, *Shielded, grounded, surrounded by love.* Our Healing Touch practitioner Janna suggested I find some words to focus on in the days around surgery. While lying on her table, eyes closed, letting her smooth and fill my energy field (which was getting easier to imagine and maybe even to feel), those words and their rhythm came into my mind. To me, the words meant I would be protected from fears and from the negativity or worry of other people, or like saying "Shields up," on *Star Trek*. I would be grounded, like the deep, deep roots of an old willow tree, and grounded like my hair dryer near a wet sink so I wouldn't freak out and flip a breaker switch. I knew I was surrounded by love coming from our family-friends-neighbors, our email following, and all the churches of people who had Scott on their prayer chain.

Shielded, grounded, surrounded by love. It had a nice ring to it.

The nurse wheeled Scott into a preparation room where clattering drapes encircled empty gurneys like ugly shower curtains. Another nurse took over, pulling up a rolling table full of supplies.

"Here, you can help me," she said, handing me a paper covered with thick, foamy green dots, the same way I would let Wil play with stickers. "These are called fiducials. We're going to stick them to Scott's head in a grid. First I need to measure out the grid and make marks. Hey, Scott, your shaved head will make it go faster."

She used a tape measure and black magic marker, while I peeled off one sticker at a time and pressed it to Scott's scalp, as she directed. "This is fun," I joked. It was easy to laugh, and Scott laughed, too.

A little girl was wheeled into the pre-op room then, with her frightened parents behind her. Her nurse complimented her on the beautiful lacy white dress she was wearing, and I heard her parents say she wanted to dress up to get her tonsils out. She was very brave and only whimpered. She left before we did.

When we were done, the nurse said it was time to say goodbye. She asked if Scott had any family waiting who might want to come in for a hug. I went out to find our family, and minutes later, two at a time, they came in.

First came Lance and Amie, her eyes red from crying. She gave Scott a hug and didn't want to let go. He closed his eyes and hugged her back. Bill and Linda came in next. Reverend Jane came in with them, to pray with us at the final minute, just like the first surgery. I barely heard her words because I was focused on feeling shielded, grounded, surrounded by love.

It was time to take my leave. I wouldn't say goodbye. I was almost giddy with courage. I gave Scott a hug, a kiss, and a sincerely bold smile. "It's gonna be great," I said. "I love you." Then, with one hand in my pocket, I gave him a high-five as the nurse wheeled him away. Alanis Morrissette had interrupted my mantra to sing in my head, and I had to agree with her, *I'm brave but I'm chickenshit*. Then she was interrupted by Shawn Mullins who confirmed as he had been doing for months now that *everything's gonna be all right, rock-a-bye, rock-a-bye*. Then Scott was gone, down the hall, behind the swinging doors, and I turned to join my family in the waiting room.

Shielded, grounded, surrounded by love. I kept up the silent mantra in my brain for most of the day. We sat in a very crowded waiting room on that Friday morning. Amie had staked out a corner and pulled together a circle of chairs. She handed out mindless magazines to read. I didn't read much— I was in my own world, shielded, grounded, surrounded by love.

The patient care coordinator from the CNI Brain Tumor Team came to say hello, meeting everyone in the family. She gave me a pager, so that I could take a walk through the hospital complex or go to the ice cream shop across the street and still be reachable. When we noticed the pager's lights were not flashing properly, she emptied the batteries from her own pager and put them in mine.

"That was so nice of her," Amie said after she left.

More visitors came and went. Uncle Mac sat with us awhile, saying Aunt Kathy would stop by after work. Then Mr. Barry arrived, bearing a brown paper bag of chocolate chip oatmeal cookies, delivering hugs and prayers from his wife, Alfreda. In my family's twenty-eight years on Corona Street, the Barry family lived in the big house on the corner with their six kids, including my best friend, Jane. As I saw him walk in and bear-hug both my parents, it was as if he brought Jane, my kindred spirit since kindergarten, to sit with me today. He brought me memories of countless cookies and milk, his sneezes we could hear down the block, trips in the back of his extra-large station wagon to Mother of God for the short Mass on Saturday afternoon. My hug from Joe reminded me how I worried all day through seventh-grade classes while Jane had surgery on her spine, until finally a relieving phone message note was delivered to me in Social Studies. On this day of Scott's surgery, Mrs. Barry was working and couldn't come visit, Joe said, but she made us these cookies.

I caught eyes with Amie again, *So so nice* she mouthed, her eyes full of tears and her hand over her heart.

Jane wrote an email the next day, "I know Dad came to visit. I hope that was okay." Okay? It was much better than okay. Joe's jovial gesture of cookies inspired Scott's sister, Amie, six months later to propose her idea of The Heartstrings Project to CNI, a way to connect brain tumor patients and families. Part of her plan was for volunteers to bring cookies during surgery, a small simple kindness on a very hard day. Mr. and Mrs. Barry's cookies had tugged at her heartstrings, she said.

In the early afternoon, I went to the cafeteria with my mom to escape from the waiting room angst and get a snack. We sat at a table by the south window, overlooking the snow-covered crab-apple trees down below. (Memories are funny. Whenever I remember that moment, I see those trees covered with snow on pink blossoms, though in truth the trees bloomed a month later. My brain believes spring arrived that day.) The sun came out and the slushy snow was dripping and shining. I could see the mountains over the neighborhood roof-tops.

Our neuropsychologist found us there and pulled up a chair. He'd been dropping by all day to give me updates on Scott's surgery. "I just wanted to say the awake part is over. He did great. He had the surgeons in stitches of laughter. And it's not easy to make those guys laugh."

"Really? That's great," I smiled back, and my mom squeezed my hand with a grin. I wish I had asked him for details that day, while it was fresh in his memory. What had Scott said when he was awake that could have made the surgeons laugh? It's a mystery I'll never know.

"It'll be awhile still, before Scott is done, but I just wanted to let you know that he's doing fine, much better than he was when I was testing him yesterday."

"What a relief," I said to my mom after he left. "What a nice guy. What a contrast to the first surgery, huh?"

"Yep, I have a good feeling about this," she said, and we walked back to the waiting room with a spring in our steps.

It was still a few hours before one of the two neurosurgeons came to the waiting room to say they were done and all had gone well, really well. Wearing blue scrubs beneath a white coat, the neurosurgeon looked tired but satisfied that the team had done a good job. He gave me some details that I wrote in my notebook.

The rest of the day was a blur. After that, I stopped thinking *shielded, grounded or surrounded by love*, though the intention rippled onward for days. My mantra did its job, ushering me through the day. I stumbled to the ICU Waiting Room to settle in a chair until I could see Scott. I called Kathy Matsey who, just like before, would send an email to our waiting friends. This is what she wrote:

6:45 pm, Friday

Dear friends of Scott and Shelly,

I know that all of you have had Scott in your thoughts and prayers today as he underwent his second surgery. I have just spoken with Shelly who called from the hospital and she reports that the surgery went extremely well. "Amazingly well" were her exact words.

The surgeons were able to remove a lot of the tumor and because Scott was awake during that part of the operation, they were able to monitor his cognitive and motor functioning. Some areas of function may even have improved. Scott has experienced no loss of peripheral vision, one side effect of the surgery they were expecting. Finally, he appears to be far more responsive than they would have expected at this point in the post-operative recovery phase. This is all very good news.

Scott will be in the ICU for a day or two with restrictions on visitors, noise, light, etc. Shelly wanted all of you to know how much your support means and that she has loved hearing from you, even if she is not able to respond.

I will send more updates as I am able.

Yours,
Kathy Matsey

I had an experience I can't prove. I can't even explain it,
but everything I know as a human being,
everything that I am tells me that it was real.
—*Ellie Arroway, in "Contact" by Carl Sagan*

20
Mystery After Midnight

This is the chapter where I get to tell you what happened to Scott when I wasn't in the room. I'm his mere scribe, his absent witness to what happened one night. Of all the things he forgot, he still remembers this night. He told me and I'm telling you.

Surgery was Friday and over the weekend, Scott amazed everyone at how well he was doing, like a laboratory chimpanzee who had learned to speak, shave, solve differential equations, and dance the tango. I went home Sunday night to sleep in my own bed, the house to myself, content that Scott was safe and sound. I kept waking up throughout the night, though, with worries I couldn't define.

Back at the hospital, it was the middle of the night and the ninth floor was dark and quiet. The second shift had come on duty, made their rounds, and retired behind their desk at the end of the hall. Scott was in room 916, one room away from the nurses' station. In his private room, with paper over the windows to prevent even indirect daylight from burning him after his photodynamic therapy, Scott couldn't see the city lights or the stars.

It started out as a mild headache and he buzzed the nurse, who brought him some pain medication. He slept, but then woke up feeling cold, shivering, shaking. Then his head started to fill, not with thoughts but a fog so thick that he couldn't see out. Pain was plodding thickly through his body, toes to knees to guts to heart to neck to head, squeezing him tight. Splotching pockets of energy were draining away all over his body. The pain was deafening, strangling, bringing the walls closer to his bed and death even closer. At that point, he couldn't call the nurse because he no longer knew who or where he was, or why he was here in this room.

"This is it. I'm going to die," Scott said out loud through his tears. He was shaking and felt submerged, as if underwater.

This was, without a doubt, the worst pain he had ever experienced, a pain that defied reason. The pain took every ounce of his willpower and then demanded more. Purple splotches punctuated the black that was beyond black. Scott knew he was dying and there was nothing he could do about it. It was not a question of giving up, but of letting go. And so he let go.

A sudden rush of heat and mist and a sheet of white light crossed his body in a horizontal wave, covering him from head to toe as he lay in bed, almost like a flowing cloud or a patchwork all-white quilted blanket. He wasn't powering the controls anymore and couldn't explain what had just happened, "Except to say I suddenly felt peaceful and the pain was gone. Just like that. I do know it had nothing to do with me. I opened my eyes. Looked around. Sat up. Then I walked to the nurse's station and told my nurse everything."

The nurse recognized the mystery and grace of what had just happened. She said to him, "Scott, you have to remember this and tell other people."

Scott walked in the hallway awhile, looked at the city lights out of the window by the elevator, and went back to his room where he left me a note and crawled back in bed. And slept.

Back at home, restless, I rolled out of bed about 7:30, showered and dressed for another day at the hospital. I forced myself to eat a slow bowl of cereal, but I was anxious to get back and check on Scott.

When I arrived at the hospital, I could tell something was wrong. Scott was disoriented and the light in his eyes was almost out. My spiral notebook was on the window-ledge above the radiator, open to a new page on which I found his handwriting. In letters more than one-inch high, taking up the full page, he had scrawled, "Hi! Don't worry I'm fine" and at the bottom of the page, as if signing off or addressing the note, he wrote "Mom Dad Wil." My worry skipped a beat to take an irrational pout in my head, *Geez, he wrote a note in the middle of the night but he wrote it to his parents and Wil, not to me?*

I wanted an explanation but now wasn't the time. He dragged his IV pole into the bathroom and came out again, shaking. "Get me a nurse," he whispered. He sipped some water, then lost his grip on the cup. His right hand started twitching, first the thumb, then all his fingers. He rested his head on his left hand, gripping his forehead, alternately hyperventilating and holding his breath.

I pushed the call button to summon a nurse. After minutes when no one arrived, I pushed it again. And waited. Veins on Scott's forehead pulsed and his face was turning purple. I pushed the call button again. No one came. And I panicked. I walked into the hallway and yelled, "We need a nurse!"

A young girl-nurse came running in the room. I was in tears, saying "Scott needs help." She calmly gave him an anti-nausea pill, and few minutes later some Percoset for the pain. Thirty minutes later, he was still in pain, and I asked if she could page Scott's neurosurgeon. As if to determine whether Scott's status warranted paging the doctor, she took his pulse and asked, "Do you know where you are?"

It took Scott a long, excruciating minute to hazard a guess that he might be at Swedish Hospital.

I count it as a miracle that our lead-neurosurgeon and his physician's assistant walked in the room then, without summons, and quickly assessed the situation.

"You're having some swelling," said the doctor, his voice like a salve as he looked at Scott's chart and at Scott. "Right on schedule. Remember? We talked about the likelihood that seventy-two to ninety-six hours after surgery you would experience some brain swelling. From this morning's lab work, it looks like your Dilantin levels are too low. We'll set you up with an IV, and you'll feel better soon."

The doctor gave directions to the nurse, who I wished he would fire for her neglect (while the rational part of me knew she had other patients, maybe in the same dire straits as Scott had just been). After he left, the nurse said, "Boy, how lucky he showed up like that. He wasn't due to make rounds for two more hours."

That was a God thing, I thought, but I was too drained to say it out loud.

Scott's mom came to the hospital a few hours later. She encouraged me to crawl into the second bed in the room, and I slept for awhile. Linda left when I woke up.

Scott dozed throughout the day, not eating or even able to carry on conversation. But, by seven that night he woke up, walked without help to the bathroom, asked for a sponge bath, shaved, and asked for some dinner, every step of which felt like a miracle.

In between Jello slurps, he told me his story.

"So when I came back to this room, I wrote that note," he said.

"Why did you write it to your parents and Wil?" I asked, not able to keep it in longer.

"I meant you, me, and Wil," he laughed. "I was writing it to all of us."

"Oh," I said, sheepish and relieved at one mystery solved. I was in awe and weirdly jealous that he had experienced a mystery I could only imagine...not that I would trade places with him for a million.

After another long moment I asked, "So, do you think that was God?"

"I don't know," Scott replied, "Maybe."

I couldn't exactly describe his mystery in an email, but I did include a clinical update about his swelling-scare in my next email, and I ended with amazing news about his surgical success:

Subj: Update on Scott - 3/16
Date: 3/16/99 8:03:14 AM Mountain Standard Time

Dear Everyone,

...To leave you with some GOOD NEWS, the MRI taken on Sunday showed excellent results from the surgery. **This sounds almost too good to be true, but as of Sunday, they actually COULD NOT SEE THE TUMOR!!!!!!!** We only expected and hoped for 80% removal, but it looks like much more was possible, thanks to Scott and our neuropsychologist having such a good rapport and talking their way through the tumor resection. The surgeons just kept picking away at it -- far more than they ever would or could have with Scott asleep. This doesn't mean that the tumor is all gone, because even 1% left means a billion cells and it only takes one cell to keep growing. But, this also means that the photodynamic therapy will be able to reach a lot more of the unseen tumor cells, and POSSIBLY, just possibly, we can go with a less toxic chemotheraphy regimen (still gotta do that). The other good news is that the peripheral vision loss that every doctor said was inevitable did not fully happen -- another miracle! Scott only lost a very little vision on his very lower right quadrant, like peripherally seeing down and to the right when looking straight ahead, but it's very subtle!

So, Scott is not out of the woods yet, but it appears that the surgery was a huge success. I haven't seen the MRI films yet or spoken directly with the doctors on all this, so take it with a grain of salt. But, we're happy, grateful, hopeful, and really know we are the lucky recipients of some tremendously AMAZING GRACE!

Will keep you posted. Thanks for all the prayers and messages! Please pray that Scott's swelling recedes rapidly and his recovery gets back on track. It's great to know you're all out there helping us along!

Love,
Shelly

If women's stories are not told,
the depth of women's souls will not be known.
—*Carol P. Christ*

21
Vote for Mackenzie

Here's one thread of truth I never revealed in my email updates during Scott's brain tumor treatment. It's the one thread I wove into the fabric of our journey in silence because, to me, it was too precious and personal to expose to the scrutiny and judgment of anyone, something I could not bear to broadcast to our ever-growing email list. But my story isn't complete without it.

That thread was my long-standing desire for another child, my hope to overcome years of infertility and become pregnant. Just because Scott had cancer didn't mean I could turn off my own hopes like a faucet. Believe me, I tried.

One of my first tasks after Scott's brain tumor was diagnosed and his surgery scheduled for November 14th, was to open my desk calendar and cancel commitments. I still remember the phone call. I stood in my office, flipping week by week's pages in my Mary Engelbreit calendar. The appointment was there, circled and starred: "Dr X 10 am" and the phone number. I booked the appointment almost three months earlier, despite no insurance coverage for infertility treatments. I had been waiting over eight weeks already, conscientiously collecting data by charting two more cycles of my daily morning temperature, to see one of Denver's top-two infertility specialists who had worked miracles for several women I knew.

This wasn't my first visit to an infertility specialist. It took two years of trying and six months of Clomid, a prescription pill, to jumpstart my ovaries and become pregnant the first time. First time.

That was six years earlier, when the pregnancy test stick turned pink in two spots on Mother's Day. I was finally pregnant! My due date was Christmas. All-day morning sickness cursed me throughout May, June, and half of July. If it hadn't been for the Georgia peaches that summer and fortified breakfast cereal, plus the kitten-toe-tickling of movement inside me, I'm not sure I could have endured the all-day morning sickness. It wore me out and forced me to swear, *Never again — I'm adopting the next child!*

That August we had the midway ultrasound that showed all the baby parts in the right places and confirmed we were having a son. I dreamed that month of meeting my new boy, telling him the names we were considering. In my dream, the tow-headed baby vetoed one name and voted instead for William. In his dream-baby words, he said, "I want a name that will last." I didn't know what my dream-baby meant by that remark, but I did know the dream meant we were connected already.

A week before Christmas my sister flew to Oak Ridge, half-joking that I better wait until she arrived to have the baby. She came in on Friday, and, as if on cue, I woke after midnight to strong contractions and The Beatles singing in my head, "Here comes the sun." My son was on his way.

I managed an IV-free, all natural birth, fearing needles but believing my doctor who said, "Don't worry. Your body will know what to do." It did, and I brought an eight pound, eleven ounce son into the world by squatting, breathing, and screaming. My left arm wrenched Scott's neck as I pushed.

"You nearly broke my neck," smiled Scott, not minding at all. Later that day he sat in the hospital chapel to tell God thanks for his son and for keeping me safe.

Turning an egg into a person, transforming my body to grow a new soul, and delivering Wil through the ring of fire was the most painful, powerful task I ever accomplished. If I could do that, I believed I could bear anything.

A year later, head over heels in love with Wil and motherhood, I felt the growing urge to enlarge our family. I hoped one successful pregnancy meant my body knew what to do and would conceive easily the second time. I didn't worry too much during six months of "just trying," but with each failed attempt, I grew more anxious. I tried six more rounds of Clomid, to no avail.

Twelve rounds of Clomid is the lifetime recommended maximum, I was told. My mother's ovarian cancer was reason enough to stop. I tried alternatives, like deep- tissue massage, herbs, and wild yam cream, even Chinese herbal tea I had to brew from chunky leaves, seeds, berries, and twigs! I dealt with my hypothyroidism with traditional medication, which felt like a welcome shot of espresso. I had covered all the bases with years of graph paper and basal body temperature charts, even sleeping with the blinds wide open during the full moon hoping to naturally regulate my cycles according to ancient lore. All for naught.

One thing I never tried in all those years was reversing, releasing my desire for another child. I felt a palpable hole in my heart like a person was missing from our family, an undefined guest whose place was already set at our table. I wasn't ready to consider adoption yet. I still believed in my body.

The day after Scott was told he had a mass in his brain, one of my first selfish thoughts was *Maybe that's why I haven't gotten pregnant. Maybe it's his fault, not mine.* I hate to admit that.

"I need to cancel my appointment. No, I'm not sure if I can re-schedule. My husband has a brain tumor and is having surgery this week. We'll have to wait and see."

I hung up the phone and cried—for everything.

Sometime during the six weeks of radiation—in December and January—we began talking again about how to go on living. Do we go on with our life as we planned, intending to live as fully as possible, tumor be damned? Was I feeding a desperate hope to create one more genetic copy of Scott, a part of him to hold onto in case the tumor damned him? I confessed to some of both, plus heightened (perhaps transferred) anxiety for Wil not to grow up alone.

We asked the doctor, "Will radiation to Scott's brain in any way affect his sperm production?" The radiation-oncologist practically laughed that no, we needn't worry. If the radiation were for testicular cancer, that would be a different story. The brain wasn't involved.

Before I could think of conceiving, I had to get over my fears that sex could cause Scott's brain to hemorrhage. After his November surgery, the hospital gave him laxatives so straining on the toilet wouldn't make his brain swell. I mean, who knew what kind of pressure sex caused? Our neuropsychologist reassured us that the endorphins from sex, for both of us, far outweighed the risks. After that we made love like there was no tomorrow.

As part of our renewed attempts, Scott agreed to reschedule the fertility appointment for mid-February, during the waiting period between radiation and the next MRI. We went to the doctor's office in the same building as Scott's neurosurgeon, and it felt strange for me to be in the patient's role. As Scott left the room to make a deposit in a specimen cup for his part of the test, the nurse looked over my chart.

"I see you cancelled an appointment in November. So you're ready now, huh?"

"Yes, this is our last attempt. My husband has a brain tumor and will start chemotherapy soon, so we're going to try one more time."

The nurse's face registered shock and pity. "Have you considered sperm banking?"

"We've talked about it, but Scott doesn't want to."

She didn't ask me anything else. Scott refused to bank any sperm, not wanting his current genetic material or his poor health to be stored for posterity. I felt he was being irrational, as if banked sperm would be any different than what we were relying on now. But it wasn't up to me. In our many conversations earlier that winter he would say, "If it's going to happen, if it's meant to happen, it will have to happen naturally—at least on my part and for you with the Clomid. If it doesn't happen this time, we'll consider adoption. Do they even let cancer survivors adopt? Let's just wait and see," he said, thinking *Let's see if I'm still alive to even be a dad. She's young enough to remarry.*

The doctor saw under the microscope that Scott's sperm was good to go. I was jealous that even with cancer Scott could probably get any woman pregnant. It was all up to me. I had to undergo a dye test to confirm that my fallopian tubes were not blocked. Afterwards, the doctor said, "You seem to be great. Let's get you pregnant." I had the green light and one last round of Clomid. Just to be sure, he prescribed a double dose.

Later that afternoon, I told my Healing Touch practitioner, Janna, that I was excited but nervous to try the Clomid once again, my thirteenth round. "All the other times," I said, "I could really feel it in my ovaries when they were trying to pop off an egg. I'm afraid of the pain and whether I'm pushing the limits. I don't want to end up with ovarian cancer."

"I can help you with that," Janna said. "You can energetically bless the medicine and set your intentions for it to do its job, but not cause harm. Here's how you do it. First, open your hand chakras by pressing gently with your thumbs in the opposite palm. Hold the pill in your hand, and cup your other hand over it. Send your energy into the pill. Say something like, 'I intend for this medicine to enable me to welcome a new life into my body and into our family, without any pain or harmful side effects.' "

I did as she suggested and I added a disclaimer, "If this is in the best interests of the universe." Placebo or real, the medicine-blessing seemed to work. I experienced absolutely no ovulation *middleschmertz* pain from the double dose of Clomid. On February 18, I had an ultrasound at the hospital —the one where Scott had his first surgery—and it showed a bulging egg follicle ready to pop. The doctor decided I didn't need a shot of hormone to make it release. It appeared to be ready and willing without an extra push.

I was full of confidence after that. Even the universe seemed to be on my side with the planets aligned. No kidding. That same week, Venus and Jupiter were slated to appear so close to one another that it would look like one large, very bright star in the southwestern sky. It was a celestial event that wouldn't happen in the same way again until 2085. Some astronomers and historians revived a long-standing debate that the star of Bethlehem was in fact the same close meeting of Venus and either Saturn or Jupiter. *Well, if that's not good karma?* I thought.

Astronomy magazine said the event should be "spellbinding," with the double evening star and a crescent moon. Even our lucky moon was showing up to cheer us on.

The very next day we discovered Scott's tumor had doubled. Shocked to the core, it took all I had to keep hoping. Were we creating a new life or losing one? Could we have both?

I put all my energy into seeking second, third, and fourth opinions. I ovulated before our trip to M.D. Anderson. We tried our best to make love not just for a baby but for holding onto each precious day. If true love were the crucial ingredient, our love would have been plenty. Scott, all the while, was getting sicker as his brain swelling increased.

Throughout the week in Houston and before surgery, I continued taking my temperature before getting out of bed each morning. The graphs showed a rise in basal body temperature, just as it should with Clomid at work, promising that my body had the right hormones to host a baby.

Every day when I drove to Swedish Hospital to visit Scott, I passed through the Englewood neighborhood of tiny post-World War II houses, sporting campaign signs on the lawn for the springtime elections. "Vote for Mackenzie" signs mocked me. Mackenzie is the name we picked—before getting married—to name our daughter someday. I took the yard signs as a good omen, a reminder to hold onto hope.

Three days after Scott's 99.9% brain tumor resection, I walked into the ICU to find Scott sitting up in bed, shaving with his electric razor. He looked good, very good, a big contrast to November's post-surgery. I walked in and said, "Well, my temperature is still ninety-nine point six," expectantly waiting a thumbs-up of encouragement.

"Sounds like a radio station," Scott grumbled, not caring one bit, or more likely, not knowing what I meant in his post-surgical neurological state. He just sat there, shaving his face.

Poof. Pop. I had been holding my hope like a metaphorical bouquet of helium balloons. Scott's response shattered one of those balloons. Kerblam!

The next day I had lunch with my sister at the ice-cream sandwich shop across from the hospital. Jenéne was flying home to Cincinnati that afternoon, having traveled yet again to help me during surgery week. Leaning forward in a whisper, I shared my secret hope that I was pregnant.

"Oh, Shel," she said in a voice deep with concern, not excitement. Pop! Another balloon exploded. "How can you think you're ready for that? That's asking too much of yourself to have a baby right now."

"We could do it. We'd have lots of help," I rationalized, but it sounded sad even to my own ears. It felt like my sister was praying against me, and so would everyone else.

That night I had a dream. *Kevin, Scott's friend, is pushing Scott up the street in a wheelchair. They both smile and wave at me, then turn a corner as if to leave. Kevin has taken over my job to care for Scott. Scott smiles and willingly goes. He points to the stroller I'm pushing and blows us a kiss. "No!" I yell. "No, I'll take care of Scott, not you, Kevin." Scott waves again and says, "No, Shel, it's okay. You have the baby now"*

When I woke up from that nightmare, I was bleeding. My period had arrived, full fledged. I was not pregnant. Our last-ditch effort had ended. Pop – pop – pop went three more of my hope-filled balloons. Only one pink balloon, still full, floated up in the sky. The last of my hopes for Mackenzie disappeared into the blue of the morning sky, not popped, not shattered, but gone.

When I was three years old, and Jenéne was four, she had a red balloon. It was from a gas station grand opening, not a circus. She let go of the string by accident and cried when it blew beyond reach and away with the wind. Later that day, maybe the next, we were playing outside and watched, amazed, as that same red balloon, it had to be, landed in our yard. It came back!

Maybe mine would, too, someday — but not that day.

Weeks later Janna asked me, "What do you think the dream meant — of Scott leaving with Kevin?"

"That Scott didn't want the baby," I said, pouting, sad and angry at the failure of our last ditch effort, blaming Scott for everything on so many levels. Wise Janna smiled, just barely, and steered the conversation elsewhere.

It was years, *years*, before I realized the power of my dream, that perhaps I made my own choice. Did my dream show me the consequence of having a baby at that point? Perhaps I wasn't willing to add another soul to my list of responsibilities, not if it meant giving up the role and commitment to care for Scott and Wil and myself. Was it my disclaimer letting the universe decide if pregnancy was in anyone's best interest? What if my body knew best?

Since that time, I've often pondered the thought of people "praying against me." What if I had asked for prayers to support us? What if everyone rose to the occasion, praying for our wish to come true? Was it too much to ask for Scott's brain to be healed and for me to get pregnant? How many miracles does one family deserve?

It's harder than hard to let go of your dreams just because cancer shows up.

As it turned out, all the months of Scott's brain tumor treatment were in fact about creating a new life, just not the life we expected. *We must be willing to let go of the life we planned so as to have the life that is waiting for us.* Still, I struggle to find the grace to accept it.

I have to believe that the Garth Brooks song is true: "Some of God's greatest gifts are his unanswered prayers." Sometimes God's answer is "No. Trust me, but *no*."

Times got harder, and months down the road I crashed in caregiver burnout. I look back now to see it took all I had, and then some, to simply survive. Had I been a sleep-deprived new mother as well, I don't know how any of us would have found the resiliency to survive, much less thrive.

I have to trust that all prayers are answered in whatever way God deems appropriate, in Her own time, not mine.

I sometimes wonder if somewhere my lone pink balloon still floats over mountains, traversing the sky. Maybe Mackenzie's soul has a middle name. Hope.

In spite of everything, life is good.
—*Hendrik Willem van Loon*

22
Decompression

Subj: Scott's at Home Now
Date: 3/18/99 6:23:31 PM Mountain Standard Time

Dear Everyone,

Just a quick note to say that Scott rebounded pretty well after Monday, so they let him come home. He had a restful, uneventful, not-in-much-pain kinda day today, with plenty of love and healing attention from Wil. We're just laying low with no visitors yet until Scott gets some strength back.

We confirmed with the neuro-oncologist that Scott will need to continue fighting the remaining tumor with the full-strength chemotherapy (a 4-drug cocktail), but he at least gets to wait until Monday, March 29th, to begin. This regimen will mean 4-5 days in the hospital every 4 weeks (3 days to drip in the drugs, 1 day to flush them out again, and 1 day to monitor his reaction). This will continue for 5 months as long as Scott can tolerate it -- meaning no hearing loss, no severe blood count drops or bone marrow impairment, not to mention overall fatigue and nausea. Pretty scary stuff, but it's Scott's best shot at the total cure.

I'll write again soon. For now, know that we're home safe and healing has begun.

Love and Much Thanks!!!
Shelly & Scott :)

P.S. I'm still working my way through the emails, but keep 'em coming.

The prospect of enduring five months of chemo cleared my mind of most everything else. We had two weeks in which Scott was allowed to recover from surgery before beginning chemo. Scott had dropped into what I thought was deep depression, despite the surgeon's report of removing 99.9% of Scott's tumor. That first week home I saw no laughter, no smiles, and the barest of interaction with me or Wil.

One night when Wil was having a sleepover at Bill and Linda's house, I saw a chance to talk. I turned off the TV and sat cross-legged beside Scott, hand on his knee.

"I've been really worried about you this week," I said, "You've been so quiet and sad. I'm worried that you've lost your will to live and I don't know why. You just can't go into chemotherapy in a funk like this. What's going on?"

"I didn't lose my will to live," Scott said, surprised at my interpretation of his silence and taking a long moment to gather his thoughts before speaking. "But I did have a lot of thinking to do. I had to come back from a deep, dark place. That night in the hospital...I realized how small and insignificant I am. I've always been able to rely on my mind, my brain, my intelligence, to figure out life. That night, I knew there was something so much bigger and I wasn't in control. I had to get over that.

"The other thing," Scott continued, weeks of worry pouring out now that his silence was broken, "Is that I have way more deficits now than before, and nobody seems to notice. I feel dazed and confused. It's hard to concentrate. The proprioception is worse—half the time I don't know where my right hand is. And when I look in a mirror, the far right side of my face disappears. That freaks me out.

"Plus, I feel like I can't be a parent to Wil anymore because I don't have the energy to discipline him and so I feel like I've lost my clout, my credibility. Wil has been pushing my buttons all week, and when I try to deal with him, you interrupt and change the rules, and then he ignores me."

I couldn't help getting defensive about Wil, but I knew he was right. I knew much of Wil's acting-out was a reaction to our long surgery week in the hospital following a long weekend in Houston and all the pre-surgery preparations, not to mention the months of upheaval since November. Wil's separation anxiety was no match for mine, and I was trying to be gentle, subjective, with both of us. I wasn't following the advice from the conference seminar on parenting, about consistent discipline during these scary times because children need to feel safe in their boundaries. I was finding it tough to be a single parent and a medical caregiver at the same time, sometimes feeling like I suddenly had two kids. I am sure that since Scott's diagnosis, I began second-guessing his parenting "interpretations" and blaming the tumor for what I thought was poor judgment. I avoided talking about it. It's hard to face conflict over normal life-issues when you're dealing with cancer, but I've learned it's even more important than ever. It just takes guts.

Thankfully, our inner grown-ups had come out to talk that night. We talked a long while.

"I don't want you to think I'm losing hope," Scott said. "It's mostly cabin fever, just being stuck inside. But otherwise I really am optimistic. I know I need an attitude check, but it might come slowly. Surgery wasn't the end of all this, just because they got so much tumor. You know what we learned in Houston...what Dr. Arenson says. Just because we can't see any tumor doesn't mean it isn't there.

"I have to say I'm scared shitless to think of facing five months of chemo. It's going to be damn toxic."

"Are you having second thoughts about going through with the chemo?" I asked.

"No. We've done our research. You know me, once I make a decision I'm ready to go for it without any regrets. I don't want the standard treatment protocol, because it's really not working for anybody. It's not the cure. I'm willing to try something new and more aggressive, even if it is damn scary and risky. I'd rather die trying."

At each step in Scott's treatment we balked at the aggressive approach, did our research, weighed options, listened to doctor's advice and asked questions, then thought even more. I think at this point in our conversation, neither of us wanted to be talked out of chemo, but some words needed spoken out loud.

"What scares me is that I won't know what side effects I'll have 'til I have them. Yeah, we know in general what can happen. It's the long-term costs I'm wondering about. What price will I have to pay for all this treatment?"

"Well, paying the price later on is something we'll just have to deal with." I choked on the future and couldn't continue this dive into worrying about things we couldn't control. "Let's just plan on having long-term worries, which is better than losing in the short-run."

My inner Pollyanna was never far away, trying to put a positive spin on any situation. Scott was used to her; it was a love-hate relationship. Pollyanna couldn't help adding, "And look, it's already been five months since your diagnosis. Let's hope the next five months go just as fast, with good times in between."

"Yeah," Scott agreed, "Time flies whether you're having fun or not."

"You know what you need for your cabin fever?" I asked, trying to salvage our conversation. "You need some company. You've been alone in the dark of this house for over a week. Let's call some friends to come over."

"Okay. That sounds good."

That very night I emailed several people, asking that they come for a visit. Within days, they did. Scott hosted some co-workers, some college buddies, and friends since high school. What he needed was guy talk, shop talk, kidding around, and little mention of cancer. Each visit did wonders for his mood. Add to that a birthday dinner for Scott's dad that included Aunt Nancy from Michigan. Finally I saw Scott resurfacing. He was playful with Wil, joking with me, just more awake overall. What a relief.

We also had a good follow-up appointment with one of Scott's neurosurgeons, who gave us the thumbs up to see a matinee at the mall. "Malls are all fluorescent lighting," he said, "So you'll be safe from sunburn walking around in a mall. Get some exercise, some fresh air. Celebrate. You're doing great."

That helped me feel chipper enough to send out an update.

Subj: Update on Scott 3/25
Date: 3/25/99

Dear Everyone,

Here's the latest on Scott's recovery from his 2nd brain surgery, which was two weeks ago today. He is doing pretty well overall. It seems that he is recovering as quickly from this surgery as the first one back in November, maybe a bit better. It is hard to concentrate on conversations, at times he feels "dazed and confused" and he's been pretty tired. But his balance, walking and strength are good, his scar already looks well healed, his hair is growing back from the radiation baldness and pre-surgery shaving, and his blue eyes are still twinkling. :) He wishes he was doing even better, but we just have to have patience. The surgeon says the swelling can take 4-6 weeks to subside, and by then we'll have the effects of chemotherapy to deal with. It will be hard to know what symptoms are related to what procedure.

We saw the surgeon on Tuesday this week for the follow-up visit and removal of stitches. That day we also saw the MRI's comparing the morning of surgery with the big old tumor there, plus two days after surgery with the tumor gone. It's true that they really did remove all the visible parts of the tumor. It was great to see that blank area instead of the tumor we've gotten used to. The surgeon did emphatically caution us against thinking it was ALL gone -- with this kind of tumor even a few cells can quickly and aggressively come back. So that's why it is important to keep on fighting with chemotherapy. Interestingly, an MRI taken on the Wednesday after surgery showed a margin of what looked like re-grown tumor, but the surgeon assured us that was cell-death and surgical healing already taking place. So it's a good thing we had that immediate MRI on Sunday after surgery for our true baseline.

We are adjusting to the requirements for fluorescent lighting and no direct sunshine as a result of the photodynamic therapy. It is so hard, with spring-time budding outside our door. It's surprising how careful we have to be -- even a few minutes watching a behind-the-clouds, almost-done sunset quickly gave Scott a burning sensation! Rest assured we are taking walks around the neighborhood after dark for exercise and fresh air, and I have found a few good hats to help cover up Scott when we go out for appointments. (You have no idea how many websites there are for "hats & sun protection"!)

Thank you so much to everyone who is helping with the cost of the light bulbs. It truly honors us that you would be so generous. We want to let you know that we plan to start a light-bulb-pass-along tradition for future patients of photodynamic therapy, so that others will benefit from your help, too. In another 4-6 weeks we should be able to open the shades and let the sunshine in! Then we'll send the lights to the next brain tumor patient.

Chemotherapy starts this coming Monday, March 29. We will be back at Swedish Hospital from Monday-Friday at least. The 4-drug cocktail takes 3 days to drip in, one day to flush out, and another day to monitor Scott's reaction. We have no idea what to expect, but hope for the best. I'll try to keep you posted next week so you know how Scott's faring. Current plans are for the chemo-week to be every 4th week, with 3 weeks off in-between, lasting a total of five months! We'll see.

All the prayers and positive thoughts you are sending to Scott are so vitally important to supporting him. We appreciate the many prayer chains around the country (& even the globe), not to mention the wonderful support we are getting from our neighbors, friends and family. I also want to give a special thanks to our Healing Touch practitioners, Janna and Carol, who really helped Scott before, after and since surgery. We continue to be amazed and grateful at the powerful healing they can facilitate by helping Scott focus his mind on healing his body.

Everyone reading this message is dear to our hearts. Thank you so very much for helping us on our journey. We will keep you posted.

Love,
Shelly, Scott & Wil

No pessimist ever discovered the secrets of the stars,
or sailed to an enchanted land, or
opened a new doorway to the human spirit.
—*Helen Keller*

23
My String Theory

On par with his pattern for months, Wil continued his 2:00 a.m. trips into our bedroom. As suggested at the "Parenting During Cancer" seminar in Houston, Wil and I made up a pallet of foam and blankets on the floor next to my side of the bed. Our deal was that he could come to our room, touch my elbow to let me know he was there, and then he could stay on the floor through the night. I didn't want him to get used to it forever, but it was a good compromise for now. I needed my sleep.

I had to prepare the logistics of caring for Wil during the week of Scott's first chemo, which meant Monday through Friday in the hospital. I wanted to stay with Scott as much as he needed. I decided to juggle sleepovers for Wil with our parents and neighbors. Wil knew I was making plans and kept asking, "When are my sleepovers going to start?"

I gave Wil the game plan of everywhere he would be for the week. Monday night he would be with Wucherpfennigs who lived on our left. Tuesday night, with Dahms who lived on our right. The rest of the week he would stay with both sets of grandparents.

On Tuesday night I didn't get home from the hospital until almost ten. Living room lights were still on at Dahm's house, so I knocked on the front door. Diane greeted me with a hug when she opened the door in her pajamas and asked how Scott did on Day Two of chemo. I was too tired for details and only said, "It went okay today. Not too terrible. How's Wil? I brought him a surprise."

I was holding a toy Siamese cat from the hospital gift shop, fluffy and soft, the same size as our two pet cats. My mommy-guilt got the best of me. Wil had seen the stuffed animal on his pre-surgery tour and without a promise from me to buy it for him, he named it Rosie (a name he'd been saving for over a year) and asked me to visit the cat in the gift shop.

Diane admired the softness of the toy cat with one finger, as if petting it, and said, "Tonight was the first night in all these months that Wil cried at bedtime and said he wanted his mommy. We all gave him extra hugs, though, so it didn't last long and he went to sleep happy. Do you want to go upstairs to give him a kiss?"

Wil was deep in his sleeping bag on the floor next to Drew and Noah's bunk bed. I resisted my urge to wake him so that I could get a tight hug. Instead, I tucked Rosie into the sleeping bag next to his pillow and kissed his forehead. When I went downstairs, Diane hugged me again and kissed my forehead before I went home and sunk into my own bed.

Wednesday night, after a long Chemo Day Three, I met Wil at my parent's house. "Mommy!" he yelled and ran down the hall to greet me, Rosie the cat in his arms. "I was so surprised to find Rosie this morning. Diane said you brought her last night. He helped me sleep really good. Are you staying here tonight?"

"I sure am," I said while we hugged. I replenished myself by reading Wil and Rosie bedtime stories and snuggling all night long. I didn't even mind when Wil snored and nudged me throughout the night. When he wasn't kicking, his arm was flung over my chest.

In the morning when I kissed Wil goodbye, I told him he'd be going to Gramma Binny's house for the next two nights. "I'm not sure when Dad gets to come home from the hospital, but it won't be too much longer. Easter is on Sunday so maybe you can decorate some eggs for us," I said. "I'll call you tonight."

Wil asked, "When will my sleepovers be done?" At first I thought he meant he was having fun and didn't want them to end. Then I realized he was really asking, when will chemo be over and my life go back to normal?

I could only answer, "I don't know."

Scott finally came home on Saturday, so that's when his mom brought Wil home, too. Wil arrived with two baskets of Easter eggs, jelly beans, two chocolate bunnies, a basket from each grandma. He was happy to be home, but tentative about getting too close to Scott. Scott was hooked up to an IV bag of saline solution for eight hours on Saturday, and he needed another eight on Sunday to continue flushing the chemotherapy drugs out of his body. A home-care nurse came both days to make sure he was set up properly. It was my job to disconnect the pump and flush his port with a syringe of saline. I had not bargained on being a nurse myself during his treatment. It was starting to get a bit too up close and personal for me.

Throughout the afternoon while Scott was sleeping, Wil was my shadow, off and on asking random questions like pulling them out of a hat.

"How do people get brain tumors?"

"Nobody knows," I said, telling the truth. "But they aren't catching. And it's nobody's fault. A brain tumor just happens."

Shit happens, I thought to myself for the umpteenth time. I know my answer was unsatisfactory, but I wasn't sure how much else to say. It wasn't the first time he asked. I sensed he wanted to know that it couldn't happen to anyone else in our family, more than – as adults sometimes do – needing someone or something to blame. I thought then that he was too young for lessons in the epidemiology of environmental causes or even to understand that brain tumors aren't hereditary. I didn't realize that in asking the question he was showing me that he *was ready* to process more of an answer.

My hindsight tells me I could have said something more hopeful and substantial, such as, "It is a mystery that scientists are working on. They're looking at ways that chemicals on farms or factories might cause brain tumors if they're used the wrong way. They're studying other possible causes, too. But we do know that it isn't something Daddy did to himself that caused it. Nobody made it happen. I wish I had a better answer for your today, but it makes me feel better that there are scientists trying to find out for us someday."

"I'm scared about Dad when he goes to the hospital," Wil said more than once that day.

I wish I knew how to extrapolate Wil's deeper worries. I could only answer, "I know. It is scary. But remember, we like this nice hospital. They have super nice nurses and doctors, and they're all taking really good care of Dad."

It was later still in the day when Wil asked out of the blue, "What does a dead person look like?"

"Like they're sleeping, I guess." I wish I made it clearer that dead means no snoring, no moving, no waking up.

"Can you keep their eyeballs?" was Wil's follow-up question.

"Um, no. No you can't," I said and couldn't help laughing. Where did he get that? Maybe Wil's five-year-old self suspected that our souls peek out through our eyes and his budding inner scientist was trying to solve that mystery in a practical manner.

"So how many carrots should we leave for the Easter Bunny?" Wil changed the subject. "Will he hide the eggs inside or outside, do you think?"

I was exhausted by bedtime from five days at the hospital, driving back and forth, worrying about Scott and Wil, not sleeping much myself. It was a relief to have all of us home, but part of me wished to have the house all to myself again. Wil was glad to be home, too, but grew clingier as the evening wore on. He seemed a bit soothed when our nighttime ritual began. First, we put Scott to bed, tucking him in with a kiss. Then we closed our two cats in the laundry room so they wouldn't carouse through the house all night. Then after a short bubble bath, Wil and I tucked ourselves into his bottom bunk to read bedtime stories. He picked out *The Kissing Hand,* by Audrey Penn, about the raccoon who doesn't want to leave his mom when he goes to school. Then we read about the watercolor-brought-to-life rooster, pig, and mouse in *Friends,* by Helme Heine. On the last page he chimed in with me, "Sometimes even good friends can't be together."

We said prayers next, "...the angels guard me through the night and wake me with the morning light. God bless Mom and Dad and me and everyone we love in the world. Amen."

It was time to turn out the light and leave. Wil grabbed me and said, "Don't go. Stay with me."

"I'll stay for a while," I succumbed. "I'm sleepy, too, though, and need to be in my own bed tonight."

"Okay," he begrudged as if crossing his fingers. I could see it coming, his stubborn refusal to fall asleep on his own. I felt stubborn, too, and tried to get up again, too soon. Tears exploded.

"I don't want to be by myself," Wil cried. Those weren't power struggle tears, I could tell, they were overwhelmed too-tired-to-be-alone tears. I lay back on the bed and put my arms around Wil, his head on my shoulder while he shed heart-wrenching sobs. I wanted to weep, too, not just for Wil's angst, but mine. I was out of answers and patience, but I wasn't willing to go to bed mad or create a big scene that would wake up Scott. I wasn't seeking peace at any price, but a peace that would last.

I looked up at the underside of Wil's top bunk bed. The red-metal tubing that held the upper mattress was still intertwined with Christmas twinkle lights, now unplugged. In between the slats we tucked in photos of Scott and Wil, me and Wil, and various snapshots of Wil and his friends playing outside. Back in December we tied a thimble-sized antique brass bell to his bed and pretended he could ring it to call on his guardian angel. That worked off and on. A porcelain guardian-angel nightlight flickered in the low outlet near his door. The street light in the cul-de-sac also lit his room, but in Wil's heart it was much too dark to fall asleep by himself.

As I lay there letting Wil's crying settle, my mind started to brainstorm. If we had walkie-talkies we would be talky all night. I wished I could tie a string to his wrist that would reach all the way to mine, which we could pull on long-distance to stay connected in the dark. It would figure, though, that one of us would trip on the string and fall headfirst down our steep stairwell. That wouldn't work.

I wished I could explain to Wil everything I was coming to consider the truth. I wished I could convey my whole lifetime of coincidence, synchronicity and brainwaves, of love at first sight, of letters crossing in the mail, and long-distance phone calls out of the blue from friends I thought of that day. I wished I could tell him how connected I felt with the email messages coming over the Internet from childhood friends, former co-workers, cousins and neighbors, and even the total strangers who were touched by a forwarded message and felt moved to respond. I wished I could explain how much better I felt after sending one of my emails and then finding my inbox flooded with loving replies. I wished I could have cracked open a golf ball and shown him all the miles of rubber string inside, which is how I pictured the support from our friends encircling the earth. I wished I could find words to describe the quantum physics of energy and all I was sensing in my own Healing Touch sessions. I wished I could have told him about Scott's midnight mystery, which hinted at something miraculous and real.

Even now, I wish wisdom arrived all at once. I looked for a way to explain what I knew to be true—that we're connected to the people we love, no matter how far, and we're never alone.

Author Phillip Pullman once said, "I think we should act *as if.* I think we should read books, and tell children stories, and take them to the theatre, and learn poems, and play music, as if it would make a difference...We should act as if the universe were listening to us and responding. We should act as if life were going to win."

This was one of those times. We would have to pretend, and a story started to form.

"Did I ever tell you about our heartstrings?" I asked Wil, interrupting his tears. He sniffed and shook his head, then opened his eyes as if asking for details.

"I haven't? Well I don't know why I didn't think of it before now?" I said in mock disbelief.

"What are heartstrings?" Wil asked.

"Heartstrings are invisible strings of love that reach from one heart to another," I told him, patting his chest and mine. "Everyone we love is connected to us by heartstrings."

"Where do heartstrings come from?" Wil asked next, and words poured from my imagination out of my mouth in reply.

"Your first heartstring comes from God when he sends you here from heaven. One end of the heartstring starts at God's heart and the other end attaches to your heart." My fingers reached out into the air and then plunked on Wil's chest like I was attaching that heartstring myself. And then I continued.

"Your next heartstrings are connected to me and Dad. You were born and had two more heartstrings."

"Like my belly button?" Wil grinned in a rhetorical question.

"Yep, only invisible, and higher of course," I tickled his tummy then patted his chest again. "Not only that, but you have heartstrings with everyone you love and everyone who loves you! Gramma Binny and Grandpa Bill, Nicky and Da, Aunt Amie and Lance, Aunt Jin, our neighbors and friends, and even Hannah and Spot."

"What would heartstrings look like if I could see them?" Wil asked, buying into the invisibility but wanting to borrow a pair of magic glasses to bring heartstrings into view.

"They can be any color, or they can be all the colors. So tell me, what color heartstrings do you have with everyone?"

Wil spent some time thinking and decided each heartstring was probably that person's favorite color. "Green for Dad. Periwinkle for you. Red for Gramma Nicky. Pink for Gramma Binny. Blue for Da and Grampa Bill and Uncle Lance."

Wil went on to define that Da's would be the midnight blue of his restored 1917 Nash Jeffery car. So maybe Grampa Bill's was red instead like his Ford pickup. Then he started wondering about heartstring colors for his two aunts and then our two cats.

"Man, just think how many heartstrings you have," I said, seeing that this color-matching could go on all night. "That's a lot of love coming to you through those heartstrings right now."

Wil put his hand over his heart for minute, thumping up and down, as if testing the concept. "But can they break?" he asked.

"Well, heartstrings are invisible, but they are very, very strong. Nothing can break a heartstring."

"How far do heartstrings go?" Wil wanted to know.

"Oh, it's like magic elastic. Heartstrings can reach as far as they need to. Heartstrings can reach from room to room, going around corners, and even through walls. They reach across town, go clear across country, even over the oceans and around the world. They even reach to heaven."

"Like to Gramma Great or Kristine," Wil said softly, thinking of Scott's grandmother and our next-door neighbor's stillborn baby daughter.

To lighten the moment, I jumped out of bed and started unfurling an invisible cord from the center of my chest like a magician pulls endless silk scarves from his sleeve. "Watch. See, I'm unreeling our heartstring. I'll go around the corner and you tug on our heartstring, okay? As a test."

I went just past the door and paused, then flung myself back on his carpet, guessing he had pulled hard. He laughed and said, "Do it again."

I walked farther down the hall this time and paused, using mother's intuition to know when to let him reel me back into his room. He was sitting up in bed pantomiming the use of a fishing rod. I stumbled in and gave another pratfall.

I stood up and pretend-dusted myself off. "I think it's time to go to sleep in our own beds," I said. "But you can hold onto our heartstring if you want to."

"But what if you don't answer me when I pull on it," Wil whined.

"Well, using a heartstring to make me come running isn't the way it works. Heartstrings keep us connected while we sleep or when we're apart. Love pumps through your heartstrings all the time whether you pay attention to it or not, just like your heart beat." Wil nodded.

I patted his heart and then patted mine. "Do you think you can go to sleep now?"

"Maybe," Wil said. "Are you going back to the hospital tomorrow?"

"No, Dad's done with the hospital for a few weeks, just doctor appointments every few days, but not tomorrow. We'll be home all day. It's Easter, remember?"

"Oh, yeah! I better get to sleep so the Easter Bunny can come hide the eggs."

Oh yeah, I thought. *Shoot. I better sneak back downstairs and hide egg now rather than in the morning. Wil is sure to wake up before me.*

I kissed Wil goodnight, and he let me leave the room without further negotiations. I sat on the top stair-step awhile, just to be sure I was free. Soon I heard his deep breathing and I tip-toed downstairs to the kitchen. I opened the refrigerator to retrieve the baskets of pastel eggs, light spilling onto the oak floor. I popped a purple jelly bean in my mouth and savored its grapeness. *Thank God our moms dyed eggs with Wil this week,* I thought to myself. I hid the eggs under the futon and chair, on the fireplace mantel, next to television and books, in potted plants, behind picture frames, on kitchen chairs and windowsills. With the threat of sunburn for Scott if he went outside in the sun, due to the photodynamic therapy, I wanted him to enjoy the Easter egg hunt with us indoors. *If we're lucky, he might even join in,* I hoped.

Bunny duties done, I crept upstairs and into bed. Scott was snoring. I lay awake thinking of heartstrings, hoping the idea would work for more than one night. Finally I slept.

I once attended a weekend retreat at the Sisters of Loretto convent in Knobs Haven, Kentucky. The retreat theme asked "Where is God in your garden?" On that Easter weekend, I would say God was in my backyard whistling *Row, Row, Row Your Boat* and helping my neighbors pull up our weeds. Then by the light of the moon, God would have dressed up in a bunny costume, hiding Easter eggs, decorating fences and trees with heartstrings like party streamers, planning to delight us with surprise in the morning. The brown rabbits that lived in our neighborhood instead of squirrels would dash out from under the shrubs and frolic in the grass. A Maypole created with a shaft of golden light would emerge out of my lawn from deep in the earth, and heartstrings would sway from the top, poised to weave in and out in the Maypole dance.

If you could have seen what I imagine for that Easter morning, you would have seen heartstrings streaming from one house to another, from sunrise to mountains, and all over town. Imagine the sight.

Reply to everything someone says with
"That's what you think."
—from "Make the Day Fun" email

24
Chemo Chemo Chemo

March, April. May. The first three months of chemo passed in a blur you may recognize. It's good that chemotherapy has progressed to outpatient treatment with more tolerable drugs since 1999. For us, it was five days in the hospital every four weeks—Procarbazine, Cisplatin, Etoposide (VP16), Carmustine (BCNU). Chemotherapy was much more than the drugs. Chemo was a collage of moments:

Walking past handmade posters of encouragement in the lobby of Swedish Hospital for the kids, now inpatients, injured in the shootings at Columbine High School. Running into a guilty-looking friend in the elevator, caught visiting our friend who birthed her baby girl at Swedish. Becoming a reluctant nurse at home, sleeping on the family room floor by Scott on the futon, keeping track of his fluids in and out, managing the IV and flushing Scott's new mediport below the skin and his collarbone. Coaching him through vomiting. Neighbors wrestling our spring crop of bindweed, picking up mail, changing our kitty litter. Friends from FEMALE Care Committee bringing meals, arranging play dates for Wil. Driving back and forth across town to doctor appointments for blood-counts and tests to monitor how Scott's bone marrow, kidneys, liver, and lungs were reacting. Constant vigilance in protecting Scott's skin from sunburn due to his photodynamic therapy. Laughing, appalled, when Scott flipped off a kid pointing at him from a car in the next lane, the kid curious about Scott's Invisible Man disguise under hat, scarf, gloves, and sunglasses. Unraveling Scott's medication schedules for Kytril, Dilantin, Phenobarbitol, Decadron, Coumadin, Benedryl, Senokote, Percoset, Pepsid, Ambien, K-Phos.

It's amazing I remembered to take my own daily Synthroid, much less trim my nails or Wil's. But we managed.

No matter what happens, somebody will
find a way to take it too seriously.
—Dave Barry

25

Money Matters

Few things upset my inner Pollyanna, but insurance coverage is one of them. My inner Pollyanna is skilled at the Glad Game, saying "I'm glad Scott's company has such good health insurance." And "I'm so glad Scott's sister works for an insurance broker so she can help us fight for costs that should be covered (like with the assistant surgeon from the first surgery)." And "Wow, I'm glad we're getting a hefty tax refund this year" And "Whew, I'm glad Scott's short-term disability policy from his company is paying 100% of his salary for six months." And "I'm glad, awed, and humbled by friends sending us money. How generous!"

Pollyanna and I freaked out, however, when the phone rang one afternoon with bad news. Scott was at the hospital having chemo, kept company by his mom, Wil was at preschool, and I was in my office paying bills, cringing over copays, while Pollyanna wearily reminded me to be glad we didn't have to pay the full amount. *Brrinngg.*

"Hello? Oh, hi, Barb," I answered the phone on a first name basis with the Human Resource woman from the small company where Scott worked. She had called many times in the months since Scott's diagnosis to clarify policies. My inner executive always took a memo in my spiral notebook to keep track of our insurance matters.

"Shelly, I finally have the details about Scott's long-term disability policy for you," Barb said. I poised my pen with optimism. "Scott's short-term disability policy has been paying 100 percent for six months, so that is over at the end of April. You know that, right? Okay, so our long-term disability policy will kick in for the next six months at 60 percent."

"Six months?" I asked. "That's your long-term?"

"Yes, six months."

Steel in her voice masked an apology. This was business.

"Then what?" I asked.

"By then Scott should be eligible for Social Security Disability. Have you applied for that yet?"

"No, I didn't know we'd need to."

"Yes, you'll need to. The company will continue to pay Scott's health insurance premiums during that time. He'll be on COBRA officially, which is the law that guarantees employees can continue with their same health insurance policy after leaving a company if they pay their own premiums plus the amount that the company usually pays. But for you guys, in your situation, we've decided to pay the full amount for your family for six months, then we'll continue to cover Scott's portion. COBRA is good for a total of 18 months. At some point, you might want to buy private insurance for you and Wil. If Scott can come back to work, it will all go back to the way it was before."

As if life could go back to the way it was *before*. I didn't know what else to say so I uttered a polite thanks and goodbye. I was stunned. This wasn't what I expected. But then again, I hadn't admitted that Scott might never return to work. I could barely foresee three months of future, much less 18. What would we do if Scott couldn't go back to work? Instead of dawning slowly, it hit me on the head. *Oh shit, that means I will have to go back to work. Oh shit. SHIT!*

Do you know the scene in the claymation movie *Chicken Run* where brave Ginger begs the hens not to panic? And so they panic? Braaaaakkkk!!!! That's how I felt, all aflutter. Cussing, hands patting chest, I paced from my office to the kitchen to the living room, going in a circle. I had to tell someone! Out the front window I saw Diane and Kathy standing in Diane's driveway. I bee-lined out the front door and burst into tears.

My two girlfriends saw me coming and offered open arms as I crossed the lawn crying. I'm sure they thought Scott had just died.

"Oh, honey, what's wrong?" Diane said.

"I just got really bad news," I shrilled in a hyperventilating sob. "We don't have long-term disability insurance after all. Scott's company just called and said it will run out in six months. If I have to go back to work, how will I take care of Wil and Scott? I have to figure out how to apply for Social Security, but it won't be enough. Oh God, this sucks."

Diane and Kathy both patted my shoulder in sympathy, and didn't roll their eyes or say *It's only money*. Their inner Pollyannas (we were a cul-de-sac of raving optimists) tried calming mine, telling us it would be okay. I hoped it was true and decided to believe it, at least for that moment, be-

cause it was time for all of us to go pick up our kids from school. My inner
Scarlet told Pollyanna to stop sniveling and get in the car—we'd think about
it tomorrow.

The next morning at the hospital, I broke the news to Scott as he lay tan-
gled up in IVs. He was too drunk with chemo to care. It wasn't his job to
worry about finances anymore. His job was battling the brain tumor. Perhaps the sober part of him wondered if he'd survive his treatment to even
need long-term disability. I had to figure this out on my own. The very
thought was enough to set off the hens in my head again, so I took a walk to
the elevator lobby where I could look out the window and glimpse the
mountains. I rounded the corner into the lobby and ran into our neuropsychologist who was on his way to see Scott. At the sight of his friendly face, I
burst into tears.

He ushered me into a chair, providing a free instant session of safe space.
Scott and I visited this neuropsychologist almost weekly since January, talking about our emotional ups and downs, on top of trying to decipher what
was emotional versus a brain thing for Scott. He knew me as well as he
knew Scott, and since we'd even discussed "sex during cancer" I figured the
intimacy of money was a valid topic, too.

"I don't know how I'm going to wake up every day and not think about
this," I concluded.

"I know you feel like that today," he said, and paused when the elevator
doors opened. As if on cue, out walked the team social worker (the woman
who gave me her own pager batteries on the day of Scott's second surgery).
The neuropsychologist left me with her and went off to see Scott. The social
worker took the chair next to me, and I retold my story.

"So you haven't applied for Social Security yet?" she asked and
acknowledged the shake of my head. "I can help you with that. You get the
ball rolling by calling Social Security and telling them you wish to start the
application process. They'll send you forms, which I can review for you. I
can make sure the dates of every hospital visit are correct. Then you'll have
a phone interview, followed by an in-person interview with the local Social
Security office."

I nodded, wishing for my spiral notebook in which to write down the
process. She continued sketching out hope, adding a background of rational
facts.

"The good thing about Scott's diagnosis, with his tumor recurring at a
higher grade after radiation, and the new pathology report from the second

surgery, is that grade-three astrocytomas are on Social Security's list of approved diseases. He should have no problem being approved to receive disability payments. Has Scott worked at all since his diagnosis? No? Then that makes it even better. You have to be out of work for a solid six months before you can apply."

"No, he never went back to work from the day he was diagnosed. It will be six months at the end of this month," I said, sniffing, and hopeful again. I knew I had a lot to figure out, but at least I'd have help. I thought maybe I could breathe a bit better now.

The second half of the long-term disability equation was pure luck. Twelve months earlier, Scott and I sat in the office of our financial planner, a savvy young man, and talked of our dreams for the future.

"Sooner than later I'd like to start my own consulting firm," Scott said. "I want to start out small, doing Oracle consulting and programming like I've been doing for years. There's a big market for Oracle database work. Eventually, I'd grow, hiring a team of employees."

"If you do that," Eric advised, "You'll want to purchase disability insurance now. If you're already in business for yourself, there's a two-year wait period before the insurance kicks in. They need to know you're healthy before you buy it. You have to prove yourself. But if you buy it while you're employed by someone else, it would kick in right away if you needed it."

"I can't see why I'd need disability insurance, why I should fork out that money now," Scott said, full of immortal arrogance. "I sit at a computer. I could work even if I were paralyzed."

"Geez, you don't get to choose what kind of disability you have," I said, exasperated, exchanging a look with Eric as if to say *What ego my husband has!*

Eric spoke to Scott diplomatically, "Well, even so, I think it would be a good addition to your portfolio, just as a safeguard. You wouldn't have to buy a large policy—you could always increase it later."

"Yeah, okay," Scott agreed, still confident his consulting career could survive any physical crisis, and secure that his plentiful salary allowed for a small disability-insurance premium. "I guess disability insurance is a necessary evil. You don't want it til you need it."

The absolute irony of Scott's attitude sticks its tongue out in a raspberry now. Scott couldn't know his career would be shot down with a precision strike to his brain. It was a total God thing that we decided to purchase a private policy at that time, finding we'd need it only nine months later. (If I had to do it again, I might have purchased a disability policy of my own. For some reason, we didn't think it necessary.)

In January I filled out the paperwork to receive Scott's private disability. Eric warned us that the company would investigate the application since it had been under a year since we purchased it. Sure enough, an investigator phoned to summon medical records to prove that Scott was not having brain tumor symptoms last spring. Nope, no symptoms until a month before his diagnosis, I told the investigators, and Scott's records concurred.

Those disability checks began arriving about the same time as the rest of this panic. Pollyanna and I couldn't decide whether to be glad that the checks were coming at all, or upset that the amount was only for eighteen percent of Scott's latest salary, not sixty percent like we'd been planning (having not read the fine print). "Well, it's better than nothing," Pollyanna said, and I had to agree.

In mid-May we made it through the interview at the dingy plastic and linoleum Social Security office where we were learned that Scott did qualify. Not only that, but as a dependent child, Wil would also receive a monthly payment until he turned 18 or graduated from high school. That unexpected bonus was topped off when we learned that disability income is tax free (that is, up to a limit we would not reach).

Then I learned at a brain tumor support group that some life insurance policies will waive their annual payment when you're on disability, and sure enough, I confirmed that would be true for Scott. It would save us a bit more money.

I rode the rollercoaster of panic and peace, trying to convince myself that all would be well. One day after one of my Healing Touch sessions, I talked with Janna about my money worries. She was sensitive to the matter, having already discounted her services so that both Scott and I could have as many treatments as needed, and then offering to trade her time for mine if I sewed her some curtains for the window and French doors of her treatment room at the front of her house.

"So we have the private policy plus the Social Security disability, and since that is tax free, it's close to what Scott was earning after taxes. But I'll have to get a job to cover the rest and make sure we have enough money to pay our medical bills and get health insurance. I can't imagine going back to work full time, like a corporate job. If I do that, who will take care of Wil and Scott?"

"You know, you can think about what you want, what would be ideal, and say it out loud," Janna suggested. "Define to the universe what you need and hope for, and say 'this or better.' That's how you can manifest a future for your family. Try it."

My inner executive and I began to ponder the possibilities. What would I be willing to do? How much would I need to work? If I made a budget of fixed expenses, I could see what amount I would need to earn. I could sign up Wil for extended-day kindergarten two days a week, which would give me a few extra hours of flexibility. I could expand from my volunteer website designing for FEMALE into a freelance work-from-home situation.

Pollyanna piped up, "I'm glad you had a good career before you became a mother. You balanced being a working mom until Wil was two. You know how to do this. You have marketable skills with your technical writing and website design. Scott's disability insurance will float the financial family boat. I know you'll find a way to be flexible and creative to make up the difference. You'll be okay. And you don't have to be in a hurry. There is time to work it all out."

As always, my inner Pollyanna made me feel better. I was surprised to realize later in May that I wasn't waking up worried about money as often. My worries didn't disappear, but eventually they felt more manageable. I had a safety net and I had options.

What happens if you get scared half to death twice?
—*Steven Wright*

26
Newsworthy

Scott's successful second surgery at the Colorado Neurological Institute both angered and energized us. Anger arose because it took us months to find CNI and its new Brain Tumor Team after Scott's original diagnosis. To find this team and receive a new lease on life made us wish the same for other brain tumor patients. What does anyone do with the mixed bag of anger and gratitude? For us, the answer was to become activist advocates, at least for a time.

While Scott focused on getting through chemotherapy, Amie, and I used some of our energy to channel our anger and gratitude into a public awareness campaign, jumping into the broader river of publicity for the first National Brain Tumor Awareness Week and the official opening of the CNI Brain Tumor Program. Amie did most of the work.

Amie called a woman reporter at one of Denver's television stations as one of her first steps. The reporter said "There's nothing newsworthy about Brain Tumor Awareness Week." That only fueled Amie's fire. Ironically, another local network aired a story about awake-brain tumor surgeries the same week, but it didn't feature a Denver hospital and we wondered if anyone knew that the same cutting-edge surgery was available in our city. How could something featured on national news not be newsworthy at home?

I told friends about our advocacy efforts within the email updates about Scott's treatment updates. I pull them out here so you can follow Amie's thread of the story:

I want to mention how proud I am of Scott's sister, Amie, who has made it her mission to mobilize publicity for the upcoming National Brain Tumor Awareness Week, which is May 3-7. Amie has plans to fly to Washington, DC, to participate in a national rally and then meet with senators and representatives to encourage funding for biomedical research, especially brain tumors. Amie has also been contacting the Denver Mayor's office and Colorado governor's office to have them proclaim Brain Tumor Awareness week in Colorado. The mayor's office called her on Friday to assure her that all her letters and emails have been received and they're working on it. Amie also contacted a local newspaper, where a reporter is interested in pursuing the story.

This will coincide nicely with the official "opening" of the Brain Tumor Team at the Colorado Neurological Institute at Swedish hospital. (I've offered to help their public relations person do whatever is necessary to get ready and publicize the Team and the National Awareness Week). We're excited about getting the word out to help other brain tumor patients in Colorado. Amie and I are also going to attend the local brain tumor support group this Wednesday night at the CU Medical Center. That should be interesting. :)

Today we delivered the fluorescent light bulbs to the Brain Tumor service, who will be giving them to the next photodynamic therapy (PDT) patient. She is a single mom with two children and is being discharged from the hospital this week. We're now calling it "Project Light Bulb Pass-Along." Thanks again to everyone who started this generous tradition.

On a funny note, Scott & I treated ourselves to Chinese-food delivery about a week ago and got a kick out of Scott's fortune cookie message: "A handful of patience is worth more than a bushel of brains."

Meanwhile, Amie and I are still trying to track down media options for Brain Tumor Awareness Week. I sent a short story about Scott to the National BTAW coordinator for a booklet containing patient stories from around the country. We'll also give you a heads up to look for articles in the Denver area papers if they materialize.

Everyone's hard work paid off. The *Rocky Mountain News* coordinated with the public relations consultant for the Colorado Neurological Institute to interview two patients who received the photodynamic therapy from the CNI team. Scott would be one of them. The other was Cynthia, who we knew. She was a year ahead of Scott in her survival of a grade-four glioblastoma.

When the reporter, knocked on the door that afternoon in early May, I opened the door to welcome her inside, only to find our copy of the other Denver newspaper on our top porch step.

"Hi, come on in," I said, bending down to pick up *The Denver Post*. "How embarrassing. Guess we better subscribe to the *Rocky Mountain News* now."

The reporter laughed as she entered our house, not at all bothered. Scott shook her hand and we ushered her onto the couch in the front living room where we all sat for the interview. She put a tape recorder on the glass-topped coffee table. "Do you mind if I record our conversation?" she asked.

The interview started off a lot like a doctor's appointment in that we re-told Scott's story of symptoms, first surgery, radiation, tumor doubling. We spoke about finding CNI, going to Houston for second opinions, having the second surgery at CNI. We talked about plans to finish three more of the five rounds of chemo.

Scott half-joked about planning to live long enough to wait for the cure and the question it poses about how to live in the meantime.

"It makes me ask myself, what have I been doing with my life? Now that it may be this short, what would I do differently? I spend a lot of time going through that," he said. "It's turned into a good thing because, I think, if I hadn't had this disease, I might have gone a long time, maybe forever, without asking myself all these questions, and that's kind of a blessing.

"There's this heavy feeling about having cancer, but anybody can cash in today. But you don't think about it like that. You think it's sixty years down the road. It's hard to pull back in and say, 'Oh, forever may be pretty close.' It may be next month and it may be next year and it may be in ten years.

"I used to have a cartoon with a fish in a blender with the plug sitting there. You don't know when the plug is going to go in. That's kind of like what this experience has been like for me. When am I going to get told something that I really don't want to hear?"

Our conversation looped in circles, going back to how we told Wil that his dad had an owie in his head, speculating on all the possible reasons Scott developed a brain tumor, the blessings that came in the form of good insurance to cover the treatment (and how I recently tallied our insurance statements to the tune of $145,700, not counting medication or two sessions so far of chemotherapy).

"Well, that's about all the questions I have," she said. "I interviewed your neurosurgeon and Dr. Arenson earlier today, so I think I have all I need for the article. Just one more question. Do you mind if I have a look at your scar?"

"No, not at all," Scott said, bending his chemo-bald head in her direction.

She stood up and walked the few feet around the couch to Scott, peering down at his head. In her article, she wrote how his scar resembled a large slice of pie.

"It's been really nice talking with you," I said as she was packing her notebook and tape recorder in her shoulder bag. "I guess all those phone calls and emails from Amie finally made a difference."

"Amie?"

"Scott's sister. She's been making phone calls all over town to TV stations and papers and asking the mayor and governor to proclaim Brain Tumor Awareness Week in Denver and the state. I thought that's how you got Scott's name for the interview."

"Oh, you're not going to believe this. I have an email from Amie sitting on my desk at work. She was relentless. I've been meaning to call her and thank her for her perseverance, but then tell her that CNI gave me the name of another patient to interview instead of her brother. And you're her brother? That's priceless."

A few days later, a photographer came to our house. It was an afternoon when Wil was home from preschool so he could be in the family photo as well. Wil chose to wear his Mickey Mouse t-shirt. The photographer spent an hour with us, posing us on the living room couch, on the stairs, and then on the more casual futon in our family room. Steve interviewed us just as if he were writing the story, which I suppose loosened us up and gave him perspective on what poses would most capture the story.

"What has it been like for you?" he asked.

"A rollercoaster," Scott and I said in unison.

"So scream like you're on a rollercoaster ride," Steve suggested, and we threw back our heads screaming and laughing. Later, Steve sent us all the photos he took, and I used that one on my Christmas collage. The one that appeared on the cover of the Spotlight section, Tuesday, May 18, 1999, was of us looking down lovingly at Wil, who was stretched out sideways on our laps. Scott's bald head didn't show his scar from that angle. I noticed the broken window blind in the background, but I'm hoping nobody else did.

The headline read "Beating the Odds" in large print, with a subhead of "Patient optimistic after removal of 99% of brain tumor." Inside with the story were two views of Scott's brain tumor from the original scan in November and the doubled-tumor scan in February. It was eerie to display the MRIs side by side. I wish the post-surgery MRI with the tumor apparently gone had also been printed. Now that I knew what to look for on an MRI, seeing the size of Scott's tumor on those two scans made me grateful to CNI's surgeons all over again.

A lot happened the same day as our photo shoot— the CNI Brain Tumor Team had their Open House, Scott attended the Qualife men's cancer support group, and Amie flew to Washington for Brain Tumor Awareness week. On that day, this was the quote on my calendar:

"If you have knowledge, let others light their candles by it."

Trust, because you are willing to accept the risk,
not because it's safe or certain.
—Stephen C. Paul

27

How Aggressive to Get?
Deciding on High-Dose Chemotherapy
and Stem Cell Rescue

Subj: Update on Scott - 4/15
Date: 4/15/99 7:39:40 PM Mountain Daylight Time

Dear Everyone,

Today is our 3-year anniversary of moving back to Denver from Tennessee, so it seems proper that I write an update about Scott on this day. Scott is now 2 weeks out since his first round of chemo ended, and this is the week when his blood counts were expected to drop. Sure enough, they have, but not drastically. We went to the Dr's office for bloodwork both Monday and today (Thursday) and will return again tomorrow (Friday) morning to see whether the trend is still dropping or his levels have bottomed out. The count the doctor is concerned about this week are the platelets, which enable blood clotting. If Scott's counts are lower tomorrow, then he will get a blood-platelet transfusion. If stable, then we'll just proceed to the next chemo, which is scheduled for Monday, April 26th.

On the morning of April 26th, Scott will have another MRI. The MRI will show whether the tumor has re-grown since Scott's second surgery and first round of chemo. Unlikely we hope, but because it doubled during radiation there's a question about its growth rate now. So, if the tumor has re-grown, then we'd have to switch to a different chemo cocktail. Ideally and hopefully, the tumor won't look that much different from post-surgery. It will be complicated to tell what is tumor re-growth vs. surgical "dead stuff".

We'll cross that bridge in another week. Right now, it's enough to know that Scott has his appetite back and is no longer nauseous. He spent several days this week playing around on the computer (after replacing a hard drive and reinstalling the operating system and software). He said today he's not sure whether to attribute his recovery to Healing Touch or to being able to play one of his favorite computer games. :) Scott's hair - which grew back after surgery - is starting to fall out in chunks from the chemo, so we shaved his head as short at possible last night. Wil was petting our very-hairy black cat and said "Spot's shedding as much as Daddy." Time to get the vacuum out!!!

Wil has gone to the doctor's office with us a couple times already and since it's also a pediatric office, the nurses, doctors and staff are great at making him feel comfortable. He actually looked forward to going today. I think Wil has recovered from the first round of chemo, too.

One thing the doctor mentioned today threw us for a loop. He asked Scott to consider undergoing a "stem cell rescue" in which they would harvest some of Scott's bone marrow (specifically, stem cells which are like the seeds that give rise to bone marrow and your immune system). Then Scott would get an extra, extra high dose of chemo, then get his stem cells back in afterwards to re-grow his bone marrow. Supposedly there are good results with this very aggressive approach for recurrent, high-grade brain tumors in young people, but mainly children. It would mean probably 4-6 weeks of hospitalization after the week of chemo, during which Scott would be in a great deal of pain and be at high risk of infection and other side effects. His bone marrow might never recover and there is a 15% chance of death from the treatment itself, as well as no guarantee of success. It didn't take long for Scott to decide against this treatment, especially since his tumor is not re-growing (that we know of yet) and it's not the higher grade-4 tumor. It seems like way too much to lose for way too little gain.

It was a hard reminder that **technically there is no cure for brain tumors** and that we will always be searching for yet another treatment option in case this chemo doesn't do the job. And also that Scott's situation can change at any time. AND that **we have to trust our guts and our God** in deciding how much treatment is enough, not second-guessing our decisions, and moving forward with LIVING at the highest possible quality every day we can.

We ARE confident in continuing with the current chemotherapy regimen and pray that Scott's bone marrow can survive despite the toxicity of it all—hoping he can make it through 5 treatments without severe side effects. If we can continue on this track, his last chemo will be the week of July 19th, and ideally give him 6 weeks to recover so we can go on a family vacation in September (Wil is on year-round school, off in Sept.). That's our goal for now.

On the bright side, literally, is that Scott is nearing the end of his photodynamic therapy limitations. We drove to the mountains on Sunday for Beau Jo's pizza; Scott has been venturing out in the morning to grab the newspaper from the driveway; and he doesn't have to wear the Lawrence of Arabia with Gloves gear as stringently. That may change again when he's completely bald. :) So, we're on the lookout for the next PDT patient to donate the light bulbs to and looking forward to getting outside in the sunshine (it snowed today!).

So, that's what's happening with us. Hope all is well with all of you. Thanks for keeping us in your thoughts and prayers. Keep in touch and let us know what's happening in YOUR lives!

Love,
Shelly & Scott & Wil Vickroy

As I drove us home from Dr. Arenson's office that morning, Scott was fuming about the proposal for the stem cell rescue. "There's a fifteen percent chance I would die just from the treatment alone!" he said, shaking the protocol paper at me, "Why would I put myself through that kind of risk when my MRIs are all clear now, and I'm already having this chemo that is more aggressive than even the docs at M.D. Anderson suggested? When is enough enough?"

"I know," I agreed, "It seems way too aggressive. But do you want to look into it, just a little bit? I can send out emails to the Brain Tumor loop and find out if anyone out there has done it."

"Yeah, you can if you want," he conceded, though added, "But I just don't want to do it. It's too much."

We didn't speak the rest of the drive home. Mom was waiting for us, having watched Wil during our appointment.

Scott went upstairs to our bedroom to rest. Mom and I went to the backyard where we sat in the sun while Wil played on his swing set. The springtime grass was still brown, but the sun strong and warm for an April day. Mom sat on the bottom step below the deck. I sat on the grass a few feet away.

"I don't know what to think about this high-dose chemo," I told Mom. "We keep thinking we've already made the final decision about Scott's treatment. We think we've taken the last step, this and no further. But then the doctors come at us again with one more idea, one more drastic step that might make the difference in his long-term survival. The high-dose chemo sounds so scary, but what if it can save Scott's life? How can we know? How did you know?"

By the time she underwent surgery for stage-four ovarian cancer, the cancer had spread. "I didn't have a choice," my mom said, "It was that chemo or die. Dr. MacMahon told me, 'You can try this, or you will be dead in six months.' It wasn't an exaggeration, it was true."

"So you didn't think twice about it?" I asked.

"It was my only hope."

Six months of chemo—including Adriamycin and Cisplatin and other drugs, too—eight rounds in all, my mother's cancer was gone. It was January 1987, the same month I met Scott on my 22nd birthday.

"Just don't say no, absolutely, without giving it some more thought," Mom advised. "Do your research."

Wil ran across the lawn to give me an early-spring dandelion and a kiss. Diverted, Mom and I laughed and went up the steps, inside for lunch. Scott joined us, but with Wil there, we just enjoyed eating and didn't discuss the doctor's proposal any further. Mom drove Wil to preschool on her way home, Scott went back to bed, and I went to my office to seek the experience of other brain tumor patients.

The national BRAINTMR email discussion loop had become one of our greatest research tools. Hosted through Al Musella's VirtualTrials.org, the listserv connected more than 1,000 subscribers, patients, caregivers, and doctors, too, though I never recall a doctor responding to a message. Newly diagnosed patients sought treatment ideas and doctor recommendations based on specific tumor types or geographical location around the United States, even the world. As with any listserv, the "regulars" sent the most messages while most of us only observed. Most messages were from parents or spouses in crisis mode, writing about the upcoming surgeries, difficult treatment side effects, discouraging MRI results, nearing the end. Many parents or spouses stayed online for months after losing their loved one, to encourage and advise the rest of us—and perhaps to stay connected to the only people in the world who really understood what they had experienced.

The BRAINTMR list often contained more bad news than good, more requests for prayers and advice than success stories (which is simply the nature of brain tumors and support groups)—but still, it was the most specific support available. After Scott's successful second surgery with a 99.9% resection, combined with the photodynamic therapy, I sent a "success" email and had a few replies, people wanting to know more about PDT. Otherwise, I didn't participate much, and I tried never to read my daily digest before bedtime because it gave me bad dreams.

In the five days after Dr. Arenson's proposal and my plea for feedback on the BRAINTMR list, I received six different replies with varying opinions. Two people referred to recent study results concluding that high-dose chemo and stem cell rescue showed no greater effectiveness against breast cancer than chemo alone.

This reply came from Leslie, signed 'dau of Mary Kay, 59, dxd gbm 6/98' in the shorthand signature style of the list summarizing diagnosis and treatments.

"Maybe you could ask for copies of the studies showing that this procedure is better with astrocytomas than it turned out to be with breast cancer. If there are no study results, then I guess there must be some other evidence on which your doctors are basing their opinions and maybe they would show you that."

A mother named Renee wrote:

"Although our son was only 3 when he underwent the stem cell transplant, we consider it as a very necessary part of his treatment. He also has a different diagnosis, but nonetheless, a brain tumor patient. I, as a lay person, would recommend that you seriously consider the treatment as an option. It is obvious that your husband's tumor is very aggressive as it has already recurred, as well as been upgraded to a more aggressive tumor type. I don't think that you can take a "wait and see" approach when faced with those types of situations. However, I do know that the decision is a very difficult one to make and I wish you the very best of luck in all of your treatment."

Another mother, Robin, wrote to us about her twelve-year old son, Dash. His name reminds me of the "dash" poem about living your life between the dates of your birth and death, as the 'dash' — the important part.

"You asked for any experiences with stem cell rescue...I just want to say that I have always felt that the high-dose chemo gave Dash the best chance at fighting his tumor and obviously gave him the longest period of time of being free of disease. It was very hard on him and he was hospitalized 24 times, with surgeries, chemo and subsequent infections from low (no) blood counts.

His white count would hit 100 every time and any little infection became life threatening. If it were me making the decision I would do it again in a minute and I know Dash would too as we had talked about this. Each day of life is precious. Dash liked to quote W. Churchill: "Never, Never, Never Give UP"."

Three patients were skeptical, but asked me to forward any additional information that I might receive on my quest. A man named Ross wrote to say he survived with his grade-two astrocytoma for seven years with just surgery and radiation before it came back as a stage-three mixed glioma. He decided to at least have his stem cells harvested at NYU Medical Center and then decide whether or not to pursue the high-dose chemo approach. At that point in April, Ross was having Temodar chemotherapy and was considering the stem cell as a last-ditch effort.

"The idea of cramming one entire year of chemotherapy in one week seemed very appealing, in the fact that I could get it over with quickly. The mortality rate even at 15 percent seemed out of line but I was only 36 and in great physical shape.

"As an insurance policy, I went thru the harvesting technique. I have excellent health insurance, but ran into delays to have the procedure approved. Later realized that the harvesting procedure is quite expensive; it cost over $2000 just for Neupogen injections."

It was a message from "Mnklup" in New York that turned the tide of our decision-making. Mike's wife, Kathy, wrote details that seemed most applicable to Scott's situation:

Hi Shelly and Scott,

I saw your post on the list and had to respond (this is long - so I am responding personally rather that to the list). My husband Mike, 32, is currently undergoing stem cell rescue.

Our history: first diagnosis was 2/98 - after grand mal seizure - had surgery – his tumor was called low grade mixed glioma - located in right frontal lobe, recurrence 9/98 2nd surgery - diagnosis anaplastic mixed glioma, radiation 10/98 1st chemo was Carboplatin 12/98 more regrowth on Jan. MRI to left frontal lobe, so then 1/99 he had Etoposide (that's also called VP16) and Cytoxan, good MRI in Feb!! We had been planning to do high dose chemo w/stem cell rescue since 12/98 with our neuro-onc. The doctor at NYU advised us to continue w/ the plan. In late Feb 99 Mike had stem cells harvested then in early March, 3 days of high-dose chemo - Carboplatin and Thiotepa, then after a 3 day waiting period - his stem cells were infused back in. Then he was in the hospital for 10 days after in a specially filtered room closed off from the rest of the hosp. to protect him from germs (family members were allowed to visit).

We are now at 7 weeks after his first dose of high dose chemo - the protocol here calls for a 2nd round - so tomorrow - Friday he gets the same high dose chemo - same 3 day wait - then the rest of his already saved stems cells are given back to him, and another 10 days in the hospital. Mike has had 3 good MRIs since Feb, and we feel great about our doctor's advice to do stem cell!!!!! His tumor is now mostly necrotic!! With only a little spot of tumor left - which we are hoping to kill with this round of chemo. He has had no new growth since January - and we feel very lucky.

It is not an easy road. Mike felt really lousy in the hospital last time - extreme fatigue - but it does get easier!!! He now feels great - has good energy level and can eat anything he wants to!! So - we know he will feel lousy again for another few weeks, but we also know that he can and will recover.

We chose this because Mike's tumor was coming back again in December and it was growing fast - by January it had spread to the left frontal lobe and was inoperable - so we had to do something drastic. Our Dr. advised us that high-dose chemo with stem cell rescue could offer a long term remission and a "possible" cure - but it is a new treatment. They have been doing this for about 2 1/2 years and have never lost a patient as a result of giving them the high-dose chemo (mortality rate from treatment is zero) He also told us about the 15% mortality rate nationwide for this treatment - (this is based on mortality just from giving patients the drugs) and you must remember that this includes elderly patients that don't do as well or some patients that are trying it as an extreme last resort. He said that people under 40 who are in basically good health (besides the brain tumor of course) do better. About 2/3 of our doctor's patients are doing well with this treatment.

Anyway, I hope I haven't overloaded you with information - but if you have any questions whatsoever regarding this treatment or stem cell harvest - please email us. Best of luck to you!

—Kathy Luparello 29, wife of Mike 32

When I read Kathy's email, I printed it immediately and showed it to Scott. "Hey—you won't believe this one. Here is a guy close to your age who just had his stem cell rescue and is doing great. And guess what? He's doing it twice! His protocol calls for repeating the high-dose chemo and rescue again just seven weeks after the first time. Can you believe it?"

"Hmmm," Scott said, not as excited as me. "I wonder what it was like—the side effects."

I wrote Kathy back and asked her for the gory details. How was it, really, to recover from the procedure. What did Mike go through physically? She told me of skin falling off, mucositis, days on morphine. Then she reminded me of his recovery, "It happens fast, once the stem cells start re-growing. When the white cell counts start to rise, you start to feel better sooner than you'd expect."

If Mike could do it twice, couldn't we do it just once? Between my mother's example, Mike's courage, and Ross's idea to at least the harvest the stem cells, Scott decided it was worth exploring further.

Scott and I had a recurring conversation that we now call our lifeboat theory.

Scott put it this way, "I like the story about the man who is stranded on his rooftop in a flood. He sits on his roof, water rising past the windows below him, and his neighbor rows by in a boat, saying 'Come with me, I'll take you to safety.' But the man replies, 'No thanks, I'm waiting for God to save me.'

"So the rain continues and the water gets higher. Next a Coast Guard speedboat docks at his roofline, commanding 'Get in, now!' but the man says "Don't worry about me; I'm waiting for God to save me.'

"Finally, the man is stranded at the highest point of his roof, clinging to the chimney and a helicopter hovers above him dangling a ladder. 'Grab the ladder!' the rescue worker yells. The man shakes his head and refuses the ladder, yelling back, 'No, I'm waiting for God to save me.'

"Next thing he knows, he's in Heaven talking with God. 'Hey, why didn't you save me?' and God's reply is, 'I tried to save you, three times.' "

That story prompted Scott to keep asking out loud, "Is the stem cell rescue my lifeboat?"

When do you trust that *this* is the lifeboat that will answer your prayers?

Do you refuse the lifeboat because you're afraid? Do you need blind faith to say yes? Do you muster bravado and say "It's a good day to die"? Or "I can die, or I can die trying." Or are those statements empty clichés? When can you agree to a cancer treatment that feels like going all out, no holds barred? Sometimes you need more information before making the leap.

Scott's lifeboat analogy helped us weigh our decisions more than once through the years.

Our decision went forward in baby steps. First we talked with our neuro-oncology team and agreed to go forward with the insurance approval (the doctors said it was feasible to have the high-dose chemotherapy and stem cell only if the insurance agreed to cover it fully). Then Scott had a heart-function test as the final pre-approval step, which told us his body was ready if his mind and spirit could also agree. For about a week, Scott went as far as agreeing to the harvest, to set aside his stem cells *just in case*. We weren't quite ready to swallow our fears of high-dose chemotherapy. Our doctors seemed to understand that we couldn't decide all at once and gave us more time.

At Scott's next chemo appointment, however, we had a long talk that put the treatment into perspective. Dr. Arenson and another doctor, who was the one in charge of the high-dose chemotherapy clinical trial for their pediatric oncology practice, came into Scott's room where he was getting the chemo to prepare his body for the stem cell harvest. This was called the "primer" dose and was a different combination of drugs than the cocktail he received in the hospital. For this round, Scott went to the pediatric office instead of the hospital, which was much easier to handle for all of us. Dr. Arenson broached the subject.

"Up to this point you've agreed to harvest your stem cells and delay having the high-dose chemotherapy. We'd like you to consider having the high-dose chemotherapy this summer. First, it appears that the insurance approval is only good for six months. After that, you will have to undergo the approval process all over again. So there's a "use it or lose it" window of opportunity.

"The other window of opportunity is the amount of tumor we're dealing with, which is very small right now, as you know. You had good success with your recent surgery, and we can be confident that the photodynamic therapy helped remove even more tumor cells. And as of this week, you've had three rounds of aggressive chemotherapy.

"The high-dose chemotherapy will be most effective if it is used against the least possible amount of tumor. To wait until your tumor has re-grown would be asking too much of the chemo. You are in the best position now, after the surgical debulking, to gain the most benefit. As I've mentioned before, when a tumor comes back, it is almost always a higher-grade tumor and therefore more aggressive and more resistant to chemotherapy even at the toxic high doses.

"Plus, your body has withstood the effects of the chemo quite well to this point. If we continued with the four-drug protocol, your body might not be as strong as it needs to be to rebound from the high-dose chemo."

Scott and I looked at each other, nodding, as if we knew it would come down to this. We had spent enough weeks searching our souls that we were close to saying yes.

The other neuro-oncologist (I'll call him Dr. S for stem cell rescue) added his opinion. "We know it is difficult to ask you to undergo one more step of aggressive treatment, especially when your MRI appears to be clear. We'd like to use the high-dose chemotherapy as a 'pre-emptive strike' on your tumor now rather than as a last resort in the future. You have an excellent chance of long-term survival if we use this strategy now.

"I've been using the high-dose chemotherapy and stem cell rescue on several of my pediatric patients with good results," Dr. S continued. "You would have adult company if you do it this summer. Mario has agreed to undergo the stem cell rescue, too. He'll be here in the office today, if you want to meet him."

Mario was the young man who had surgery plus photodynamic therapy the day before Scott, back in March. He was twenty-two years old, a police officer fresh from the academy, and he wanted his career to continue. We knew he was in the hospital at the same time, but we never had a chance to meet face to face.

"So what do you think?" asked Dr. Arenson, looking from Scott's face to mine.

"What you say makes a lot of sense," Scott said and took a deep breath as if preparing to cliff dive. Scott looked to me for my buy-in, or push, and I nodded. "Okay, I will do it."

"Great," Dr. Arenson said, standing up by pushing off his knees with his hands. "I will have the transplant coordinator at PSL call you to arrange a tour of the new transplant unit. She can answer more of your questions about the process. And Shelly, be sure to ask her about the family support they offer. They have a support group for caregivers and child-life specialists, too, in case Wil needs someone to talk to."

Before we left the office that day, Scott met Mario, who was hooked up to his own IV undergoing his primer dose before harvest. They shook hands with a firm grip.

"So I hear we are going to be having our stem cell rescues at the same time," Scott said.

"Is that right? It will be nice to have company."

"Maybe we can skip down the halls together in our hospital gowns," Scott joked.

"You're on," said Mario.

Sometimes a man can only stand so much endurance.
—Our doctor's friend

28
Side Effects

It was supposed to be an easy week between Scott's "primer dose" and his stem cell harvest. We knew the next Monday that he'd be going to a different hospital where a cardiac surgeon would insert the new Neostar port in Scott's chest to accommodate the complicated needs of his stem cell rescue. So this week was all about resting, relaxing, and recuperating.

I was sitting at my kitchen table about four o'clock on Wednesday afternoon, luxuriously talking to Julie in person, while our boys played together upstairs in Wil's room. It was our first normal stay-at-home-mom playdate in more than six months, since the day I took her to her first chemo appointment (and that doesn't count). We weren't even talking about her cancer or Scott's, just mom stuff. She'd only been there half an hour when Scott walked into the kitchen, pulling a digital thermometer out of his mouth.

"We need to go to the hospital now," he said. My brain could not interpret what he was saying. Hospitals were not on my To Do list that week.

"What are you talking about?" I replied, looking at Julie with apology for the interruption and a touch of embarrassment, as if Scott were delusional.

"My temperature hit 100. I've been watching it all day."

And I thought he'd been watching TV. I tried to talk him down, selfish about my time with Julie.

"Do you really think we need to go to the hospital right away?" I asked. "Let's call Dr. Arenson first."

"I already did. Talked to the nurse. She said to go ahead to the emergency room since it's so late in the day. Remember, they said I would be susceptible to infection with this round of chemo. I think that's what's happening." He handed me the thermometer still displaying 100, offering proof.

I didn't want to believe him, and yet I knew it was true and not to ignore, not with Scott's immune system plummeting. The idea with his recent dose of chemo was that it would knock down his bone marrow quickly, to zero, but then rebound quickly, too—in theory. The stem cell harvest would take place on the upswing, those days when his bone marrow was rebounding. But first, his system had to crash. Apparently, today was the day, though it seemed a week early.

Julie understood. She'd been going through cancer a month longer than Scott and knew all about side effects, emergencies, and paying attention to signals like fevers. "I'll go get Cameron. Do you want Wil to come home with me? He can stay as long as you need him to. Will you be home in a few hours?"

"I don't know. I'll call my next-door neighbor, in case we get home late. It would probably be easier."

My pleasant afternoon with Julie was over. It was like sitting down to birthday cake and having it pulled away before the first bite. Is that how firefighters feel when the alarm goes off just before dinner? I was back in fire fighting mode, a caregiver on call, resigned to the odd hours of my job.

As Julie went home, Scott went to sit in the car, and I took Wil next door. My neighbor Kathy never said no. (I can't say enough about the grace and good luck of having nice neighbors). I drove against the flow of rush-hour traffic, everyone else going home while we headed north up Broadway to Swedish.

"I can't even think where the emergency room entrance is," I said to Scott as we neared the hospital.

"I can't believe we've gone this many months without needing the emergency room," he said, thermometer between his lips yet again.

I felt like a stranger in the ER, among staff we didn't know who didn't know us. It was odd to sit behind a triage curtain, repeating our brain tumor story and our chemo concerns. I felt impatient and annoyed at the process, at what seemed like questions of curiosity more than diagnosis. The ER nurse took Scott's temperature with an ear thermometer, popped it back out on the near-instant beep and pronounced, "Normal. You said you had a fever at home?"

"You barely had it in his ear long enough to register a temperature," I blurted out. "Scott's been monitoring his temperature all afternoon, he has seen it rising. It was 100. I saw it myself."

She looked skeptical, condescending—well, that's how I took her look. I hadn't relinquished my Julie-afternoon and driven through rush hour on a hypochondriac lark, I wanted her to know. Then the doctor arrived—a tall, athletic fit-to-be-on-TV-doctor—and took over the interview. I stopped being surly. He determined a blood draw was in order, then asked us to hang out and await the results.

Scott lay back on the narrow exam table and slept, feeling worse. It was a long wait, through the dinner hour without any food. Over-optimistic as ever, I thought it would be a short wait, so I decided against the hospital cafeteria which was too far away. Instead I brought out two packs of peanut butter crackers from my backpack, always stocked with our spiral notebook and snacks.

Hours later the doctor returned, holding Scott's chart. "Turns out that Scott does have an infection, but we can't say exactly what. I've sent his samples off for further analysis. We're going to admit you upstairs—we'll start you on antibiotics. We'd like to keep an eye on you."

"Great," Scott said, sarcastic, bitter, and relieved all at once. "What floor will I be on?"

"Back to the ninth floor, same as where you have chemo. I'll check in on you later."

A nurse ushered Scott into a wheelchair, arranged the IV pole for walking, while I shouldered the backpack. *Here we go again,* I was thinking. *Wonder what time I will get home tonight?*

I have to admit, I wasn't in the mood that night for more cancer, more hospitals, unknown side effects. I was tired. My blood sugar had crashed, as had I. I needed to call Kathy and tell her I'd be at the hospital even longer, ask if Wil could spend the night. On top of it all, I was worried for Scott.

Scott finally got settled at the far end of Ninth Floor, as far from the nurse station as could be. Coming to the hospital for something other than chemo meant he would not be the honored guest. How we had been spoiled. It didn't matter. I could feel myself settling into my hospital-caregiver role as Scott's wife, medical advocate, and absentee mom. I knew how to do this.

Once Scott was settled, I went home and dropped into bed. It was almost midnight by then.

I sent an email update the morning after Scott was admitted to the hospital, in the habit after all these months of sharing our news, good and bad. Later that night I sent another when I realized he wouldn't be coming home anytime soon.

Subj: Update on Scott 6/3 p.m.
Date: 6/3/99 9:42:07 PM Mountain Daylight Time
Hi again,

Scott is still in the hospital and may be for several more days. They have found a bacterial infection is causing the fever, but have not quite pinpointed where. It's likely the mediport in his chest (where chemo goes in and blood samples come out). And it's likely that it's Scott's own bacteria (we all have it) that he is now susceptible to since his white counts are so low. Scott has received 4 bags of new blood and several antibiotics, all of which should improve his counts in the next day or so. (Some of you have asked if you could make blood donations in Scott's name—unfortunately it wouldn't help us directly, but it's always nice for the blood banks.) Other than very tired and weak, Scott wasn't running a fever today or in pain. He just slept and snored—made for a very boring day for me. :)

The doctors say to "THINK WHITE BLOOD CELLS!" That's what Scott needs now to help his immunity and resistance to infection. I don't know yet how this affects the schedule for next week's stem cell harvest, but I hope it can still occur.

Over the next few weeks, Scott could REALLY use all the encouragement he can get from all of you...telling him that he can endure the high-dose chemo and stem cell rescue and successfully, finally, get rid of his brain tumor. I worry that he is running out of steam. If you could send him some letters of hope and encouragement, or even some good jokes, photos, stories about YOUR relatively normal lives, that would help immeasurably! I think he needs reminding that he is not alone in this fight.

Thanks a million!!
Love,
Shelly

Scott's infection, a form of e-coli as it turned out, had nasty side effects like vomiting, diarrhea, fever, and chills. On top of that, Scott had to endure nurses prodding and pricking every hour or more, then clattering food service, then lab technicians taking more blood. Scott hadn't slept all night due to the noise and discomfort. It was worse than his chemo week, maybe because it was so unexpected. He wasn't mentally prepared. His body was worn out, ravaged by chemo, with this infection to boot.

Scott's agony went on for days and still he wasn't improving. I started to worry that his infection would prevent him from getting his new mediport on Monday. What if he wasn't well enough for that minor surgery, which perhaps wasn't so minor for poking a plastic tube near his heart, plus the unexpected additional procedure to remove the infected port? Would we have to endure another round of the priming dose and risk yet another round of side effects?

I asked Dr. Arenson these questions on Saturday as he came to do rounds. He assured us that Scott would be better by Monday, that the harvest had to go on, that it could and it would.

Saturday afternoon I was still skeptical. Scott was exhausted to the point of tears. Scott's blood counts were just barely starting to recover, despite six transfusions plus two bags of platelets to help his red blood cells and blood clotting ability. His white blood cells, which fight infection, remained very low—as expected due to the chemotherapy he had. All that, plus the noise of the hospital, was taking its toll.

"I don't know how much longer I can keep this up," Scott said, his voice catching as sobs threatened to erupt. "I just want to go home, but I can't."

I don't know how the universe does this, but it happened more than once. The door opened and relief entered, in the form of Scott's neuropsychologist. He was doing rounds for his other patients and decided to stop in for hello.

"Hi guys, how are you doing?" he asked with his hand still on the door knob, his bright smile turning solemn as soon as he saw Scott's strained face. "What's going on?"

"This infection is kicking Scott's butt. He's exhausted and hasn't slept in days. It's too noisy."

Scott nodded, too tired to speak, not trusting his voice. His shrug said enough.

"I'll be right back," the doctor said.

Minutes later, he returned with a blank piece of paper, Scotch tape, and a thick black pen. He started to write as he told us his plan. "I've checked with the nurses," he said, "And we agreed it's okay to put up a note. It's going to say 'Do not disturb. Entry must be approved at nurse station.' That will at least keep the lab technicians and other interruptions out of here so you can sleep for awhile. The nurses said they will coordinate checking on you and minimize the other interruptions. Now that you're doing better with the infection, they shouldn't need to come in here as often. Let's see how you feel after you get some real rest."

"You know, we've been calling this whole chemo thing an endurance test," I said, "But I don't know how much more Scott can stand."

"I know what you mean. You know, an old friend of mine once said, 'Sometimes a man can only stand so much endurance,'" he said, taping the note on the door. "I hope this note will help."

It did. Plus I put my chair outside the door and sat there on guard while Scott crawled into bed in his darkened room, bolstered by the permission slip taped to the door. I waited two hours before going back in. Scott was still sleeping soundly, and so I went home.

As an aside, we had a bright spot of good news from the Brain Tumor Team's social worker. When I saw her in the hall, she told me that the *Rocky Mountain News* article about Scott was so well-read that she fielded twelve to fifteen phone calls a day for the first week, with more calls after that, from people not only in Colorado but around the country who had received the article from friends and family. More specifically, she said that one brain tumor patient would be coming to Denver from Colorado Springs to have surgery with the photodynamic therapy. The treatment was a perfect fit for his type of tumor, and the newspaper article was published at the perfect time for a decision. That good news perked us up.

Sleep finally seemed to help Scott turn the corner toward recovery. By Sunday afternoon, signs of his infection had improved enough that the doctors agreed he was good to go for his port-replacement surgery on Monday morning and his stem cell harvest later that week.

Scott was scheduled to show up at the other hospital for his outpatient surgery at six in the morning. Scott's dad and I arrived at Swedish at 5 a.m. to oversee his discharge and transport him to Presbyterian/St. Luke's (Denverites refer to it simply as PSL). It was surreal and lonely to be transferring Scott like this, so early that both hospitals and the whole city seemed still asleep.

Leaving Swedish that morning felt like a turning point. The hospital had become so familiar and safe, a place of successful surgeries, nurses and doctors who knew us and went out of their way in their caring. Even this week of infection, now abated, had turned out okay. To have come through this infection brought us one step closer to the high-dose chemo and stem cell rescue, all of which would take place at PSL, where I was out of my comfort zone. Trepidation was my word for the day.

It was a short drive to PSL. We checked in, swapping Scott's clothes for yet another hospital gown, and put his other clothes in a locker as if he were just having an MRI. Then I said so-long to Scott as he underwent his no-big-deal, not-brain-surgery surgery. The waiting room felt claustrophobic to me, so I wandered to the hospital lobby where I thought I could breathe.

When I found the lobby, the sun had started lighting the day, but still no one else was around. I sat by myself on a couch, looking out a tall wall of windows. Outside was early-summertime green of trees, a freshly mown lawn. It was only 7:30 and the lobby was empty, except for me.

I sat there alone with my thoughts, which veered past exhaustion, through worry, arriving at fear about Scott's upcoming treatment. I reviewed the risks in my head, the fifteen percent chance of death from the toxic high-dose of chemotherapy drugs. Then there was the slim chance his stem cells wouldn't engraft to re-grow his bone marrow. I thought again of the recent study results in the news reporting that women with breast cancer who underwent high-dose chemotherapy with a stem cell rescue did *not* increase their chance of long-term survival. I reflected on Scott's latest MRI and how the tumor already seemed to be gone. I asked myself, *What are we doing putting Scott though this when he's already gone through so much already? He could barely endure this week of infection, and that was nothing compared to what he'll be going through soon.*

An exhausted morning is not the best time to second guess the decisions that your wide awake, clear thinking, well researched stronger selves have already concluded. The universe intervened once again, right on cue. Have you noticed how hope arrives just when you need it?

The door to the outside May morning opened, and a woman in a sundress and cardigan walked beeline across the dark marble floor, sitting down next to me. She was tall and thin with fine brown hair, her blue eyes were kind. It was as if someone had sent her to find me. She asked why I was waiting here so early in the morning, and I told her Scott's story, condensed.

"I had breast cancer five years ago," she said. "My final treatment was high-dose chemotherapy and a stem cell rescue. Your husband is making the right choice. He will be fine." She patted my leg, stood up, and left.

Her words and her timing were perfect. I love synchronicity—and waiting-room angels. I tucked her reassurance into my soul-purse in case I'd need it again. It wasn't that I believed she knew without doubt that Scott would be fine, but because *she* was fine, five years later, her presence gave me hope. As I sat there alone, and the hospital came awake for the day, I too felt more awake. Our harvest week had begun. I decided to believe we could do it.

No ray of sunshine is ever lost, but the green
which it awakens into existence needs time to sprout,
and it is not always granted to the sower to see the harvest.
All work that is worth anything is done in faith.
—Albert Schweitzer

29

Harvest Week

What began as a grueling week turned out better than we ever expected. The emails I sent during the week of Scott's stem cell harvest say it all. I could not give you any more details from that week, except to say we took a camera with us to the Apheresis department to photograph the process. Scott wore a red bandana, black sweatpants, and a blue denim shirt that could be unbuttoned for easy access to his new Neostar mediport. After six weeks of being light-sensitive due to his photodynamic therapy, Scott had inadvertently developed a nice tan that, despite his bald head, gave him a quasi-healthy glow. As the week progressed, he recovered from his infection and started looking pretty cute for a guy fighting cancer.

The technical explanation, as concise as can be, is that the stem cell harvest happens over several sessions through a process called apheresis: taking blood out in a continuous loop about two cups at a time, spinning off the stem cells with centrifugal force, and putting the rest of the blood back in. If you've ever donated platelets, it's nearly the same. Each subsequent day, as more stem cells appear, more are harvested. Stem cells are the seeds of the bone marrow: basically, white blood cells, red blood cells, and platelets. The goal is to harvest a critical level of stem cells to use later for replacing Scott's bone marrow after the high-dose chemo destroyed it.

A stem cell harvest is like picking sour cherries from the last Montmorency tree in your world. It's tricky because you can only pick the ripe cherries, and must wait for more to ripen in the afternoon sun so you can pick those the next morning. Each day's batch of cherries must be washed, sorted, pitted, measured, and zipped into a plastic bag with Fruit Fresh and sugar for preserving the color and flavor, then labeled and stashed in the freezer. Finally, by the end of the week, you have picked all the cherries that tree has to offer, and you hope there's enough for your pie. Then you burn down the cherry tree, the last in your world. And you wait with crossed fingers until pie-making day.

You might be asking, with your hand snaking up in the air, "But, uhm, how are you going to replace that cherry tree?" Here's the hard secret. You savor the pie, every last bite, and then you take all the pits, and go plant an orchard.

Aside from that secret, I don't know whether to attribute our successful stem cell harvest week to Scott's fortitude, good luck, or the power of prayers. Or is modern medicine simply that miraculous?

Subject: Another Scott update 6/8/99
Date: 6/8/99 1:19:14 PM Mountain Daylight Time

Dear Everyone,

Scott had surgery on Monday morning to remove the infected mediport from the right side of his chest and then the surgeon installed a new, larger port on the left side. That port entered his chest by his collar bone, tunneled through a large vein, and then exits in the center of his chest through a tube about the size of a large McDonald's drinking straw, with three other tubes dangling from that. Thank goodness for lightweight plastic! The other procedure he had was a bone marrow biopsy, with two "plugs" taken out of his hip bones at the back on either side of his spine. As you can imagine (and I imagine many of you cringing already), he is in a lot of pain from these 5 wounds -- he says they seem like gunshot wounds. Scott is taking pain medication and has various ice packs around his body (even a bag of frozen lima beans) that are taking the edge off of his pain.

Scott's white cell count is still effectively ZERO, so the stem cell harvest has not yet begun. We will continue going to the hospital every morning at 7 a.m. this week, including Saturday if necessary, to have his blood counts taken. At the hospital they also give him another dose of the Neupogen (white-cell stimulating hormone) as well as his IV antibiotics that he needs to finish off the bacterial infection.

Technically, Scott's white cell count has to be at least 1,000 to begin the harvest and it is registering at only 100 today, which might as well be zero (normal range is between 3,900 and 10,600). They hope it will climb to 500 by tomorrow so that harvesting can begin on Thursday, with a count of 1,000 or more. Nobody is betting money on what will really happen, though. (Mario, the other young BT patient, harvested twice as many cells as needed in just one session! He's a tough benchmark.)

SO, this may sound corny but if you can, please help Scott by focusing your thoughts, love, prayers, and energy on those little stem cells, imagining them as millions of bulging flower buds bursting into bloom. By the time they "burst", imagine so many of them that it only takes 1 or 2 days to collect more than enough for his stem cell rescue. Also, to help his pain we can imagine a bubble surrounding Scott, expanding larger and larger away from him, filling it with healing light and love, and allowing the pain to escape from the bubble into the atmosphere.

Thanks for your help and encouragement! It really does make a difference!

Love,
Shelly

p.s. At the hospital this morning the nurses introduced Scott as the celebrity from the newspaper. :)

Subj: Good news for Scott 6/9/99
Date: 6/9/99 6:22:09 PM Mountain Daylight Time

Thank you - thank you - thank you!!! Scott's white cell count leaped from 100 yesterday to 1800 today, amazing the nurses and doctors! You should have seen them all scrambling to get Scott hooked up to the stem cell harvest machine, running around saying "It's a Go!" It was great. I just know that with so many of you focusing on Scott's healing, that it REALLY HELPED! He only has taken 1 pain pill today, first thing this morning. We also thank Carol for an impromptu Healing Touch session this afternoon.

We are heading back to the hospital on Thursday morning, 7 a.m. again, for Day 2 of harvesting. They don't know the amount of stem cells collected today, but regardless, they need at least two separate collections to ensure a backup plan in case anything happened to the first collection bag. It's likely that we'll need at least 2 or 3 more days, but who knows. All bets are off after today's surprise.

Several of you have asked how I'm doing (thanks for asking). I am hanging in there, thanks to much help from our family, neighbors and friends. I am making some time for myself. I've also reminded the doctors that they need to consider the caregiver aspect of our situation when "allowing us the favor" of outpatient chemo and other "homecare" (meaning I get to be nurse on duty all night). Overall, I am feeling stronger than I did last week. :)

I'll write again when the harvesting is complete. Thanks a million for helping us!

Love,
Shelly

Subj: Scott 6/10 - more good news
Date: 6/10/99 1:57:46 PM Mountain Daylight Time

Hi everyone

Just a quick note to say that Scott's white cell count jumped from 1800 yesterday to 5600 today!!!!! Again, it's amazing. He should have been able to harvest a good number today. The goal for harvest is some minimum quantity of "2" and yester-day he got as far as 0.33. Today I'm sure was much more. We're going back again on Friday for hopefully the last time, and then Scott can rest for 4 weeks. Our next MRI is next Friday the 18th, although we won't know the MRI results until the fol-lowing Monday.

While Scott's white counts are skyrocketing, his platelets (for blood clotting) are still dropping, so if you can imagine an increase in those by tomorrow, it couldn't hurt. He's hoping to avoid yet another transfusion.

Talk to you soon
Love,
Shelly

p.s. I've had too many 5 a.m. mornings, so I'm off to a nap. I'll try to answer eve-ryone's emails by this weekend. :)

Subj: Scott on Sunday - harvest done
Date: 6/13/99 9:08:41 PM

Hi everyone

All those thoughts and prayers surely helped Scott's stem cell harvest last week! Thank you sooooo much!! Thanks, I know, to your productive visualizations, Scott's white cell count went from Tuesday thru Friday like this: from 100 --> 1800 --> 5600 --> 15,400!!!! His harvest on Wed-Friday accumulated like this 0.33 --> 1.5 -->> 4.3!!

The doctors called us Friday night to say that Scott had surpassed their goal of "3" (I don't know what this number means) and how happy they were to say Scott was all done with his harvest within 3 days. We didn't have to go back on Saturday after all! I must say I was practically giddy on Saturday to not be at the hospital or worrying about Scott for a change.

Scott did get blood transfusions on Friday -- red cells and platelets, and that is helping him recover. He is still tired and sore, but nothing like the pain earlier in the week. Turns out that much of the pain was related to his bone marrow crank-ing out those stem cells, making his bones really ache. Glad to be done with that!!

So, we don't have to go back to the doctor until Tuesday, then the MRI on Friday, and the results of the MRI next Monday. We are hoping for and planning on a nice relaxing week, sleeping in and avoiding hospitals if at all possible. :)

Thanks again and again for all your support, encouragement, prayers and love.

All our love to you,
Shelly, Scott & Wil

Everybody needs beauty, places to play in and pray in
where nature may heal and cheer and
give strength to the body and soul alike.
—John Muir

30
Mountain Respite

We went to the mountains three times to rest before Scott's final leap of faith in his nine months of brain tumor treatment. Due to doctors' vacations, Scott's high-dose chemotherapy and stem cell rescue was pushed back from mid-June to the second week of July instead. At first we worried about the delay, fearing it gave his tumor extra weeks to grow. We soon re-framed the reprieve as a grace period for his body and soul to gain strength. Now I know how much I needed that respite, too.

Our first mountain getaway was to Julie's cabin near Estes Park over Father's Day weekend, following by a short trip to my Aunt Mary's cabin south of Leadville, and a reluctant drive back to Denver, too soon. Those days in the mountains were like treating yourself to a plate of potato chips, but wanting much more, so—cats fed and watered, Scott's meds and our clothing replenished—we went back to Aunt Mary's cabin again.

One afternoon while Wil played with Aunt Mary, and Dad went trout fishing again, and Scott took a nap, Mom and I snuck off by ourselves. We drove out County Road 22, going east on Weston Pass Road. Weston Pass began as a Ute trail and became a stage coach route carrying as many as 100 westbound gold-seekers a day during the rush of the late 1800's, plus farm-ers and shopkeepers who supported the miners (like caregivers). If you fol-lowed the road east over the top at almost 12,000 feet, you would find your-self in South Park at Fairplay. Going home took hours extra that way, so we hardly ever did, except a few autumns when the aspen glowed gold.

That day Mom and I drove halfway up Weston Pass to a wide spot where the road levels out before it gets steeper and the snowmelt creek runs shallow. It was a good place for our mother-daughter foodless picnic. In June the creek sparkles crystal clear cold at just above freezing. Our bare feet became bright red the instant we stepped in and jumped out. It's always a challenge, a contest, to see who can dip longest in the water. The willow branches always win.

We put on our shoes and socks and sat in the sun. Soon we felt like moving and so hiked further up the road. For awhile we held hands. We stopped and turned around, looking back to see how far we'd come. Across the valley, Colorado's tallest peaks—Mount Elbert and Massive—seemed eye-level with us. I snapped a few pictures of the scenery, wanting a magic photo to step through after I developed the film, the same way Mary Poppins could step through Burt's sidewalk chalk paintings.

We sat down in the middle of the road. Mom put her arm around my shoulder, "How are you, honey?"

I breathed a deep sigh before answering. "Good. I'm getting refreshed. It's so good to be out of town and up here."

"Here, let me take a picture of you," she said, scooting backwards in the dirt so that she was above me on the road and the photogenic long view was behind me. I grinned for the camera. Then I took a picture of her. There were no good rocks or stumps to act as tripod, so we didn't get a snapshot of us together.

We might have talked more, but I don't remember. My memory didn't keep all the words. Sitting on the warm dirt road, next to her and so close to the sky, my soul felt completely connected to God, Mother Nature, and Mom.

"I wish I could sit here forever," I said, dreading Scott's coming chemo and stem cell rescue, his countless weeks in the bone marrow transplant unit, and the uncertainty of his outcome in the short run and long haul.

Mom handed me a random rock from the road.

"Take this home with you," Mom said. "A piece of mountain until you can come back."

It was the size of my fist, angular, mica-flecked granite, shaped somewhat like an old fashioned iron or the spinner in a giant's board game, in one side a chunk of foggy quartz crystal. It looked like a rock someone might leave behind to point the way on a trail for those who might follow. It fit my palm perfectly. Its weight and warmth sunk into my skin, as if the mountain itself were holding my hand.

"I love this place," I said, "Why don't we come here more often? For all these years it's been so easy to say we're too busy."

"I'm sure Mary would be happy for you to use her cabin later this summer. Maybe Scott will feel up to it later in August when he's been home from the hospital awhile. The weather will still be nice to drive over in September. We'll come back with you if you want."

"Thanks. Maybe," I said, not willing, unable, to make plans for a month down the road. That moment, that day, from that spot on Weston Pass, the view of my mountains was as far as I could see. And it was enough.

Funny—in hindsight—how I claimed that *view* across the valley as mine. Those 14,000 foot peaks were as far away as my future. I never set foot on their summits, before then or since. This I know now: *My* mountains are not the ones I gaze upon, but the one where I sit. Like the rock I can hold in my hand. Like the moments that make up a day. Only *that* can I claim as my own—where I am now.

Mom and I sat awhile, then walked back to the truck, drove back to the cabin. Before we went back to the city, we all spent a final afternoon in Leadville, listening to an Independence Day concert in the yard of an old brick house-turned-museum at the north end of Main Street. The musician channeled John Denver, and I cried behind my sunglasses when he sang *Sunshine on My Shoulders* and *Rocky Mountain High*. I bought his autographed CD, adding it to my collection of soul-saving music.

We made it back to Denver in time to do laundry, sort school supplies, and gear up for Scott's high-dose chemo week and Wil's first week of kindergarten. I put my Weston Pass rock by the side of my bed, next to my journal. I still have it within reach. Whenever I want, I can grasp it and return to my mountains once more.

Perhaps soul-whisper is where courage
comes from for any leap of faith...
Body is stunt double, soul is safe.

31
Laying On of Hands

It was Sunday, July 11th. I thought of it as the "Beginning of the End." The next morning was Scott's first day of high-dose chemotherapy and Wil's first day of kindergarten. My sister had flown in yet again from Cincinnati and would stay with us all week, caring for Wil, cooking for me.

"I'd really like to go to church this morning. Where is the closest Catholic one?" Jenéne asked, using her big-sister clout to overrule my church-going ambivalence. After all, she was doing me a big favor to be here; the least I could do was take her to church. It would give Scott and Wil some father-son time, if only cartoons. It might do me some good, although I must admit I was skeptical.

"Umm, I think there's a new one on the east side of Highlands Ranch. We could go there. It's too late to drive downtown to St. Elizabeth's."

We looked in the suburb newspaper and found a list of church addresses, denominations, and service times. Just as I thought, we could make it to the 10:30 service at Pax Christi. The newly built church was not far from Janna's house, the big soccer park, post office, and driving range. I had not been to church since January, when we went to a Presbyterian one with Scott's parents and I cried after the service, but couldn't say why. We hadn't gone since, mostly due to Scott's radiation fatigue, then his second surgery, then his lack of immune system during chemotherapy. That, and because I was afraid I'd cry again.

I sat down in the dim sanctuary with my sister, looking around at colorful banners strung from the modern, bare-metal beams. I wished for stained-glass windows. People sparsely filled the rows of padded chairs, wearing casual clothes and friendly smiles. I didn't know anyone there and liked the anonymity, but felt out of place. I knelt on the hinged padded kneeler and closed my eyes, chin on folded hands. I tried a silent talk with God.

Hi God. Fancy meeting you here. Wasn't it nice in the mountains last week? Wish I was still up there instead of here. Um, thanks for Jenéne being here this week. Please help Scott's body deal with the high-dose chemotherapy this week. I hope it won't be too terrible. Please help Wil have a great day at kindergarten tomorrow. I hope I can get Scott set up at the doctor's office and be back home in time to take Wil to school. Please help me get through the week. Please help me...

Without warning, tears and fear overcame me. I unzipped my always-stocked purse for a Kleenex. I whispered to Jenéne, "You can stay. I'll meet you outside after."

With her brown eyes brimful of understanding, she squeezed my hand and whispered back, "I'll request prayers for Scott." I nodded, knowing from emails that our friends were requesting prayers for Scott all over the country that day. I felt weird knowing people might realize they were praying for the husband of the crying woman who just ran out. How embarrassing.

I found the ladies room and went in to pull off a long swath of toilet paper, knowing my Kleenex stash wasn't enough. *I should wear waterproof mascara this week,* I thought. Then I stepped outdoors. It was too hot to go sit in the car, so I sat on a slope of lawn, not far from the open doors. The full Front Range of mountains was hazy far to the west. A young dad in khaki shorts bounced a crying baby and smiled at me with gentle concern. I put on my sunglasses, still crying.

Crying. Crying. *God, I'm so scared. What's this week going to be like?*

Crying. Crying. *How weird that all those people are praying inside. Praying in churches throughout Denver. Praying in Tennessee, Michigan, who knows where else, as far as our emails were forwarded. Do prayers make a difference? Will prayers really help Scott survive this week's high-dose chemo and next week's stem cell rescue? What if nobody prayed?*

Crying. Crying. Scared. Tired. Really scared. *What if the statistics come true and this high-dose chemo kills him? What if chemo doesn't kill him but it doesn't work either and we have to find yet another treatment option. How long can this go on? Is Wil's entire childhood going to be overshadowed by his dad's stupid brain tumor? What will he remember? Will life ever be easy again? Forget Scott and Wil—how am I going to survive?*

Crying. Crying. Wishing I could jump forward in time, skip this shit, and see how it all turns out. *Oh God, am I scared!*

Wouldn't it be nice if we had a guarantee *beforehand* that all would turn out well? If we knew we would survive, could we face the coming dangers with more courage? We didn't have any guarantees then, nor do you in your own story. But today we're going to flout the rules and jump ahead five years. It took me that long to realize what the prayers were about, what church could mean, and how courage happens.

So, close your eyes and picture my ever-present spiral notebook, the curling wires touching the pages of 1999 plus all pages in between, linking myself and my story to the same days and dates—and us, the survivors—in 2004.

On Saturday, July 10, 2004, I woke Wil up early so we could go feed and water his chickens at my parent's orchard, dubbed St. Francis Farm when we moved over the mountains to Palisade three springs earlier. After sharing a protein-powder milkshake (ice cream in disguise), we strapped on our helmets. No other traffic shared G Road as we bicycled the two miles with the sun at our backs.

Nobody was home when we arrived—Mom off on errands, Dad in Seattle that week. As we parked our bikes on the patio, we saw a tiny, yellow oriole barely sitting up on the concrete not far from the kitchen door. Its head was listing to the side, its wings drooping by its side as if giving up. "Oh, poor birdie," Wil said, stabilizing his kickstand and tip-toeing toward the bird. The fresh smudge on the kitchen window told the bird's story.

I took off my bike gloves and helmet, debating whether to take a photo with the digital camera I brought to photograph Wil with his 4H chickens. I decided against it and walked toward the bird, too. "I can give it some Healing Touch for Animals," I suggested, already pressing my thumbs into the opposite palm to open each hand's chakra. It had been years since learning Healing Touch for people or attending one of Carol Komitor's HTA workshops, but the energy medicine techniques had become second nature, especially for first aid. I slowly sat down on the kitchen deck step and held out my hands, cupped lightly toward the bird. "Sshhhh, it's okay." I said to the bird, "It's okay." The oriole was too winded, too injured, to be frightened. He just sat there, stunned still.

I twisted my palms together maybe four times, then squeezed my hands like a short prayer. I filled my heart with love, sending that energy from my hands to the bird. I could see when it arrived a millisecond later because the bird twitched its tail, turned its head, and dropped a white splatter. "Well, at least you made it poop," Wil said, somewhat impressed. After two to three minutes, the energy was pulsing in my palms and the bird's tail was tapping up and down, nearly in tune to the beat I was feeling.

"What's happening," Wil wanted to know, "Why is he doing that? Does it hurt?"

"It's okay. I'm just sending love, and the bird can feel the energy. I'm sending the bird only what energy it needs, nothing more."

The bird hadn't tried to move its wings, but was turning around on one leg. We could see that his left leg was splayed awkwardly, toes limp and curled. Its knees looked bent backwards, but on second look I realized that's just how bird legs are. Forming my right thumb and first two fingers into a pinch like I'm almost ready to snap them, I moved them in the tiniest circular motion, imagining my fingers within inches of the bird's left foot with a laser to seal the leaking energy on its broken leg, or at least help its leg feel stronger. It was an imaginary, energetic stitching motion.

I thought to myself, *What if this doesn't work and the bird drops dead on the patio? What am I going to do with its body? No, don't think that. Just send good energy. Couldn't hurt. Might work. The bird seems more alert already.*

"Look at his beautiful feathers," I said out loud, and we marveled for a moment at the black and white stripes on his wings, contrasting with his lemon yellow body. I saw a tuft of feathers at his neck that look just like when a foxtail is stuck in my cat Spot's fur and he can't reach it, and he lets me pull out the sticker only if I pet him at the same time.

I went back to sending energy with my cupped hands, then using my right hand—again at a distance—smoothed the bird's ruffled feathers and energy field. One toe on the bird's left foot twitched, and the bird tried standing on both legs, almost. He was leaning more on the right, tail still thumping, eyes brightening.

Okachobee, Wil's bantam rooster, crowed from his perch in the spruce around the corner. The mother robin, who for months had been nursing her fledglings in the red birdhouse above the lawn, began singing. I heard more birds in the globe willow adding their voices, but I didn't dare look. I didn't want to break eye contact with the injured oriole. He'd spun around, looking straight at me. "He's not trying to fly yet," said Wil, worried.

"Here, you can help," I said to Wil, nodding at his hands. "Think of sending him your love and energy. You can do it," I said to the bird and to Wil.

"You can do it, fly away, birdie." Wil cupped his hands at ground level, open toward the bird. The tree-singers were even louder now, as if cheering. *It's okay*, we were all saying.

I said to Wil, "Let's open our arms wider, sending even more healing light and expanding its energy field so the pain can be released."

We held our arms out for less than a minute and watched as the bird stood stronger on its legs, though its wings had not yet fluttered. In a flash, the bird rose up and flew to Wil's tree house in the globe willow branches. Wil and I jumped up, too.

"We did it! Wil, we did it! Look what happened when you added your energy, too!" We hugged each other.

"That was cool. That was so cool," he was saying, walking in circles of disbelief, pride, and happiness. "That was amazing."

We were both grinning. I rumpled his hair, and we took one last look at the tree, but the bird was gone, or lost to our sight in the leafy green branches. The rest of the birds in the trees either flew off or stopped singing, going back to their business. Okachobee crowed once more. Wil and I walked toward the chicken coop, back to our business, too.

As we rode our bikes back to our own home that day, I reflected on how I had been doing a pretty good job using Healing Touch for Animals by myself, but it wasn't until Wil added his energy that the bird took off from the ground. The energy-medicine bird-moment seemed a perfect metaphor for how I pictured the combined prayers of so many people supporting Scott, especially that final week of his high-dose chemo and stem cell rescue. It was as if all the people under so many steeples were holding their hands together, focusing love and healing energy to stitch up our hearts, the same way Wil and I and the trees full of songbirds and poultry energized the oriole into flight. It wasn't for us to know if the bird would live, if he could survive his injuries. It had to be enough that our help made a difference that morning.

All summer of 2004, I had been struggling to write our stem cell chapter, still trapped in my fear on the church lawn that long-ago Sunday morning. But now I thought I could write of it, starting with the meaning of the oriole moment.

The bird story poured out on paper, but when I tried again to recreate the day in 1999, I was still stumped, unable to release my memory clamped shut by fear. So I revisited my 7/11/99 journal entry, looking for clues to my courage back then. The finger of synchronicity pointed out that five years earlier, July 11 was also a Sunday (have you noticed that with 365 days plus leap year, parallel dates rarely happen?). If printed on transparent paper, 2004's July calendar would overlay 1999's precisely, as if I could touch elbows with myself over time. I loved the coincidence and took it as a sign from the writing gods that the energy of me-today was linked in a time warp with me-then. Suddenly it all came together.

With the enchantment that tends to arise when I'm writing, I told myself to take a chance to time travel. Who knew? Like prayers, it might matter.

It is Sunday, July 11, 2004, and Scott, Wil and I are in the right-side pews of First Congregational Church, about half way back from the altar. The ceiling is ridged in seven arches with curved timbers of wood that recreate the intentional upside-down sense of the Mayflower hull. Sitting shoulder to shoulder with our good friends—Nancy, Mike and eight-year-old Ryan—we are surrounded by the congregation of perhaps ninety (a bit sparse, it being July), most with gray and white heads. Reverend Sharyl stands at the altar lectern. She has reported her list of church members and extended family who need prayers and assistance due to cancer, surgery, accidents, illness, old age. Holding her arms out wide, she asks, "So what joys and concerns do you bring today?"

Since joining the church in March, I have yet to raise my hand for a microphone to announce my joys or sorrows. Heck, we joined the church without ever feeling confident to introduce ourselves as guests. We joined because on the night of our first visit to this church, Sharyl led a "Science & Faith" discussion group on the topic of the soul and the brain, and Scott came home, flopped on the couch, and said in happy relief, "I've found my church." Up to now, I've added my own pleas in silence. But today I'm going to do it out loud. I've worn waterproof mascara and brought tissues just in case the dam breaks. I raise my hand and an usher approaches, microphone outstretched. I take it and stand up, making eye contact with a few people nearby, then with Sharyl. Scott puts his hand at the back of my knees (he knows what's coming).

"Hi. First, I have a sad thing to share. Last Sunday morning, my grandmother died—my dad's mom who was in a nursing home in Denver. It's a blessing, really, and we like her choice to leave on Independence Day. But we're still very sad. So I'd like to ask for prayers for my dad and our family. Last Sunday's service I could smell someone's rosemilk lotion just like my grandmother always wore, so it helped me to think about her that morning." I say that much, then mumble, "Not that I knew I needed to be thinking of her." I try not to choke up as I continue.

"Secondly, exactly five years ago today, July 11th, which was also a Sunday if you can believe it, was the hardest day of my life. It was the day before Scott started his high-dose chemotherapy, to be followed a week later by a stem cell rescue. It was also the day before Wil started kindergarten (we had year-around school in Highlands Ranch). We weren't church-goers back then, and Scott couldn't go anyway because his immune system was in danger after months of chemo. My sister went with me to Pax Christi Catholic Church. I started to cry as soon as I sat down and had to walk out. I sat outside in the grass, listening to the music and the liturgy because the doors were wide open. I still couldn't stop crying. I was overwhelmed.

"This is going to be the craziest prayer request you've ever heard, but I promise you'll get instant gratification."

"If you would indulge me in a bit of time travel, I'd like to ask everyone to send their prayers for peace and strength and courage and hope — to me when I was sitting there outside of church five years ago, and to Scott who was getting ready to fight the last battle of his treatment, and to everyone in our family who were all just as scared but being strong for us — and feel free to include anyone else across time whose soul needs prayers for healing.

"I have a feeling now that one reason I was crying so hard is because I could sense the love and energy of people all over the country who were praying for us that morning — and because your energy today was sent back through time, too. Until we joined FCC, I never really knew what it truly meant when friends and strangers told us their churches were praying for us. Now I know. So thank you for being part of our healing — back then as well as today."

I sat down in a rush, face blazing red, sure that everyone thought I was nuts and was shocked that I'd been so open. A lady sitting behind me leaned forward to pat my shoulder. I wanted to cry. A few other people stood up with prayer requests and I tried hard to listen, but I was reaching back to myself of five years ago, through the quantum thread and heartstrings, thinking *"Do you feel it? We're with you. Hold on."*

That's what I wrote on Saturday afternoon to visualize what I might try on Sunday, if I got up my guts to risk ridicule. Here's what really happened at First Congregational on Sunday, July 11, 2004:

Scott drove us to church that morning, while in the passenger seat I wrote bulleted points on an index card. I kept rereading the printout page three of my Word document, having shown it to Scott and Wil so they'd know what I was up to.

"You know I'll do anything to save your life, even if it means embarrassing you," I joked with Scott. "And besides, we already know it worked."

"Hey, nothing can embarrass me now," he replied.

By the time we pulled into the parking lot, I decided to leave all my notes in the car and let my heart do the talking. I still wasn't sure I would do it.

Scott and I sat by ourselves in the sixth row cushioned pew where the sun was almost blinding through the stained-glass windows. Our good friends weren't at church that day (the first difference I noted compared with my pre-written description). The air-conditioning blasts from above gave me shivers on top of my nerves, so I leaned into Scott. After the brief "time with children," Wil walked down the aisle with five other kids for Sunday school.

As I stood up with the microphone for "joys and concerns," I forgot most of what I planned to say. I did tell about the smell of rosemilk the morning my grandmother died and liking her choice of leaving on Independence Day, but I forgot to request prayers about her passing. I'll bet the congregation noticed my omission. I did ask for time travel prayers and promised instant gratification. I forgot the crucial part about how maybe I was crying in 1999 not out of fear but because I sensed the overwhelming love flowing at us in prayers around the world and from the future.

I sat down trembling and Joan, behind me, leaned forward to squeeze my shoulders and whisper, "That was beautiful."

Scott held my hands in both of his until I stopped shaking. I didn't feel like crying at all, but instead felt alert and connected. I soaked up the rest of the service as if it were meant for my 1999-self as well. The readings and lyrics throughout the service felt tailor-made for us on that day and five years before. At the piano during the offertory, Martha played a Psalm Twenty-Three in F Minor, "Shepherd me, O God, beyond my wants, beyond my fears, from death into life." My inner Catholic knew the words and mumbled-sang along in an off-tune whisper, though it was Martha's solo.

Reverend Sharyl ended the service with a quote from St. Francis, healer of birds and channel of peace. "Go out and preach the Gospel to the world — and if necessary, use words."

Some of us question the power of prayer and another some (perhaps overlapping) doubt the energy of Healing Touch. Maybe everyone is skeptical of time travel, but not me, not in the metaphorical sense. What if, like

Marty in *Back to the Future,* we could travel to the past and leave a note to be found in the future. Why not send a message to your younger self or listen for one from your older survivor? Maybe it's no different than leaving breadcrumbs in the forest or planting bulbs in October to bloom as tulips in April. Healing happens in layers of time, not always in chronological order.

I like to believe our infinite soul can reach to us anywhere, any when, and whisper that time, fear, and death are only illusions. Listen. Imagine. Trust. Perhaps soul-whisper is where courage comes from for any leap of faith. Courage is faith in the future, acting as both parachute and trampoline to soften our landing. Body is stunt double. Soul is safe.

Back in 1999, thanks to the loudspeakers, I could hear the priest preparing Holy Communion, then people walking to the altar, singing. Mass would be over soon. I stood from the lawn, sniffed, and brushed grass off my skirt. I followed the sidewalk to a standalone chapel up the hill, where I took a moment to collect myself in private. I sat in the circular space and looked up to see the chapel rafters were made of aspen. For a moment I was back in the mountain aspen groves where I'd been the week before, then back when I trimmed golden aspen branches to adorn the altar for my wedding, and back even further to childhood Sunday pancake picnics among aspens with my family. I felt calm and fortified to face the week. I blew my nose a final time, put the damp tissue in my purse, and stepped outside.

People streamed out of Pax Christi into the hot July morning. I waved at my sister who stood on the sidewalk looking for me. I wore my sunglasses, but I wasn't crying anymore. Somehow shifted, surprised, I felt at peace.

That night at my parent's house, our family shifted its focus from Scott to Wil by having a "back to school" party, complete with cake, ice cream, and new crayons. What better way to prepare us all. "Eat, drink and be merry, for tomorrow we start chemo and kindergarten."

I like going to a playground, getting in a swing and
swinging high, because I believe God lives in us
through the joy and power we sense when we swing high.
— Sister José Hobday

32
High-Dose Chemo & Kindergarten

Subj: Wil's 1st day of school
Date: 7/12/99 5:11:04 PM Mountain Daylight Time

Hi Everyone,

Scott got home from his first day of chemo today in time to see Wil get off the school bus -- on his first day of kindergarten. Problem was, Wil didn't get off the bus -- cuz he wasn't on it!!! The 5 neighbor kids all got off the bus shrugging and anxiously saying "We don't know where Wil is!" So I ran down the street to our house to catch the phone ringing, the kindergarten teacher calling to say Wil was with her at school.

We had a big misunderstanding, or call it a lack of planning/training, about what bus number to look for. Wil was convinced he was on bus #9 and I had told Ms. Mackey bus #22. Rather than risk the wrong bus, she kept him off. So, I drove to school to get Wil (and found him in the office with another little boy -- Wil wasn't alone in this fiasco). And tomorrow, we're putting a note in his backpack with his bus number on it. Wil did remember his phone number, though, so Ms. Mackey could call us right away. Gotta be proud about that.

At least Wil has a good story to tell now about his first day of kindergarten. Wouldn't it have been boring to just report that he'd gotten off the bus just fine. :)

That's all for today. Keep ya posted!
Love, Shelly, Scott & Wil

P.S. Please keep your fingers crossed that neither Wil nor I bring home any sneezy viruses to infect Scott. The doctors are more concerned about viruses than bugs that can be treated with antibiotics. And Mario is getting his stem cells back tomorrow (Tuesday morning) so think "GO STEM CELLS!" for Mario.

Subj: Scott's Chemo Update
Date: 7/15/99 9:13:58 PM Mountain Daylight Time

Hi Everyone,

This week was Scott's 4th round of chemotherapy and the highest dose of drugs ever, but amazingly he has gotten through this week easier than any other chemo week -- so far. The difference is in the drugs and what side effects they have right away. Luckily, he has made it to the 4th day with very little queasiness. BUT, it is starting to catch up with him and he is getting more exhausted and more queasy. Friday (tomorrow) is the last day of chemo and depending on how he feels, he can go into the hospital tomorrow or wait until the last possible hour on Sunday at 4 p.m.

It's really strange to be going through this high dose chemo, knowing it will be so harsh as to kill off not only the brain tumor cells but all his good fast-growing cells and bone marrow -- and to not have any sign yet of its strength. **It's like knowing you're about to be in (and volunteered for) a near-fatal car accident but don't know what hour the crash will happen.** And I must say that I'm already missing Scott's presence in advance for the weeks he will be in the hospital, especially knowing the pain he will go through to come out the other side. We're likening it to a vision quest of being at the edge of your existence, spiritually and physically, and coming back a new, whole person. I know he can and will do it.

The hospital already has assigned him to his room, on the side of the hallway with the nicer window view. Scott's stem cell rescue will be on Monday morning, about 8:30-10:00. Please surround Scott with all your love and healing energies and then focus on those little stem cells as they thaw out and are returned to Scott's bloodstream. Tell them to wake up and get growing! :)

Wil has had a fun week of kindergarten and, except for that first day, has made it on the bus successfully (thanks to our neighbors' daughters!). He is going on a camping trip this weekend with Aunt Amie and Uncle Lance -- his fun just never ends.

Thanks to all of you for helping us through this, and thanks especially to my neighbors -- the mighty maids -- for offering to get and keep our house clean, and to my friends in FEMALE (formerly employed moms at the leading edge) who are bringing us meals. More than anything, thanks for your love and prayers for Scott and our family.

Love to all of you,
Shelly

p.s. We hear that Mario is doing just fine with his stem cell rescue this week.

My emails say about all I can remember about Wil's first week of kindergarten and Scott's week of high-dose chemotherapy. I alternated between the efficient caregiver, driving Scott to his chemo each day, the cheery mother who listened to kindergarten news in the evening, and the weepy wimp on the verge of tears, anticipating the worst for what was to come.

Several nights I dreamed about being in trailers and mobile homes. Maybe unsettled, huh?

Thursday night, I cried in the car before going into Trailblazer Elementary for Back to School night. Partly I was tired, but mostly I was sad at going alone. I sat by myself in a gymnasium full of chattering, happy, carefree parents, listening as the principal outlined the various ways parents could be involved. Many other parents sat alone, too, spouses traveling or at home with the kids, no big deal. I know Scott would have been overwhelmed by the noise if he'd gone along. But what saddened me most was not signing up to volunteer for PTO or room help, as I would have, as my friends were, because I couldn't commit to anything else but Scott's cancer. Times like that made me hate Scott's brain tumor for changing what kind of mother I was and wanted to be. I wished life was normal again.

When Scott's chemo ended Friday afternoon, it was like being followed by Captain Hook's crocodile amplifying its ticking alarm clock. When it rang it meant it was time to take Scott to the hospital. The mean trick was, nobody could say when the alarm would go off. It felt a lot like nearing your pregnancy due date, waiting to go into labor, scared to death of how painful delivery might be.

My sister left on Saturday, having taken care of us all week. When my parents came to take her to the airport, Jenéne gave me a long, tight hug, and I burst into tears. Only then did I realize how I wasted that week by not letting my guard down to receive more of her hugs. I think my body turned into a fragile glass pitcher that week, filling, emptying, filling, emptying, trying not to topple over, not willing to let anyone too close lest I crack and crumble.

Wil left on Saturday, too, to go camping with Amie and Lance and a friend's son, named Aaron. Scott napped off and on, allowing me a nice quiet day all to myself. I spent six and a half hours sewing the tree curtains for Janna to cover the picture window in her Healing Touch treatment room. Sewing was contemplative meditation for me, pinning, ironing, the whirring stitch of the machine. I almost finished the curtain that day, happy with the way it was turning out. I wish you could see it, white on white muslin, this huge tree trunk, branches and narrow oval leaves sewn in layers with my new Elna. When it hung in the window, daylight would reveal thread-sap flowing beneath the muslin bark. I made two more similar panels for her French doors.

At 8:30 that night, with the summer sun nearing the mountains and me looking forward to an early bedtime, Scott came into the dining room.

"Time to go," he said.

"What? Now? Why?" He didn't look that sick to me. I thought sure he could wait until morning.

"I don't know when I'm going to crash, but it seems like it must be getting closer. What if it happens in the middle of the night? I'd rather get to the hospital and be there, checked in, ready for it. That's better than having some emergency at home."

"Well, okay. I'll call Dr. S to let him know we're on our way." I phoned the on-call answering service. When the doctor phoned back, he sounded surprised but accommodating.

"I'm sure he'll be fine at home until tomorrow, but if you want to come in now, that's okay. I'll meet you there."

"Sorry. We do."

Rushing around packing Scott's bags and my backpack reminded me of the night Wil was born, heading to the hospital in the middle of the night. While Scott checked me in at the hospital, I remember holding my sister's hand as I paced through contractions in the hallway, crying because I was so scared about the pain that I knew would begin soon. Feeling the same way now, I choked back tears and kept moving.

By the time we arrived at the hospital, it was almost ten o'clock. We went straight upstairs, up the long elevator in the quiet lobby, to the bone marrow transplant unit. The nurses were ready for us and showed us to Scott's room. He would have a wall of north windows overlooking a neighborhood of turn-of-the-century brick homes. We could see out over the lower rooftop of the emergency room below.

Soon after, I left Scott tucked into his bed at the hospital and drove home alone in the dark. It seems like I should have spent the night, since I'd be back first thing in the morning anyway. I was torn between wanting a good night's sleep before the unknowns of the week began and not wanting to leave Scott alone. I opted for my own bed. *Let the nurses take care of Scott overnight. He'll be fine,* I convinced myself.

Sunday was uneventful. Still waiting for the side effects of chemotherapy to descend, he lay in bed all day, watching TV or napping. I sat in a chair, reading, and waiting.

Amie and Lance brought Wil to the hospital on Sunday evening. He came with a bunch of helium balloons, which he placed in strategic singles around the room, corner, chair, table, bedside. Then he wrote a note for Scott on the cardboard that the balloons had been tied to, a series of Xs and Os. Wil seemed cheery enough, but when it was time to go I had to remind him to say goodbye. It was as if Wil had formed his own protective wall against this scary version of Scott.

"See you tomorrow morning, first thing. Love you." I said with a kiss as Wil and I left.

"Bye, Daddy. Love you."

"Bye, guys. Love you, too."

The next morning would be Scott's stem cell rescue.

I'm wondering what there is to do in this
one-dimensional town we've built for ourselves.
— Scott Vickroy on Morphine

33
Zero to Fifty-Four Hundred

Monday, July 19, 1999. Scott's new birthday, according to the medical staff, because the day of the stem cell rescue is counted as Day Zero. A new beginning. Hopefully.

Scott's stem cell rescue started at 9:20 in the morning. Dr. S and a nurse named Audrey came into Scott's room at the bone marrow transplant unit, after washing hands outside the door according to protocol. Dr. S toted a red Igloo cooler as if ready to share a picnic. Scott sat in a chair by his bed, and Dr. S knelt on the floor next to the cooler. It reminded me of the salesmen who help you try on new shoes. I stood beside Scott, my hand on his shoulder. Scott wore blue scrubs-pants under his hospital gown, which was open to the front so that the nurses could access his Neostar port with its three dangling plastic tubes. Audrey swabbed one of those tubes in preparation.

When the doctor opened the lid of the cooler, we should have heard drum rolls. Clouds of liquid nitrogen billowed over as he pulled out the first of six small metal folders, maybe half an inch thick and the size of my journal. Inside each hinged aluminum case was a plastic bag of Scott's stem cells that he harvested in June. He placed the metal case in a plastic tub of warm water to thaw. After a few minutes he transferred the rosy-pink bag of stem cells from the metal folder into a large Ziploc-like bag, then back in the warm water to thaw further. It looked like frozen cherry slush, but the room began to smell like garlic tomato paste. The doctor explained the aroma was DMSO, the preservative in the cells, and that we should expect the smell to linger for a few days.

Dr. S connected a syringe to a plug on the plastic bag, drew it full of the stem cells, then connected the syringe to one of the plastic tubes dangling from Scott's chest. He squeezed the syringe, pushing the slushy stem cells into Scott's bloodstream. "I can feel the cold," Scott grimaced.

"You might get an ice-cream headache," the doctor cautioned as he continued the slow infusion. Scott received the first three bags just fine. On the fourth bag, Scott began to hyperventilate in pain, his tongue, mouth, neck, and jaw reacting to the DMSO (as the doctor explained).

"Heart rate and pulse are normal," Audrey reported.

"Do you want to stop for awhile and do the rest later?" asked Dr. S.

"No way. Let's get it over with," Scott said, bracing himself for the last two bags. Audrey gave him some anti-anxiety Ativan through one of his other port tubes to help Scott relax. Whether it helped or not is uncertain. I held Scott's hand for the last three bags and then a little bit longer.

And that's all there was to it. That was the stem cell rescue, on the outside.

On the inside, I imagine the hearty stem cells shaking off frost as they flowed through Scott's veins, continuing to thaw with the warmth of his body. I see them as if in a Disney-esque health film introducing themselves like perky superheroes to the existing, exhausted blood cells. "Hey there. Hello. We're here to help. Can you point us to the bone marrow? We need to get settled and start growing new blood cells. Gosh, this man's immune system has been completely destroyed, but we'll grow him a new one. Give us a few days and we'll report back."

I also think of the stem cells like miniature seeds being sown in the slush of spring snow—like Yellowstone after the fire. Seeds take time to germinate. The medical term is "engraft" which is like a seed splitting open, fragile roots taking hold in the soil, reclaiming the land as its own, while a sprout points up through the dark soil looking for light. Until Scott's stem cells engrafted, his immune system would hover at zero.

Dog Days

The side-effects of high-dose chemotherapy are not a pretty sight. One of the high-dose chemo drugs is expelled through the skin, so Scott began to look and feel like he had a nasty third-degree sunburn. Mouth sores were starting, too, as the high-dose chemo wiped out all of Scott's fast-growing cells—not only tumor cells but also skin, hair, and the fragile cells that line his mouth, sinuses, throat, and gastro-intestinal tract. The only remedies would be several showers a day and some lotion, then morphine for pain.

We expected the dog days to hit even sooner. Scott didn't need the morphine until Wednesday, to the surprise of his doctors and nurses, and he didn't start running a fever until Thursday night. Our Healing Touch practitioners, Janna and Carol, came to the hospital as a double-dose team to help ease his pain and pump up his energy field. The hospital had a Therapeutic Touch department which delivered trained volunteers to anyone's room on request, so the staff treated our practitioners like part of the team. I told our friends about it in an email update, asking, "Please add your prayers and healing white light to expand Scott's energy field and help get him through this rough time."

Our friends and family sent help in more tangible ways as well. Email encouragements. Cards and balloons. One family sent a package of drawings their kids made to decorate Scott's room, with a letter saying how they had become closer-knit, aware of life's precious meaning more than before. One of Scott's friends wrote to say he found himself changing his fatherhood style to spend more time with his young sons.

People literally gave of themselves to try and help Scott by donating platelets. Several days that week a nurse knocked on the door to Scott's room to tell me a visitor was waiting. On Day Zero, it was Scott's manager-friend from work. She spent hours in the Apheresis Department, offering up any and all of her veins, to donate platelets for Scott. She was bruised and dejected for being unable to get her blood pumping enough.

Another day, I went to the visitor's room for the bone marrow unit, wearing my pale-green linen jumper Scott's mom bought for me and looking, I'd say, prettier than most days. I found myself in a bear-hug from my friend's husband, who donated platelets that day on his lunch hour. He burst into tears at the sight of me, saying, "Oh, look at you. I can't stand to think of you and Scott going through all this. You know we're all praying for him." Flabbergasted, blown away, I felt humble to my core.

Years later, a friend of my parents said how he considered donating platelets for Scott as one of the most important contributions of his lifetime. I often think about those platelets Scott received, which our friends donated with so much love and compassion from the depths of their own bone marrow. Not only was Scott rescued by what was inside him—his own stem cells and strength—but by the heartfelt intentions of each platelets donor and each person who prayed.

Often on my way through the visitor's room into the HEPA-clean air of the bone marrow unit, I would see Mario's mother sitting there, taking a break. She would give me an update on her son, which I would include in my email updates. "Mario also has mouth sores and his skin is now coming off on his chest. And he's grouchy, says his mom." Mario was a week ahead of Scott in his stem cell rescue, and he set the benchmark. It was the ultimate buddy system, to know someone else in the lifeboat.

Scott grew worse by the day because his confusion increased in direct proportion to the dosage and strength of pain medication.

As part of his daily checkup, Dr. S would ask Scott if he knew where he was ("Well, it's not Sloan Kettering...") and if he knew the day ("Uhmm, summer?"). Dr. S asked, "Do you know who I am?" and Scott said, after much thought, "Dr. Richards? Chris?" I have no idea who he was talking about. By Friday, when asked who this pretty woman was standing next to him, Scott looked at me with a blank stare and couldn't come up with my name. After some long moments he guessed "My wife?"

I could have been crushed. Part of me felt like going home until he was better, as in cured, but the other part of me couldn't care less. The universe thought it was funny. All week, whenever I drove home on Downing Street, I saluted the ironic movie title on the Esquire Theatre marquee, *An Ideal Husband*. Another day, driving home on University past the Denver Country Club, an automatic speeding-ticket machine took my snapshot. The photo ticket arrived by mail, proof of an exhausted woman in sunglasses slumped over the steering wheel of her Honda Civic. Cameras don't lie.

Thank goodness Scott's parents came to relieve me of duty each day. Linda would arrive at 3:00 p.m. so I could be home in time to meet Wil at the bus stop and hear about his day at kindergarten. Around dinner, Bill relieved Linda and stayed well past midnight, sometimes later. Amie came after work and kept company, too. Scott, oblivious, provided comic relief.

Late one night, Scott said to his dad through the haze of his pain meds, "I'm wondering what there is to do in this one-dimensional town we've built for ourselves."

"Why don't you sleep," Bill replied, not missing a beat.

"Okay."

Another night, Scott said out of the blue, "We should have everyone over here for a sleepover and talk about what we're going to do."

During the days, Scott lay propped on his pillows, vacant bleary eyes, with a suction tube in his mouth, vacuuming out the thick mucus from his mouth and throat. I know—very gross. He was too far gone to care when we pointed to the television to show him a young cancer survivor who was making his cycling comeback by racing in the Tour de France, even favored to win. Not even when we said, "That guy survived testicular cancer and

brain tumors." Scott wasn't alert enough to care, but the rest of us were inspired by Lance Armstrong.

Scott looked like a human-snake mutant in molting season, losing layers
of skin from every inch of his body and every single hair. I helped him rub
Desitin lotion all over, as if he had diaper rash or a chemical burn, which is
in fact what he had. I wondered if his skin would have sloughed off to the
same degree if he had showered more during high-dose chemo week. Once
that amount of poison soaks into your body, the only way out is the skin or
the liver.

Scott's liver was toast. His eyes and what was left of his skin turned yellow, jaundiced with the effort to detoxify his body. I found out later that
when the liver is failing, the brain swells, and so some of his confusion
could have been that. Due to his mucositis, Scott couldn't swallow anything,
only ice chips. He was getting bags of "total parenteral nutrition" (a.k.a.,
TPN) and all other pain meds intravenously. The one medication to help
Scott's liver could only be taken by mouth—it was a horse pill.

On Day 7, the second Monday, the doctors decided Scott needed a feeding tube since he could not swallow the liver medicine. It was a procedure
that would mean leaving his safe room in the bone marrow unit and going
somewhere else in the hospital. An aide brought a wheelchair and we
helped Scott move into it. I wasn't going to let him do this alone and told
the aide, "I'm coming, too."

I won't go into even more of the gory details, but let me tell you just a bit
more because it's the part Scott actually remembers, and for me it was the
rock-bottom moment. If the nine months since Scott's diagnosis had been
pregnancy and our week since high-dose chemo had been labor, this was
delivery.

The day our son was born, I held Scott's hand nearly crushing his bones.
In the final moments, as he whispered *Push*, I wrapped my left arm around
his neck and squeezed as I screamed. That day with the feeding tube, our
roles were reversed and he lay back on the table, tilted at an angle, his left
arm clenching my neck. The tube went up his nose and needed to go down
the back of his throat, but it wouldn't. The medical team kept saying, "Swallow. Try again. Swallow."

"If he could swallow, he wouldn't need this feeding tube," I said, omit-
ting the obvious cuss word to focus on Scott and encourage him to relax
enough to take the tube down his throat. "You have to do this, Scott. Try
one more time. You can do it, honey."

I could see a flicker of light in his eyes that told me the Scott I knew was still in there. Scott's inner samurai accepted his fate and his duty and swallowed. Then he lay back and closed his eyes, unable to say anything more.

We returned to Scott's room to find his mom waiting for her afternoon bedside shift. Scott was so worn out, he didn't even say hello. I'm not sure he even recognized his mom, as his confusion continued to worsen, in part due to the amount of pain meds we gave him to get through the tube swallowing. A few minutes after he crawled back in bed, we found out just how confused he was. He thought he had just endured preparations for another awake craniotomy.

"Please tell them I can't be awake for brain surgery today," Scott said through tears. His gurgling voice made him sound like a toddler. "I can't do it. Don't let them wake me up during surgery."

"Honey, you're not having brain surgery today," I said, completely surprised.

"Yes, I am," he replied, glaring past me to his mother like she was my accomplice in lying.

"You had a feeding tube put in so you could have the medicine you need, and now you're all done," I continued, telling Linda with my eyes that I was sorry she had to see him like this. "There isn't anything more. You're done for today. Really. No surgery."

"Bulllllll...SHIT!"

It took some time to convince him of the real situation. I explained over and over. By the time he accepted my reassurance, it was time for me to leave to pick up Wil. "I have to go now, but I'll be back in the morning," I said.

Linda shot me a look of pure panic and said, grabbing her purse as she stood, "Why don't I go get Wil today. He can spend the night with me and I'll take him to school in the morning. I think Scott would be more comfortable with you tonight, Shel."

I had to agree. I spent the night on a cot in the room. The next morning I wrote and replied to emails on my laptop and went home mid-afternoon. Scott slept through a blessedly uneventful day and didn't miss me when I left.

Thirty-two hours after the feeding tube went in, Scott pulled it out. He woke up in the night, still confused, while his dad dozed in a chair by the bed. Scott wondered what weird thing was up his nose, so he yanked it out. He looked at the tube in his hand and said, "Oops."

Remember, along with no white cells, Scott had no platelets, no clotting. His nose gushed. Bill woke up and called the nurses, who ran in to stop the bleeding. The doctor arrived and assessed the situation, still dire for the state of Scott's liver and complicated by his lack of platelets. He didn't want to risk bleeding by reinserting the feeding tube. The liver medication had helped Scott turn the corner, so Dr. S decided Scott could go without the tube. Scott remembers it this way, with the doctor saying, "I'll give you a choice. We can put the feeding tube back in, or you can swallow this pill."

"Give me a cup of water. I'll swallow that pill."

And he did.

Resurrection

Scott's white counts had begun to rise—from zero on feeding-tube Monday...to 80 on Day-8 Tuesday...to 300 on bloody-nose Wednesday. The numbers meant his stem cells had engrafted and were starting to grow. We were told that if Scott's white counts could stay at 500 for a few days, then he could be weaned off some drugs and come out of his delirium. It had been a terrible week but now I could see his recovery was right around the corner. Mario went home on his Day 15, so that gave me hope.

Subj: Scott - Day 10
Date: 7/29/99 5:14:17 PM Mountain Daylight Time

I know it's a lot of emails I'm sending this week, but I just have to keep you posted on this rapid turnaround for Scott. Yesterday his counts were at 300, and today they are up to 1800! He's able to drink liquids now!! And he's able to speak again with a normal-sounding voice. What a change 24 hours makes! What a relief.

They told us the healing would be rapid once his white cells started to grow, but it's amazing to see the changes overnight.

Scott now needs to work up some strength to do laps around the hallways and just get stronger by the day. He'll be weaning off the pain meds and also the broad-spectrum antibiotics, which should help in all ways to make him feel better. His bones are starting to ache, like they did with the stem cell harvest, but it's a very tolerable kind of pain to know that it's productive, cranking out new bone marrow.

So that's where we made it to by Day 10. At this rate, the doctors say he'll be home in a week. I said he had to wait until I had time to clean the carpets, then he can come home. :)

Will keep you posted on this great progress.

Love,
Shelly

p.s. Luckily it seems that Scott can't remember how bad it was this week. Thank goodness for THAT!

Subj: Day 11-Leaps & Bounds
Date: 7/30/99 10:45:14 AM Mountain Daylight Time

If you thought yesterday's message was exciting, today's news is even better. Scott's counts are up to 5,400 from 1800 yesterday and this morning I came in to find him eating Rice Krispies with milk. The doctor actually votes for Monday to send him home, with the caveat, of course, that it could be much later in the week if we have any setbacks. He's putting Scott on meds by mouth tomorrow to get him off all these IV pumps. We'll be doing laps in the hallways later today (the nurse made Scott walk down the hall to the kitchen to get his own Jello last night, and he just cruised away).

Thanks to my good friend Anne, the carpets are getting cleaned tonight and we should be ready for Scott whenever he wants to leave this lovely place.

We'll see . . . .
Love,
Shelly

p.s. Even if we do go home Monday, we'll be back at the Dr's office daily next week and at least 3 times a week for awhile to get checked and for more platelets. But still it's better to sleep at home. :)

Anger is just as irreplaceable as sadness, fear, joy,
or any other emotional state.
— Karla McLaren

34
It's Okay to be Angry

With guardian angels and heartstrings, I had tried giving Wil a way to cope with his fear and worry. *The Human Body* book gave his mind images to dissect, diffusing the mystery of what's inside our skin. But as the months unfolded, on nights when he crawled into bed with me or I fell asleep in his bed after he did, I discovered he was grinding his teeth in his sleep. During the days, he would sometimes complain of a tummy ache for which there was no answer.

I hadn't faced the idea that Wil needed a way to cope with his anger, maybe because I was still trying to figure out what to do with my own. July had been so very long for us, with Wil's first days of kindergarten obscured by Scott's first day of high-dose chemotherapy. Wil's first month of kindergarten, when he had so many stories to tell me, was diluted by too many nights apart while I stayed at the hospital with Scott, while Wil stayed overnight with grandparents, aunts, or our neighbors. At the end of July, while Scott was still in the hospital waiting for his stem cells to re-grow his bone marrow, I woke up to how the nine months of treatment were taking a toll on our son.

One Monday morning when I was at the hospital, Wil was with my mom. He asked her to help him illustrate a story he wanted to write. Wil called it, "Sarah and the Wicked Boy." Wil directed her to draw the pictures for the first part of the story and write the words, while he drew the final big picture. In Wil's story, a girl named Sarah has two cats and two kittens that get lost. A wicked boy finds them and tries to stab them. Then Sarah comes to "scrape and pudge" the boy, putting him in jail and saving the kitties. Then she takes the cat family home for a tea party.

The picture Wil drew of a bloody knife and angry faces was the most frightening picture I'd ever seen him draw. When Mom showed it to me, seeing my shocked expression, she was quick to say, "I thought you should see what he's working on. This is a healthy way for him to express his anger. It was a way for him to be the wicked boy and be saved by a nice girl. Wil has been trying so hard to be good, because you've insisted on that from him. He needs a physical way to let go of some anger. Maybe we can spend some time kicking the soccer ball, or swimming, or give him a tennis racket to pound a pillow, or just roughhouse with other little boys. Don't worry, though, he'll be okay. He is okay."

I wanted to be sure. The next day after school, I took Wil with me to Janna's to deliver the curtains I had sewn. Upon hanging the fabric trees in her Healing Touch treatment room, I was dismayed to find that the one for the big window was an inch and a half too long, so I promised to take it home and fix the hem. Then I patted her massage table and said to Wil, "Jump up, buster."

He crawled up on the table, using a step stool, and Janna playfully spread a large and colorful silk scarf over him, like the parachute game we used to play in gym as little kids. Wil wasn't ready to play. He pulled the scarf over his face and turned to lay facing the wall, his back to us. Janna spoke softly to him for a few minutes, warming him up to ask him the real question.

"Hey, Wil, do you ever get angry?" she asked. His head nodded beneath the scarf. "And who do you get mad at?"

Wil's left hand snaked out from under the silk scarf and, as if his index finger had eyes, pointed at me without a word. I looked at Janna in surprise, not so much at his answer as his honesty.

"It's okay to be mad at me, honey," I said.

"Sure it is," Janna added. "Why don't you come out for a minute?" and she gently pulled the scarf from his face, while he rolled onto his back, cheeks blazing red. He glanced at me warily, and I grinned back and squeezed his shoulder.

Janna tickled Wil then and he laughed. She tickled his feet, his knees, his belly, then his neck, subtly tickling open his chakras. While she rubbed his tummy in soft circles, she said, "How about you practice saying this...Say, 'I'm mad.' "

Wil giggled then pursed his lips, refusing to say it. With Janna's encouragement, he whispered it, then repeated it a few more times until his voice was stronger and louder. He was still giggling, but his cheeks weren't flushed with embarrassment anymore and had returned to his typical rosy glow. His eyes were bright, and he looked me in the eyes with a big smile.

In less than ten minutes, Wil sat up, climbed off the table, sliding down between the table and wall rather than off the front. He was done, and ready to play with Riven, Janna's new kitten, and her daughter and son who were upstairs.

The next two nights, Wil slept through the night, but by Thursday he was grinding his teeth again. I had stayed at the hospital until 8:30 that night and had a short time to cuddle with him before bedtime.

"I'm mad you didn't come home sooner," he said to me as we shared space on his pillow.

"I know. I'm sorry. I'm doing the best that I can," I said, kissing his cheek. *Well, at least he is saying it out loud*, I thought to myself.

"That's okay. I love you," he said, and then he fell asleep.

I didn't get to see him at all on Friday, leaving for the hospital before he woke up, my mom on duty at our house that morning. When I spoke to him on the phone later that morning, he was his silly self again. The plan was for him to have a sleepover with his buddy, Aaron, who gone camping with Amie, Lance, and Wil on the weekend Scott entered the hospital for his stem cell rescue. It was the first time he'd be sleeping over at Aaron's and I wasn't sure he was game.

"I'm not going to see you tonight since you're going to Aaron's house," I said, anxious about his reaction.

"That's okay, Mom," he replied, "Remember our heartstrings."

And so we hung up the phone, with him comforting me maybe more than I comforted him. Earlier that day, I learned Scott would be coming home the following week, which meant we were getting closer to a normal existence again. That would mean more time at home for Wil and no more hospitals in our foreseeable future. If I knew Wil was coping, then I could cope, too.

For all that has been, thanks.
For all that will be, yes.
—Dag Hammarskjöld

35
The End of the Beginning

Subj: Day 14 - Heading Home
Date: 8/2/99 9:56:19 AM Mountain Daylight Time

Dear Everyone,

Scott is heading home later today! He was weaned off the IV pain meds over the weekend and isn't in very much pain anymore. He's swallowing pills just fine and managing to eat more Rice Krispies each morning. His stomach is in shock trying to digest food after nearly 3 weeks without eating, so he will slowly work up to eating real food again. At least through this week, Scott will have IV nutrition at night.

It's scary to leave the safety net of the bone marrow transplant unit, but there's not a lot to worry about, really. We'll have to keep our house very clean (which is no problem thanks to our very wonderful neighbors!). Still no flowers or live plants, which could harbor fungus and mold. Scott is allowed to go outside walking, but we'll have to avoid large crowds and limit our visitors —especially little kids— for a few more weeks to avoid unexpected viruses and flu. Also, if anyone has recently had a live vaccine, you'd have to avoid Scott (like a chicken pox vaccine). Hand-washing will be our biggest ally.

We'll go to the doctor's office daily this week to check blood counts and possibly get platelet transfusions. Next week we might go daily or only 3 times.

Now that the high dose chemo and stem cell rescue are over, it's a "wait and re-cover" game. It will take 2 to 4 months for Scott to get his energy level back, and maybe his hair will grow back by then, too. In 4 weeks, Scott will have a follow-up MRI and another at 12 weeks post-rescue. It will take several months for the brain tissue to process out the dead cells, so MRIs won't be a definitive picture of the stem cell rescue's success. In our hearts, we have to believe that the brain tumor cells are completely gone, never to return.

For now, we're just relieved that the worst part is over and that Scott can focus on recovery. We will take it a day at a time, but also look forward to the future. Thanks for helping us get through this time. We'll definitely stay in touch and keep you posted. But consider no news as good news. :)

Love, Shelly & Scott

Part Two:
Dark of the Moon

I wish I could tell you that life was instantly better, that we began Living Happily Ever After as soon as Scott's stem cell rescue was over. I wish I could tell you that life after cancer was easy and great. I wish I could tell you that, but I can't. And those who have been there would know I was lying. But it wasn't all bad.

This phase of our cancer journey was the dark of the moon. I always thought the crescent moon was the new moon. Now I know that when the moon goes dark you call it the new moon, which blends the end with beginnings. We don't question when the moon wanes; we take for granted when it waxes. But if you follow its phase through the month, like me, you notice the nights it is gone.

Let me tell this part of our tale, about the hard months after Scott's active treatment ended, but not because I want to complain. Let me tell you how hard it was so that you understand about caregiver burnout and life after cancer. Let me show you how we got through that dark night of the soul, how we spent fall and winter in the dark forest before we emerged in the spring. Let me tell you how grief and anger and exhaustion slowly decompose and regenerate.

Let me tell you this part of our story in layers, like how aspen leaves first turn a brilliant gold shimmer, how more faded leaves flutter and fall to the ground, how the pile grows deeper, until the branches are bare, and darkness falls before dinner. Let me tell you this part of the story like making a bed, one layer at a time, until finally it's done, and instead of admiring the tight sheets with no wrinkles, we allow ourselves to pull back the covers and crawl in, sleep deeply through the night, and pay attention to our dreams.

☙

What if we thought of ourselves like the moon
and had equal faith in what is ready to fade away
and what's invisible as we do in what is shining?
—Dawna Markova

36
Fall Color

The end of Scott's stem cell rescue, leaving the bone marrow unit on Day 14, would be a nice way to end our story—full of hope and potential for a permanent cure. It was the end—but only in the sense that delivering your baby is the end of your pregnancy. It's the beginning of a brand new life with a new focus and stress and many unknowns. You might say that the first year after cancer treatment is like having a colicky, high-maintenance baby, when you feel so tired you'd kill for a nanny or a shot of tequila. And yet you wouldn't give back your baby for anything. Not that you could.

When Wil was born, he had jaundice, so every day for two weeks we went back to the doctor's office for bilirubin bloodwork. Wil's treatment was wearing "twinkle lights" in a belt around his belly, which lit him up like a Christmas tree.

Likewise, every day after Scott's discharge from the bone marrow unit, we drove back across town to our doctor's office for bloodwork, which usually revealed that Scott needed a transfusion of platelets. After two weeks, we reduced our trips to every few days because Scott's white cell counts and platelets continued their slow upward climb. His immune system was beginning to recover, but it would be months, years, before his counts reached the normal range.

One night I dreamed that Scott was done with his stem cell rescue and was going to a graduation ceremony, but we were trying to figure out how to avoid the germs of a large crowd.

As Scott recovered, the rest of us suffered our own fallout from so many months on the edge. Scott's mom crashed and stayed in bed sick for days. Then Wil brought home strep throat from the raging epidemic at elementary school. Scott steered clear of Wil, although the doctor said it was too late for quarantine—we'd all been exposed to Wil's germs four days before. Poor Wil lay on the couch, whining, "Can't you see I'm sick, too."

My throat was scratchy, but I kept telling myself *I am not, I cannot, I will not get sick.* I piled on the Vitamin C and echinacea and made sure to take my multivitamin. The day after Wil came down sick, I felt asleep on the couch after dinner, and then hobbled upstairs to the guest bedroom to avoid breathing on Scott overnight. I woke up delirious with a fever. I wanted to dial the phone and say "Help" but there wasn't a phone in the room. Besides, I didn't know what number to dial or how, and I was too tired to move. I was aware of Scott bringing me hot tea, but I couldn't open my eyes. My parents came over to take care of Scott and Wil, while I slept all day. At some point, my dad took me to the walk-in clinic, where the rapid strep test turned positive in an instant.

Antibiotics are miraculous, aren't they? I recovered in a few days, after much sleep and TLC from my parents. The irony is that I had staved off colds and strep for the past nine months, not letting my body succumb to any illness while I was needed as Scott's caregiver. It was as if by the end of Scott's active treatment, my body caved in, begging for deep, uninterrupted sleep.

Scott had an MRI at the end of August, the first since his stem cell rescue. As usual, the test was scheduled first thing in the morning, so we left home as the late summer sun was rising. On the drive to the hospital we saw the moon on the opposite horizon, a sliver shy of full. It was the opposite of the crescent moon that appeared for both of Scott's surgeries as well as the stem cell rescue. I couldn't decide if that meant our MRI luck might flip or we had moved to the survivor's side of the moon, so to speak.

Dr. Arenson showed us the films of Scott's brain, comparing it to June. The black cavity left after surgery was shrinking. The white rim of enhancement around the border was slightly narrower. A white bump he called a node was still there but a bit different.

"There's no reason to believe that node is tumor," he reassured us. "It's more likely dead tissue. We will keep an eye on it next time and see if it grows or decreases."

Great, I thought, *we will never stop worrying about what shows up on these MRIs.* Most disconcerting was hearing Dr. Arenson talk about starting yet another aspect of treatment. My mind put up a flat hand at his words to say *Oh-my-god-will-we* ever *be done?*

"We can put you on high-dose Tamoxifen," Dr. Arenson said, as he made notes in Scott's chart. "That would be ten pills a day for two to three years."

"Isn't Tamoxifen what breast cancer patients take?" I asked, knowing my friend Julie was taking it for the next five years.

"Yes. It's an estrogen interrupter, which is why it works for breast cancer. We don't know why it works against brain tumors, but it does, in high doses. Breast cancer patients take one or two pills a day. We use the high dose.

"Or there's Thalidomide," he continued, "Which is considered biological therapy, anti-angiogenesis. You remember hearing about Thalidomide babies in the sixties? Babies born without limbs? That's because thalidomide prevents blood vessels from forming, which feeds the growth of arms and legs in a fetus, but in the brain would prevent the formation of new blood vessels that would feed a tumor. The downside of Thalidomide is that is makes patients very sleepy. So we'll wait until the next MRI, twelve weeks out from transplant, to see how you're doing. That will be a more conclusive picture of your situation, so we will make a decision about more treatment at that point. Tamoxifen has fewer side effects, even at the high dose, so I'm inclined to prescribe that for you first."

Scott didn't seem too concerned at the moment, basking in his relief at the still-clean MRI. "What's a few more pills," he said, "That's nothing compared to what I've already gone through."

With the first post-treatment MRI under our belt, it felt like permission to continue breathing, at least for two more months until the next MRI. We continued our baby steps back to normalcy, or at least a new normal. We fell into a rhythm of kindergarten for Wil, continual doctor visits for Scott to monitor his blood counts, and for me—cleaning, laundry, grocery shopping, cooking (we stopped our meals from FEMALE, wanting to go back to our own familiar recipes), driving, reviewing Wil's homework, paying insurance copays, fighting and winning over unpaid claims, filling out disability paperwork. Our next-door neighbor Fred continued to mow our lawn for us. I looked forward to weeding and deadheading my sunflowers. We drove to the mountains several times, with a few days back at the cabin in Leadville. The aspens delivered a stunning yellow-gold that autumn, as they always did—but in past years we didn't make time to notice.

The best part of Scott's treatment ending was that I finally felt comfortable leaving him alone for awhile. It was such a luxury to leave the house for an occasional girl's night out, which I'd been missing so much for nine months. I was surprised to find how my timeouts affected Scott. One afternoon, out of the blue, he came into my office and blurted, "I feel like you don't want to be around me anymore."

"Huh?" (My standard reply to Scott's surprise announcements.)

"It seems like you can't wait to get out of the house and away from me. Am I that repulsive now, all bald and skinny?"

"Oh, no! It's not that, not at all." I paused a moment to gather my thoughts. "You have no idea what a big step it is for me to feel like *it's okay* to let you be alone for a few hours at a time. It's progress for both of us that you're doing better."

"Oh."

After that, I tried to make sure we had date-time, like lunches together and more family time. I realized how isolating life had felt for him, now that the focus was off. He wasn't the recipient of cards and emails anymore. Plus I told everyone in our emails that it was time to lay low, resume our daily activities, regain our energy. But I didn't think about the impact on Scott. His comment helped hatch an idea for a follow-up birthday party, come November, to celebrate his one-year anniversary since diagnosis and turning thirty-four.

For me, though, I wasn't ready to relinquish my newfound freedom to get out of the house and have time to myself without cancer worries. I went out with girlfriends to a movie (*Runaway Bride*). I got a haircut and color, going to a new stylist because the one I'd been seeing all year wouldn't stop talking about everyone and anyone she knew who had cancer. I also signed up to walk in October's Race for the Cure on the "Friends of Julie" team to celebrate her one-year anniversary; she was now in remission.

Inevitably, I found myself at the paint section of The Great Indoors, feeling a need to reclaim my life with a big wall of color. During that summer, I saw a friend's dining room painted a deep, rich red, all four high-ceiling'd walls. I started scanning my house for just one wall that would look good in red. Our oriental rug (a Scotch-guarded version we bought as newlyweds) had a background of rosy brick red. Then my parents offered to give us their upright piano, a white turn-of-the-century piece with carved flower panels, which had lived through a flood in the '20s and was a survivor itself. Part of the plan was to provide a creative therapy for Scott's brain to coordinate his hands playing the keyboard. I knew right where the piano could go—in our front living room—with a red wall behind it as backdrop.

The one drawback was that the paint chip I picked, Martha Stewart Rodeo Drive, which matched the carpet threads perfectly, happened to be the exact color red as the six bags of Scott's stem cells.

Scott's reaction? "Spare me! I couldn't stand to walk downstairs everyday and see that color, that much of it. It would be as bad as smelling lasagna, reminding me of that terrible tomato-paste smell."

"Why can't you think of it as a nice reminder of the stem cells that saved you? It's a great color," I said, feeling stubborn.

I debated with myself for a week, tucking the paint chip in my purse. I would pull it out, match it to the rug, hold it up in the light, and wish for a sign, yes or no. I didn't think I could live with that wall being white, now that my inner decorator had imagined it red. And no other color would do.

By mid-September, Dr. Arenson announced that Scott's white count, hemoglobin, and platelets had risen "just a hair" over two weeks. It wasn't as much as the doctors had hoped, but it was moving in the right direction. The upward trend meant Scott wouldn't need any more transfusions and he wouldn't have to return for a checkup for another four weeks, which felt like a lengthy reprieve.

Better yet, Dr. Arenson agreed it was time to remove the Neostar port from Scott's chest. Every day, doctor appointment or not, I had to help Scott swab and flush each of the three dangling tubes. It was a constant reminder of the stem cell rescue and cancer in general. When my mother finished her treatment for ovarian cancer, confirmed by clean bloodwork and a second-look surgery, her doctor recommended she keep her port in "just in case." She told him "No way!" She wanted that port to be gone, because she believed her cancer was gone and didn't want anything suggesting otherwise. Sure enough, she had it removed and her cancer never came back, defying statistics and Murphy's Law.

Scott went to a cardiac surgeon to have his port removed in a simple office procedure. I decided, for once, that I didn't have to be in the room. I scanned a magazine in the lobby, assuming Scott was simply having stitches clipped and snipped. As even Lance Armstrong will tell you, removing a chest port is one of the worst surprises at the end of your treatment. Scott's skin had grown around it and didn't want to let go. As Scott tells it, "The guy literally put his foot on the table to pull that thing out of me. Tug! RIP!"

Ouch! Port gone! A milestone! Scott's blood counts were rising. He was on his way to recovery. I took that as my sign, so I painted my wall.

When I opened the can of paint, I was appalled at the pinkness. But I trusted the truth that paint always dries darker, so I painted away. I used a full gallon and saw I'd need more. I ordered Scott to withhold judgment until I was all the way done, wishing he would hold his breath and told-you-so scorn until I returned from the paint store with the second gallon. He looked skeptical. After the second coat, which dried into the perfect shade of red, we were both relieved.

"It looks pretty good," Scott said. "I like it."

The antique piano arrived the next week, needing its own coat of fresh paint, satin white. My mom came over to direct its delivery, watching it inched into place on our carpet. We stood there admiring the old work of art, a perfect contrast to the red paint, and welcomed it to its new home.

"It will definitely need tuned," Mom said as if leaving us directions for babysitting along with the sheet music of my childhood, annotated with Mrs. Steven's penciled teachings.

"And remember to tell the piano tuner that because of being warped in the flood, the piano can't maintain a perfect middle C. It has to be tuned to itself."

"Don't we all?" I grinned back as she walked out the door.

The first song I taught Wil to play was *Heart and Soul*. We banged out happy variations for half an hour. I only wish I knew all the words.

Next I played Bach's *Minuet in G*, amazed that the faded book stayed open to the page of the piece I memorized for a recital in fifth grade, even more amazed that my brain and my fingers remembered each note. Scott, disgruntled with *his* brain, left the room, disappointed, "I can't read music anymore." I kept playing, determined to enjoy making music beneath my new red wall.

When Scott's first brain tumor symptom appeared on that October Saturday, I was painting my periwinkle wall in the bedroom. Eleven months later, painting with Rodeo Drive red, was like putting the second bookend on the survival-shelf of our year. I wanted my second colored wall to represent the completion of our journey. Color—ten feet high by fifteen wide—was my way to reclaim happiness, to insist on living a full-spectrum life.

I didn't know then how many more walls of my life would demand to be painted.

Only two questions matter: What color next and which wall?

I love having paint chips to ponder.

Mi shebayrach, avotaynu, m'kor ha-b'rakha l'motaynu.
May the source of strength, who blessed the ones before us,
Help us find the courage to make our lives a blessing.
                              —Debbie Friedman

37
Survivor Guilt

Another layer of life colors how we recovered from nine months of treatment. Summer turned into September, who reminded us how there is a time for every season. While we waited for Scott's next MRI at twelve weeks "post-transplant" to tell us whether his brain tumor was shrinking or growing or stable, we were faced with the news of many friends dying. Autumn's soft light and shrinking days flickered in the harsher light of mortality statistics for brain cancer patients—only one in three people survive past five years.

Our fears and grief combined into vivid dreams that gave us a sense of the mystery in death.

First we found out that Reverend Clyde MacDowell lost his brain tumor battle. Nobody told us when he died in June, perhaps because they didn't want Scott facing his high-dose chemo under a cloud of grief. When Scott did learn the truth, his soul sent him a dream.

"I was in the mountains on a summer day." Scott told me. "I was standing in a valley surrounded by mountains. Clyde was there, looking completely healthy, wearing a yellow parka and Levis. He smiled at me, then started walking across the valley. That's all it was, but I knew he was healed. It almost felt like I was awake and not dreaming."

One evening I had a girl's night out that felt like a gift from Reverend MacDowell for me. The two women who told us about him in the first place (who still went to Mission Hills Church where he had been the senior minister) invited me to a women's faith night that would feature Christian comedienne, Chonda Pierce, a perky blond stand-up from Tennessee. I enjoyed an inspirational gut-busting night of laughing until I cried. I sat in the church with my neighbor, Judy, and hundreds of other women listening to Chonda's stories of family and faith. What I remember most is Chonda's story about both of her sisters dying in a short time, followed by her father (a preacher) leaving the family not long after he performed the wedding for her brother. At her second sister's funeral, standing at the cemetery, Chonda yelled across the open grave, "Momma, we're droppin' like flies."

The topic of death must have hovered at home because even Wil was affected. At bedtime one night, Wil picked out *Just In Case You Ever Wonder* by Max Lucado, a Christmas gift from his cousins. The last page ends with a line about being together even in heaven, and Wil choked up and then so did I. Wil closed the book without a word and didn't want to say prayers that night.

But on another night, which gave me hope that Wil would be fine, I overheard Wil videotaping Scott. He narrated his home movie, "This is my dad, who had a brain tumor, which is a bad thing. But now he's all done going to the hospital, I hope—*I hope you know.*"

The next morning I received an email from my high-school boyfriend (long since married and a father himself) to tell me his father, Doug, was in the hospital with yet another brain tumor metastasized from skin cancer. Doug was like a second dad to me during the years I dated his son, and in a small-world twist, our parents had gone to Lakewood High School together in the mid '60s. In the early 1980s our families spent many happy summer days and winter weekends at the cabins in Leadville, fishing, hiking, cross-country skiing, laughing over card games after dinner. You can move beyond a teenage love affair but your heart remembers the connections.

"Dad is hemorrhaging," Jake's email read. "It may only be a few days. He's being moved to hospice tomorrow."

Two nights later I dreamed of attending a funeral in a forest. I couldn't remember the details, but I woke to find an email from Jake saying Doug had died at 3:30 a.m. The memorial service would be in Leadville the following Saturday. I cried.

The next night I had the big dream—in which Scott died—the one time in all of Scott's treatment or since that I dreamed he was dead. *In my dream, he's already gone and I'm just starting to realize I'll never see him alive again, that death is not temporary. A disembodied dream, being aware of your thoughts as you float, with only your thoughts as the dream. I am dream-thinking that I haven't let myself cry yet but I probably need to, especially before Scott's funeral. I'm pondering, now that he's dead, whether I truly believe in heartstrings, the idea that love connects us all the way to heaven, as I've been telling my son. I cry out in my dream-thought for a sign or a visitation from Scott to let me know we're still connected. No reply.*

When I awoke (and confirmed Scott was still breathing), my inner prag-
matist speculated that if we really did have to face Scott's funeral, we
wouldn't have a priest or a reverend who knew Scott, or even a church we
could call our own. I didn't feel the urge to pull out the Yellow Pages or decide on a church. I wondered if my own relationship to God was strong
enough to bring me peace and comfort, with enough to give Wil.

The night before Doug's funeral, my mom and I took Wil and two
neighbor boys to Elitch Gardens, Denver's oldest amusement park since
1890 which had recently been moved downtown and renovated. We'd been
planning the night at Elitch's for weeks and decided to go, then decided to
stay even when an brief afternoon thunderstorm threatened to ruin our fun.
I do not like amusement parks, as a general rule, because the rides make me
barf and the noise gives me a headache. That night, with the three boys, I
didn't ride any rides (except the swings which made me feel like flying
without wings). My mom and I stood watching as Wil, Sammy, and Jake
rode the miniature roller coaster, hooting and howling and grinning. Then
Sammy and Jake rode the Tower of Doom. I stood at the bottom, squeezing
Wil's hand, grateful he was too young for that ride, while we watched the
two older boys ascend to the top, awaiting their twenty-two-story vertical
free-fall.

"Oh, God! Their mother will kill me for letting them go on that ride,"
Mom whispered behind her hand. "But they *are* tall enough."

We stood there, looking up, clenching and bending our knees, screaming
and laughing each time the ride plummeted to the ground. It was as if our
own stomachs were on that ride. I never laughed or screamed so hard, nor
had so much fun just watching. What a gift, amusement parks are, to let us
experience fear and joy at the same time. Our night at Elitch's somehow set
the right tone for Doug's funeral the next morning, as if reminding me that
life is a wild ride, brief, scary, well worth the price.

In the middle of September, my grandma had a stroke. My mom did not
expect her to improve, so we drove over the mountains to Grand Junction to
visit her in the hospital. By the time we arrived, she was talking and moving
her left arm and hand, but her dementia had progressed. It was very hard to
see her, so shrunken and confused, not knowing who or where she was. I
gave her a long hug when I left, surprised by the force of her clear-hearted
love hugging me back. I swear her soul touched me in our embrace, telling
me, *Don't worry. I'm fine in here. Everything is all right. I love you.*

Gramma offered these semi-lucid words when she saw the tears in my eyes after our hug, "We've had a good life, haven't we? Not too much bad? We're all healthy, right?"

Surprising everyone, Gramma didn't die that year. We all wondered why.

As the weeks went on, we learned of more brain tumor deaths: Allie, who Scott met at radiation where she told us about Dr. Arenson's team at the Colorado Neurological Institute. If not for Allie, we might never have found CNI. My heart broke for her husband, John, who told me last time we saw each other at a chemo appointment how he had first fallen in love with Allie. He sounded so small when he called, saying he wanted to bring over something Allie left for us. He never did.

My college-friend Krista called to say her father, Jim, died with his family at his side, a peaceful goodbye. Jim surpassed the survival rates for lung cancer by years, but then the cancer metastasized to his brain. He lived even longer thanks to multiple successes with gamma knife treatment, but eventually his brain metastases were beyond treatment. I put myself in Krista's shoes, as a daughter, and in her mother's shoes, as a wife. I hoped I would be lucky, someday, with a peaceful farewell.

Scott's sister told us that her penpal's brother Jerry died, losing his brain tumor fight. Amie met her penpal through the American Brain Tumor Association (ABTA), providing sister to sister support. Amie wondered who she would talk to now.

Every brain tumor death felt like a parallel existence, a version of ourselves, dying, too. They were us, at a different phase of life. They were our Richards and Leslies, like in Richard Bach's *One*.

And then Mike Luparello died. Mike, the young man from New York who did his stem cell rescue twice, six weeks apart, who gave Scott the courage to do it once. This news hit closest to home.

I had not heard from Mike's wife, Kathy, for over a month. I was no longer reading the national BRAINTMR listserv and missed her email to the online support group. When I sent out the email inviting friends to Scott's November birthday party, she wrote back with the news. Mike had died not because his tumor outgrew any treatment but because he contracted *Pneumocystis carinii pneumonia* (PCP), an infection to which immune-suppressed patients such as with AIDS or cancer are susceptible.

I couldn't bring myself to tell Scott the news, not when we were coming close to his twelve-week MRI which would tell us whether his stem cell rescue had worked. We'd been holding onto Mike's success story as proof that Scott would survive, too. On top of all the other brain tumor deaths, I wanted to protect Scott for a few more days. I wanted some days of denial myself. But it was hard.

We found out another brain tumor patient, Craig, who we knew from the local support group, was in hospice. I wrote a letter to his wife, Bev, telling her how sorry we were. A young man, Brian, wasn't doing so well, his wife Angie told me by email, his tumor growing by twenty percent in three weeks. Yet another man, David, found out he was no longer a candidate for surgery with photodynamic therapy because his brain tumor had re-grown. We had not met David yet, nor his wife and their son, but Dr. Arenson had hoped that we could to give them encouragement. I wondered if we would ever meet in person after that. Then Julie's younger sister was diagnosed with breast cancer almost exactly a year after Julie.

Heartbreak, denial, not telling the truth, gave me bad dreams. I dreamed Scott's MRI showed new tumor growth and that Scott refused further treatment. My inner optimist rationalized the dream, writing in my journal, "In my heart I can't believe this MRI will show any re-growth because Scott seems to be doing so well."

When a friend emailed to ask how I was coping in this period without doctor appointments, waiting for the next MRI, I told her it wasn't so bad, trying to make it true by putting it in writing.

"We haven't been waiting, so much as finding our new stride, a new normal routine," I wrote back. "I know this MRI is supposed to be more conclusive about the success of the stem cell rescue, but how can that be when we haven't seen any definite tumor since Scott's surgery in March? For all anyone knows, since they haven't been back in his head to see it, that white 'enhancement' on the MRI is just necrosis, cell death. That's my belief, anyway, and my hope."

Scott's next MRI was in mid-October. Dr. Arenson showed us the films lit up on his office wall, the previous MRI next to the new one for comparison. Our eyes were becoming accustomed to the image of Scott's brain, the black hole left behind after two surgeries, edged by the hazy white nodule of unknown pathology, possibly tumor but more likely dead tissue.

"See there, the area of enhancement is shrinking and so is the cavity. That's a step in the right direction. I'm pleased to see this progress, and that's without any additional treatment since July. We'll hold off on

Tamoxifen or Thalidomide for now. Let's do another MRI in eight weeks. I'll see you at four weeks in between."

Scott and I smiled at each other, relatively calm at this good news—until we got in the car, me behind the wheel. We turned to each other after buckling our seat belts, before I started the engine, and gave each other a spontaneous high-five. Then I burst into tears of relief.

"I was so scared!" I said.

"Me, too. Whew."

We celebrated at the Fourth Story restaurant above The Tattered Cover, which had become our standard post-MRI tradition of gourmet lunch and a new book, both soul food. It felt bittersweet to celebrate when so many we knew had died or were dying. I wanted to toast them all—Allie, Mike, Doug, Jim, Craig, David, Jerry. I could imagine their spirits beside Scott at the table, toasting him in return, not begrudging us life. I couldn't make a toast without the whole truth.

"I have to tell you something. Mike Luparello died…back in September." As I gave Scott the details, his smile stopped and his breath fell out of his chest.

"I'm sorry I didn't tell you right away. It's been so hard this past month hearing of so many people who have died."

"I know. It makes the statistics seem so much more real."

"Do you ever feel guilty, you know, for still being alive?"

Scott sat in silence for several minutes before answering. He sipped his ice water with lemon, wiped his mouth with the red linen napkin. If our friends had been there in spirit, I know they would be shaking their heads, patting his shoulder. He looked at the books on the shelf next to our table, which decorated the restaurant, as if an answer might appear on the pages.

"No, I don't. I don't want to feel guilty—it seems like a waste of energy. I don't know why I'm still here. I'm nothing special, no more special than anyone else. But I can't feel guilty to be alive. I'm grateful to be here, for whatever reason. It's humbling to be alive when others don't make it. I guess it means I better make the most of the days I have here."

"Yep. If you're still here, I think it means you're not done yet."

It wasn't a book from The Tattered Cover that day, but one I found years later at a friend's mountain cabin that best describes what I have come to believe about death. It wasn't my book, only borrowed, but the words I found made me want to mark the page by turning down the corner. Then I noticed the corner was already creased into a tiny triangle. This is from *The*

Chosen by Chaim Potok, first published in 1967. He died of brain cancer in 2002. *I learned a long time ago, Reuven, that a blink of an eye in itself is nothing. But the eye that blinks, that is something. A span of life is nothing. But the man who lives that span, he is something.*

What else could we do but go on with living? As with each MRI, we felt a renewed ability to breathe a little deeper and plan a bit further ahead. I made plans in earnest to have a party at our house to celebrate Scott's thirty-fourth birthday and his one-year anniversary of survival. The caveat in my emailed invitations was that if anyone was sick or recently vaccinated with a live virus that could infect Scott, we hoped they would keep their germs at home instead of coming to Scott's party.

Scott's sister came up with an idea to help other patients, proposing "The Heartstrings Project" to the Colorado Neurological Institute. Her idea was to form a peer support group who would provide cookies during surgery, housecleaning, sidewalk snow shoveling, dog walking, or driving. Amie's original inspiration was my friend Jane's dad, Joe, who brought us Alfreda's oatmeal chocolate chip cookies during Scott's second surgery.

Amie didn't know about my heartstrings theory with Wil or how I was trying to translate my idea into a children's book. When she told me her plans over the phone, my first reaction was, "You can't use that word, that's mine." The next instant I realized our joint choice of words was a God thing. So of course I supported her, designing a logo and volunteering to help however I could. The Heartstrings Project was Amie's way of making sure that other sisters had someone to talk to and feel less alone.

Events conspired to set the Heartstrings Project in motion on a personal level. Brian's wife, Angie, sent me an email telling me about another Colorado couple facing a brain tumor. With another email I connected to Amy, whose husband Charlie was interested in what Dr. Arenson and the CNI team might propose for his tumor, and she mentioned they were new parents to a baby boy, Matthew. As we were leaving Scott's next checkup, there they were in the lobby of Dr. Arenson's office, same age as us, wearing Levis and sweaters and backpacks: Charlie, Amy, and Charlie's brother who was there to take notes. It felt like seeing ourselves if Scott's tumor had arrived when Wil was a baby. For all the connections that seemed to be ending, here was a new one.

In my post-birthday email, I mentioned that bright spot in our next step toward healing:

We had a nice gift from the universe last week to remind us just how far we've come—meeting one more newly diagnosed brain tumor patient. It is truly a gift to be in a position to now help others just stepping on this arduous path, able to empathize with their emotions and hopefully help them sort through some of the treatment decisions by sharing our story. In one year we certainly went through the full range of treatments and emotions and feel so blessed & lucky to still be here to talk about it.

I love my family, my children…
but inside myself is a place where I live all alone
and that's where you renew your springs that never dry up
—*Pearl S. Buck*

38
The Middle and Mexico

I don't want to talk about it. The middle. After Scott's one-year anniversary and his birthday.

The middle was the dark part. I didn't like it. I was tired. I was done.

It was hard. Harder than the months during Scott's treatment.

That surprised me.

Unexpected. Depressing. Exhausting.

The middle was the part when I wanted to run away.

I had a passport. By 1999, I didn't look a bit like my 1991 passport-photo self, my former self who wasn't a mother yet, who worked a fulltime career and flew overseas once a year, who wasn't burned out by cancer caregiving.

In 1999 I still had that passport and I wasn't afraid to use it.

Yes I was. I was afraid to leave and go too far. I was afraid I would never come back. What kind of horrible mother and wife would I be if I left? I was afraid if I left there would be an Emergency back at home and I wouldn't be there to fix it. What if I went somewhere and broke a bone or crashed a car on the wrong side of the road. Or even worse, what good stuff would I miss by not staying?

Such were my thoughts, like the song wondering *if I go there will be trouble; if I stay it will be double.*

What can you do, short of running away and not coming back? First, you have to tell someone how you feel, if only yourself. In my journal I admitted that I was starting to sag from the weight of the year. I wrote a brief note to myself:

I feel wiped out and on a very thin line, a shaky edge between being fine and completely burned out. I try to be thankful for being so busy with normal concerns, like Wil in school. But I'm also sad at the lack of time I've had to rejuvenate myself, to have time for writing the kid's and adult books, for journaling, for being with my friends.

As one remedy, I tried to step back into my old life of gourmet dinner nights with girlfriends. I signed up through FEMALE to join the next open group and found myself in a beautiful house at a dining room table with women I barely knew. They knew me because all year they'd been reading my Scott-update emails. One woman was new to our chapter, however, and didn't know my whole story. As much as I thought I wanted to move past my cancer-caregiving year, I found myself telling the story.

I talked from the first glass of wine through dinner and into dessert. I told about Scott's treatments from surgery to radiation to another surgery, chemo, chemo, chemo, then high dose chemo and his stem cell rescue. I told how Wil was wary of Scott now, how Wil was grinding his teeth, angry at me. I told how Scott could not work, probably ever again, about the paperwork for disability, about his deficits like a lousy short-term memory.

I was used to hearing the ohs and wows and "you've been through so much" kind of comments. But then the hostess asked me a question I didn't expect.

"So, can you live with what's left?"

I paused, stunned. Anger flared in me like the candle sputtering in the floral centerpiece.

"Well, of course," I replied. But then I wasn't so sure.

That was the last gourmet dinner I attended through FEMALE.

I can't remember why I was driving across town one afternoon by myself, but I've never forgotten the moment. I was heading west on Iliff Avenue over I-25. I fantasized about turning north at Colorado Boulevard and driving straight to the airport, wondering how much it would cost to buy a ticket at an airport counter for immediate departure, without any luggage. Where would I go, if I had the guts and reckless abandon to leave?

As I pondered this notion, something like an invisible backseat driver urged me to look out the passenger window. Walking along the narrow gravel-strewn sidewalk was a bearded young man wearing a backpack, carrying a sleeping bag, and holding hands with a little boy the same size as Wil. If I'm not mistaken, they were homeless.

Seeing the pair extinguished my flight-fantasy as quickly as stepping on the brakes to avoid a collision. *That wouldn't happen to Scott and Wil if I left,* I told myself.

How do you know? myself replied.

Can a cautionary tale be told by a man and a boy on the side of the road?

The truth about wanting to run away is that I wanted an escape, but I didn't want to leave my life forever. I just needed a vacation, a true vacation. I needed a rest based on honest self care, not a reckless decision based on panic or hopeless despair.

What gave me perspective was a memory from the previous spring, one evening at the brain tumor support group at University Hospital. The support group always began with patients and family in one room, and then we caregivers breaking out to a separate room of our own where we could speak freely, unshackled. I remember on that particular night the words of a tall woman with long, straight blond hair, pretty without makeup. In her Levis and plaid blouse she looked like a wholesome farm girl who could have lived a carefree California surfer-girl's lifestyle if given the chance. Her husband had been going through brain tumor treatment for over a year.

"I went home, back to Iowa, to stay with my parents on their farm for a week. It's the first time I felt like I could sleep through the night without worrying about my husband. I knew I needed to get away for a break, but I never imagined that a simple week back home would be so refreshing. I feel like I grounded myself where my roots are. I had time with my mom, my sister, some of my childhood friends. It was so nice to be taken care of and gather my energy. I feel like I can keep going now."

She looked around the room, seeming almost guilty at her reprieve, probably because the rest of us looked so jealous. She added, "I highly recommend it."

After remembering that woman who took a short break from caregiving, I wrote in my journal, testing out travel options in private, framing my options as a positive step. But in my dreams that night I still felt guilty.

I am far away from home, being chased and hiding from a posse, The Law, who look more like a dusty gang of bad guys in a B-rated Western. First I am walking through town, just avoiding them, and then I am inside a bungalow with a group of girlfriends trying to be nonchalant. Then I panic, laying on the floor to look out a low window. As the posse comes up the sidewalk of the house, I run into a small hall closet, afraid that the dogs in the house will sniff at the closet door and give away my hiding place. The closet is so shallow that I lean against the back wall and my knees, shaking, are braced against the door. High on the wall is a lace curtain and I think perhaps the curtain might hide me. I think that if I were shot dead through the door, at least I wouldn't know when to expect it and then death would be easier to accept. I wonder if I could hide in the guacamole dip on the kitchen table and I ponder, "If I was the guacamole and they ate me, would I disappear?" Is that my escape

plan? Soon the posse is gone and I emerge from the closet to go talk with my friends,
pretending that nothing is wrong.

I blamed the dream on late-night reading of *Like Water for Chocolate*, but I
knew my desperate dream was saying I better try telling the truth. I had a
chance to do just that over dinner one night. Julie, Kathy, and Debi sat with
me at the Tres Margaritas on County Line Road. I ordered cheese enchiladas
and, since I wasn't driving, a frozen margarita. As had been happening lately, my angst seemed to dominate the conversation. I said I didn't want to
talk about it, but I couldn't stop talking. In between mouthfuls of tortilla
chips and guacamole, I talked about the December MRI, how the next one
would be in March. How we had three months between deadlines, three
months before we could know whether it was safe to keep living.

I took a long sip through the straw. The tequila tasted good. What I said
next surprised even me.

"Some days I'm so tired I wish he would just hurry up and die."

I can't blame the tequila. I looked deep into my margarita so that I
wouldn't see their silent gasps and shocked glances. I will always be grateful they didn't admonish me.

"God, I can't believe I just said that."

Julie, Kathy, and Debi put their hands out toward mine over the near-
empty plates on the table, all for one, one for all.

"You need a vacation," Julie said, with Kathy and Debi nodding.

"Where would you like to go?" Kathy asked.

"Hawaii?" I said. "I don't know. A tropical beach sounds good. In Hawaii I wouldn't have to worry about speaking another language. But that's
really too far. I'd freak out to be an ocean away, and it's too expensive."

"You could go to my cabin for as long as you want," Julie offered.

"Thanks. I've thought of that, actually. But I'm afraid one call from home
and I'd be back again before I even had time to relax."

"We will figure out something," Julie said.

A few days later, Julie called me with the solution.

"Remember how we were going to come up with $100 from 50 friends to
cover the copay for Scott's stem cell rescue? Well, just because you didn't
need that money doesn't mean we can't do the same thing to help you.
What helps keep you sane also keeps Scott healthy, right? So here's my idea.

"I've sent an email to twenty or so women who know you well and
we've come up with enough money to send you to Mexico for a week.

We're sending you to Puerto Vallarta to a hotel that I've been to a bunch, an all-inclusive resort where you won't have to think about anything once you're there. The food, drinks, room—all paid for. The beaches are beautiful and the pool and the rooms. Then you can totally relax."

"No way. Are you kidding?" I was shocked by the generosity of my friends and her initiative to find a way to help me. "Really?"

"Yes, really. I will book it through Apple Vacations, which includes cheap airfare. You pick a date and I'll make the arrangements."

"Wow. You're the best. Wow. Let me think about a date. Maybe in January for my birthday. I have to tell Scott. Ask my mom and his if they will help take care of Wil while I'm gone."

"We can help with Wil. Any of us are happy to make play dates or take him to preschool or anything. We can even make dinners for Scott while you're gone. We don't want you to worry about a thing. Just go and come home refreshed."

My mom concurred when I told her. "If you don't go now, I can see a day coming when you leave and don't come back." She knew me so well.

I contemplated asking someone to go with me, but I wanted them to take care of Scott and Wil more.

And so it was arranged. I left in mid-January on a pre-dawn Tuesday morning. Kathy drove me to the airport, after I said a stoic farewell to Scott and Wil, who both sat in tears and pajamas on the bottom stair by the front door. I borrowed bikinis and Fresh Produce dresses, packed my floppy straw hat, my laptop, and $100 in travelers checks, believing that would be plenty.

As I walked through the airport, I remembered my first outing after Wil was born. I wondered if anyone could tell by my tired eyes, my impressive chest, or my still-sore hobbling walk that I was a new mother. That day in the airport wearing my beach hat and dress, I wondered if anyone could tell I was a burned-out wife escaping cancer caregiving for a week. Of course they couldn't. I was glad to be anonymous. I was looking forward to it—a whole week of not knowing a soul, not having to talk or do anything except what I wanted. What would I do?

I woke up the first morning at the hotel to discover that the lids to the water bottles in my refrigerator were not factory-sealed but broken already, fake and refilled, that my balcony was on the north and would never see sunshine, and that my left eye had pink eye. I was pissed. What did I do to deserve this? Would I get sick from drinking the water? Should I ask to move to a sunnier room? Did I pick up a germ at the airport bathroom (why couldn't I wait?) and then touch my eye? Where would I find medicine? What would happen if I poured tequila in my eye as antiseptic? *Bad idea, don't try it,* I cautioned myself.

I walked downstairs to the pool, sat there a minute trying to read but fuming instead. So I went back to my room, by way of the stairs, and found on the landing that I stood at the door to the hotel physician. I went through the door and the doctor greeted me. "Pink eye," he said as soon as he saw me. He gave me a tube of ointment and an invoice for $80 U.S.

"Eighty dollars?" I asked.

"Do you want the medicine or not?"

"Fine. Do you take traveler's checks? I have to go get them in my room. I'll be right back."

Twenty dollars left of my traveler's checks. So much for souvenirs.

That's how my week in Mexico started. It got better after that, and worse. I spent the days on the beach, reading *Welcome to the World, Baby Girl* on a towel in the warm sand. Then I saw a spot on my arm that looked like ring worm. I blamed it on the beach and thought it lucky that Scott and his immune system had not come to Mexico, too.

I ate every meal alone and didn't care when noisy families looked my way in pity. I made up silly stories in my mind about the four kittens that frolicked on the restaurant patio and the slow iguana under the palm tree. In my hotel room I set up my laptop and tried writing various versions of my heartstrings story. I organized my year's worth of email updates on Scott into files, preparing to someday write a book, but I couldn't bring myself to reread the ones during his stem cell rescue.

At night I cried. I called Scott collect and wished I were home, missing him and Wil, mad about my pink eye and the resulting lack of cash to do anything fun like snorkel or shop, wishing I hadn't come alone. Scott said I should come home early. I wasn't ready for that, despite my angst. It dawned on me that I wasn't in Mexico to party. It was okay to be there to grieve and be sad.

I wrote in my journal: *Funny to have gone through the crisis in my Pollyanna mode and only now when everyone thinks it's time to celebrate, I am finally ready to be sad and tired and angry. Angry?*

Angry. I didn't know what to do with that. So I went to sleep asking to wake up peaceful and rested. I slept without waking. The bags under my eyes were deep, but I almost felt a smile on my face all the next day. At breakfast a big sigh escaped me. I had a massage (charged to my room not cash) that unknotted my muscles as I consciously let go of my responsibilities and fatigue and everything that had been resting on my shoulders. *Release, revive, relax, renew,* I said to myself as I surrendered my knots. I walked up the beach. I floated in the water. I saw a whale jump. I watched a movie in my room (*Ever After*) and ordered filet mignon from room service.

One day toward the end of the week I went to downtown Puerto Vallarta. I rode a bus from the hotel with two other tourists, Marion and Ivan, who helped me find a bank where I could charge my VISA for $50 worth of pesos. I bought string puppets for Wil, a t-shirt for Scott, and tampons for me (necessity not souvenir). I walked up the street past tourist shops, not wanting to haggle with vendors, and down side streets, looking for the bus stop back. By the time I returned to the hotel I had a raging headache, a raspy cough, and wanted to scrub in the shower. The day drained me.

On my last day in Mexico I lay in the sun all day long, soaking up every last bit of solitude and releasing every last grain of stress into the sand. I ate hot French fries and a cold Corona for lunch. I splurged for another massage. I bargained with a fat local woman to spend the last of my dollars to put braids and beads in my hair, though she didn't believe it was really the last of my money. I finished the third mindless paperback book I brought with me as if that were the signal my vacation had ended.

That night I called home to check in with Scott and Wil before my next-morning flight. As I had on every phone call, I told Wil how much I missed him.

"Well, it's already tomorrow that you'll get to see me," he said.

I couldn't wait to get home.

Turns out, that was the whole point of my trip to Mexico—becoming ready to go home again. I had my week to escape, to experience angst at aloneness, to begin to grieve, to relax, to rejuvenate. I could always have another short break—I was allowed more than one. But I needed that break in Mexico to remind myself why I was willing to be a wife and a mother, and even a caregiver. Being home again with Wil and Scott, and the remnants of Scott's brain tumor, wouldn't be perfect, but it was better than being alone. Love was worth it. And so was vacation.

39
Welcoming Grace

I came home from my week in Mexico revived and ready to face the new year. We survived Scott's cancer treatments, we survived Y2K, and as far as I could tell, I survived a nasty bout of acute caregiver burnout. Every three months we would repeat the MRI process of waiting, wondering, and holding our breath to see what showed up on the scans. If Scott's brain scans stayed clear, it felt like life could proceed. If the scans didn't...well, I couldn't think about that.

With the new year, new millennium, and new lease on life, it was time to get organized for whatever came next. It was time to get back to reality.

Scott kept busy with physical therapy appointments, a follow-up neuropsychological evaluation to see how his brain was functioning (better than last year but not back to normal speed yet), and his own handyman project in our basement. In the fall, we received a lump sum of cash from Social Security, the back pay for six months of permanent disability. Since we had not expected the money, we considered putting it all in the bank, but instead, we decided to finish our basement. It felt like a decadent act to pick up our life where we left off before Scott's brain tumor. The basement became an unspoken metaphor for rebuilding our life from the foundation up.

The practical fact of the metaphor was that a finished basement would mean (1) a desk of Scott's own for his computer and bookshelves of programming books — allowing me an office to myself again, (2) space for Wil to be rowdy with other kids, (3) a private guest bedroom and bath, (4) a higher resale value if we found ourselves unable to meet the mortgage, and/or (5) a feasible option to rent the basement as a garden level apartment with its own entry in case our financial situation grew dire with our lump sum depleted. Scott's dad, master builder that he is, took care of the subcontractors for framing, drywall, and electrical. My dad, architect and renovator, along with my Uncle Mac, took care of the plumbing in the crawl space under the floor and hooking up sinks, toilet, and tub.

Finally, the men had something constructive to do.

I started planning in earnest to open my own one-woman website design company. I couldn't face the thought of returning to a full-time corporate job, being gone all day. I figured a home-based business was my best option for having flexible hours to still take care of Wil and Scott. My goal within a year was to be earning enough money to afford health insurance. My biggest concern was the $946 monthly cost for Scott's high-dose Tamoxifen, which Dr. Arenson prescribed for two years, 10 pills a day. We'd have prescription coverage on COBRA, but once Scott went on Medicare he would not have any prescription coverage (in 2000, Medicare did not yet offer drug benefits). Really, prescriptions and COBRA and health insurance are topics for which caregivers should seek expert advice. I only mention the whole messy deal now to put my financial concerns in perspective.

A friend and financial author asked me to help him build a website for his upcoming book, and with that I had my first client. My second client came right out of our cancer experience with the Colorado Neurological Institute. I submitted a marketing proposal to CNI that outlined all the ways, including an overhaul of their website, to make sure the Institute didn't stay Denver's best kept secret. I was awarded the job after demonstrating my skills to disprove some concerns about giving the website work to a patient's wife.

On March 15th, I signed the corporate license papers to open Brainstorm Communications Corporation.

The irony did not escape me and Scott that I was the one opening my own computer consulting company, which Scott always wanted to do, while he had all the time in the world to play around the house, which I loved to do. I couldn't dwell on that irony. Learning more about website design invited my brain to focus on something creative and fun. Starting my own business was like adding a new member to the family, one that would need nurtured and demand much of my time.

Through all those months of putting life back together again, my mommy pangs never ceased. I couldn't help hoping for another child—no matter how irrational, inconvenient, and literally inconceivable. I still felt that desire for a sibling for Wil, another soul for our family to love. I tried to let go, yet every month I found myself wishing for a miracle despite Scott's high-dose chemo that was said to cause permanent sterility, not to mention my own troubles with getting pregnant again. I might as well have been wishing for Immaculate Conception. I wondered how many miracles our family might get. While part of me hoped it might happen, another part of me did not ever expect my wish to true.

I didn't consider that my wish might come true in another form. Kathy Matsey, nearly nine-months pregnant, called one Monday mid-March with an invitation I couldn't refuse.

"I was wondering if you would like to be with me in the room when I deliver the baby," she asked. "We set the date for Friday to induce labor. I've invited Julie, too. Jim and I would love for you both to be there."

"Oh, my gosh! I would love to. Are you sure? That would be completely amazing."

"Yes, really. I'd love for my Ya Ya's to be there to welcome her into the world," Kathy said, referring to our recent favorite book. "You and Julie will be special aunties to her. She's going to be our Petite Ya Ya."

Kathy knew just how to put frosting on the cake of our past year. Julie had come through her own year of breast cancer, and I came through my year of caring for Scott. Kathy was key supporter for both of us, fielding phone calls, listening to our private worries and wishes, taking care of our little boys along with her son, J.J., whenever we asked. Now she was offering us a chance to be present to celebrate life at the very first breath. Heck, this wasn't just frosting; this was one big candle to light and blow out with a wish.

On that Friday, I leaned shoulder to shoulder with Julie as we witnessed a new life emerge into the world. Jim stood next to Kathy's side, coaching her through contractions and holding her hand. Julie and I stood a few feet back from the hospital bed, out of the way of the nurses and doctor. We kept looking at each other, beaming at our luck to take part in the moment.

"You can send us out anytime if you change your mind, Kathy," I offered, and Julie nodded agreement.

"No, you're fine. Will you take pictures when she comes out?"

Kathy breathed bravely through her contractions, and her body knew what exactly to do. At six minutes past noon, a head of dark hair appeared, then a nose. The almost-here baby peeped open one eye, as if checking to see she was in the right room, and then she closed both eyes tight for Kathy's final push. And voila! She was out. We knew a girl was on her way, but we couldn't know how much love would flow into the room upon her arrival, like a whoosh of wonder and light streaming from the tips of her perfect ten tiny pink toes.

As the nurses cleaned and weighed our new baby girl in a clear plastic crib on a cart, she cried a minute, filling her lungs, and then she was contentedly quiet. She looked around the room with old-soul eyes and seemed to smile at the nurses as they measured her: seven pounds, six ounces, twenty inches long, head diameter thirteen and three-quarter inches. Apgar score, a perfect 10.

Jim carried the flannel-clad baby to Kathy, who snuggled and kissed her beautiful daughter.

"Hi Grace Danielle," she whispered.

Jim took Grace, whispering secret dad-love stuff. He handed her first to Julie, then to me, as he took the camera to capture the moment for us.

"Gracie, this is your special Julie and your special Shelly," he said. "They're going to take good care of you as you grow up."

We all grinned at each other. I thought in my head I would hear the tones of *Amazing Grace*. Instead, I kept hearing the strolling melody, *My girl, my girl, my girl...talking 'bout my girl.*

That night, I created a website for Grace, posting her debut photos to share with her relatives across the country, around the world. I found a tinny-sounding midi file of *My Girl* to serenade the pink and yellow daisies in the background.

Every night for a week I had baby-girl dreams. In none of the dreams was the baby my own, but I was helping to feed and care for her in each one. One night I dreamed of holding Grace and twice she spoke my name out loud. I loved her already, and I believed she loved me.

One year before, I mentally let go of my last pink balloon, my metaphorical version of hope. With Grace Matsey's arrival on earth, my pink balloon landed.

Why did the chicken cross the road?
To show the raccoon it could be done.

40

Victory Tour

I love road trips, but I dread the long drive. The second summer after Scott's brain tumor, we went on our Vickroy Victory Tour. Four thousand miles in less than three weeks. Twelve-hour days on a mission to get to the next friend's house in time for dinner. I did most of the driving because Scott was still recovering his stamina from his nine months of brain tumor treatment.

Yes, we could have picked just one state, or two. Yes, we could have flown and rented a car. Or we could have gone on a cruise and told all about it in our next Christmas letter. But while Scott was starting his last round of chemo in June 1999, we set the goal of taking a trip the following summer. We needed to physically hug everyone who had been so supportive, spiritually and emotionally. We needed to make contact.

I visualized our 4,000 mile loop like this: *It was like putting out your right arm and spinning in a big, slow circle, scooping up love and positive energy from everyone we saw and everywhere we went, storing it up until we saw them again.*

I can tell you the states we traveled on our Victory Tour—Colorado, Kansas, Missouri, Alabama, Tennessee, Ohio, Michigan, Wisconsin, Minnesota, North Dakota, South Dakota, Wyoming, home again. Just like I could tell you the route of Scott's brain tumor treatment from the day he was diagnosed—surgery, radiation, tumor doubled, second surgery (awake), chemo, chemo, chemo, high-dose chemo and stem cell rescue.

Long way to go, huh? Impressive in a "glad it was you-not-me" kind of way. But it doesn't tell you much about the fun we had, the people we met, or what we learned along the way. I won't bore you with a slide by slide show.

Instead, here's what we learned about road trips (and cancer survival).

1. Always bring your own pillow and a box of your favorite necessities from the medicine chest in your bathroom at home.

2. Don't trust Mapquest or GPS to always know the way. Mapquest doesn't chart all the roads and Ivan, the GPS voice, stutters when you don't follow directions, "Nuh, nuh, nuh, no." Besides, where you're going might not even be on the map.

3. Whoever is driving gets to pick out the music. You should agree in advance to sing along to *Do, Re, Mi* at least once, but not not-at-all.

4. You should enunciate if you say "Let's have lunch at Arby's." Your Airstream-fanatic kid might think you are lunching at a dealership called RVs.

5. Listen to the camera salesman when he suggests the digital camera that uses AA batteries instead of the rechargeable type. That way, in case you leave the battery charger at your last stop, you can just go buy batteries.

6. If you leave the camera charger at your first stop, remember that you can buy disposable cameras and get a CD of photos, if you must, when you get the film developed. (Have the charger—and also that swimsuit and sock—shipped straight back home, because it will never catch up with you on the road.)

7. Recovering brain tumor survivors should not drive in big cities. Give them the straight-aways, but never ask them to find a parking place amid a construction zone at the St. Louis Arch.

8. Most big landmarks, museums, and tourist attractions have long lines and expensive entry prices. If you have only thirty minutes because you're due down the road in six hours for dinner, just go to the gift shop. Or call and say you'll be at dinner tomorrow instead.

9. Pay attention to the color and species of flowers along the highways. It appears that each state's highway department plants flowers to match their football team colors.

10. Take a turn buckled in the backseat. You will have a new appreciation for how kids feel without control of the wheel. Look out the windows while snacking on gingersnaps to avoid getting carsick.

11. Don't start hating the driver. You must realize, in most cases, it's the road, those bumps, grooves, cracks, potholes and patches, not the driver. A side note to drivers: If you slow down even a little, everyone in the car will feel better and the road will feel smoother.

12. If going sixty you pass a stack of canoes in twelve different colors, gleaming with morning dew, stop, backup and take a picture. Ironical-

ly, if you never take a photo, it may still be your most memorable image, but you'll never stop looking for the four-by-six glossy.

13. Be sure you have the correct area code and driving directions for every person you plan to visit. It's better than driving around in the dark, lost and hungry, with the wrong phone number.

14. It's always okay to stop and ask for directions. But be sure to ask someone who knows.

15. If a cuss word escapes past your lips and does a demon dance on the dashboard, roll down the window, swat it out in the breeze, tell everyone that's what you're doing, then apologize. Let fresh air enter the car.

16. Bringing two bottles of wine as a hostess gift is a great idea because you can offer to uncork one on arrival. Then say, "Oh yes, I'll have some. Biggie size it!"

17. Watch your kid's fingers when closing car doors and doors to any popup campers ya'll enter.

18. If you visit someone you may never see again, spend all day asking them every question you've always wanted to ask. If you see them again, you'll have more to talk about. If you don't, you'll have peace about leaving nothing unsaid.

19. Hug hello, hug goodbye, and hug often while you visit.

20. Schedule in lazy days with nothing to do, nowhere to go, nobody to see.

21. Accept detours as adventures, even if it means 400 miles out of your way.

22. If you find yourself on the coastline of Lake Superior, 200 miles north of where you expected to be, get out and take a family photo. Wade in the water, even if it's freezing. You will warm up again, but you may never return to that beach.

23. If you find yourself in a disgusting and overpriced resort, don't stay. Leave right away. Insist on a refund, or eat the cost and tell yourself it's cheaper than the price of regret.

24. If you're eating spaghetti in Fargo but the waitress says, "The tornado and flash flood will be here in fifteen minutes. Can I get you anything else?" and you say, "A tornado shelter?" and she says, "We don't have one, just the restroom," ask to see the dessert menu, then get it to-go.

25. Don't drive under flooded highway underpasses. Let your aunt from Fargo do it.

26. Let yourself laugh til you cry. Two points for snorting. (When we saw an old porcelain stove sitting out in the middle of a farm field, with no farm buildings in site, Wil quipped, "Somebody must be cooking out.")

27. If you get to Mount Rushmore, but your neck is so twisted from sleeping on the bad pillow at the most expensive, disgusting hotel on your trip, it's perfectly okay to skip the gift shop, skip the tour, give a wave to Abe Lincoln and the rest of the heads, and head home.

28. Make the brain tumor survivor drive the last twelve hours home through Wyoming. After all, if it wasn't for him, you would be on a beach in Hawaii right now.

29. Don't be surprised if by the time you get home, you begin thinking about where else you could live if you were ready to go somewhere new.

Let's get the clichés out of the way: life is a highway, cancer is a journey, what a trip, there's a long road ahead. The thing about road trips is that you have chosen to take that trip, even though you may swear never to do it again. I recommend a cross-country drive at least once in your life to see the states up close and personal. With cancer, you don't get a choice but if you find yourself on that road, you might as well pay attention and find something that makes the trip worth the expense and your time.

Cancer is like going on a cross-country road trip with one day to get ready, not knowing when you'll return. Cancer caregiving is like being the one responsible to make the lists, to pack the car not only with clothes, but snacks, maps, and music, and to arrange for cat sitter, lawn mower, putting mail and newspapers on hold, and to do most of the driving, and to pay all the bills, develop the film, restock your fridge and find a place for the souvenirs when you get home. Cancer caregiving is like going to see his relatives, not yours, and even if you love them, it's exhausting to be on your best guest behavior.

Cancer survival is like realizing you've done all the fun things on your itinerary and you're as far out as you intended to go, but it hits you: You still have to drive all the way back. And you can't get home without driving through all the Great Plains. The farm reports on the radio don't mean diddly to you, you're out of touch with the national news, and you're ready to fling every CD out the window. You realize everything, everyone, smells a bit odd. You realize, when the fun part is over, that it's just you and your immediate family still in the car (unless they jump out near an airport and fly home without you, or they ditch you at a gas station and sing *Do Re Mi* all the way home).

Caregiver burnout is like getting home from that road trip, too tired to tell anyone if you had any fun, dreading laundry and Monday.

Acknowledge your end-of-vacation blues. It takes time to adjust to your home time zone again. If necessary, start planning your real dream vacation.

I propose this roadworthy advice because I've been on more road trips since then. It's all easier said than done. I didn't know then that the challenge with cancer survival, and coming home after a long trip, is to find ways to love the life you're left with, to trust that the best is yet to be, to realize you're free to make changes. The transition back takes longer than nursing the last mosquito bite, shaking the last sand from your shoes, removing a seashell from a suitcase, framing a postcard, finding shelf space for a quirky souvenir, or climbing back into your own bed at last. Perhaps when you wake up one day, you'll see life through new eyes.

Ask yourself, now, where would you like to go next? Of course, staying home is a valid answer, too.

The real voyage of discovery consists not in
seeking new landscapes but in having new eyes.
—*Marcel Proust*

41
Late Summer Surprises

That summer after our Victory Tour, it was hard to be back home in reality and even harder to see into our future. Every week it seemed I was being disappointed further by the sad state of Medicare and the cost and availability of insurance coverage for someone like Scott with pre-existing conditions, on Social Security disability, and under 65 years old. I was finding out that only seniors qualified for the Medi-Gap plans to cover prescriptions and other items that Medicare wouldn't—even the insurance consultants who came to our house full of confidence in selling us a plan were dismayed to discover that fact. I didn't know how I was going to manage financially, even with my growing website design business. Our mortgage and utilities alone would eat up the entire amount of Scott's monthly Social Security check. The private policy he had would cover the other basics, but didn't leave much for leftovers.

With our basement almost finished, Scott was running out of things to do. The first day he mowed the lawn in the spring, Scott cried happy tears because during his chemo the summer before he didn't think he'd ever mow the lawn again. By mid-summer, Scott remembered that lawn mowing was overrated. He wanted to go back to work, yet every six months he had to sign a form testifying that he had too many neurological deficits to be working. It is a cruel aspect of long-term disability paperwork—looking for all the signs that your brain is rewiring itself and improving, then having to sign a form saying it's not true. Social Security doesn't ask—grade three brain tumors are on the "approved" list. But private policies want to confirm every six months in case you're faking a backache—but who fakes a brain tumor?

Summer's high point was our three weeks on vacation, out on the road visiting friends and seeing new places. The rest of the summer went downhill. What I remember most is how Scott got a hair transplant in July, followed by his shingles in August. I wasn't allowed to tell anyone about the hair transplant, except our immediate family. The statute of limitations has expired on that secret by now.

The newspaper article published in May 2000 about Scott's status as a cancer survivor, as a follow-up to the article the previous spring, resulted in a surprising phone call from a head and neck surgeon. "I saw your story in the newspaper and thought I could help. I do hair transplants and would like to offer one for you at no cost to yourself. Perhaps we could cover up some of your scar. I've never done a hair transplant for someone who had radiation, but I think it should work just the same."

The surgeon gave Scott a website to view for more details on the procedure, asking that we not tell anyone because he wished to stay anonymous and not become known as the doctor who did this procedure for free. He had helped a popular local television newscaster, he said, whose hair looks much fuller now.

Scott had to think about the offer for a few days, weighing in on his desire for better hair. Scott couldn't see his scar above his left ear toward the top of his head. Unless he looked in two mirrors at once, he couldn't see how his male-pattern bald spot had slipped off lopsided to the left where radiation zapped it. During his year of treatment, Scott wore a blue corduroy ball cap, which covered more of his head than most caps. But, even though we lived in Colorado, land of hat-wearing men, Scott couldn't wear it everywhere. He couldn't help feeling self conscious at restaurants, at the grocery store, anywhere people would sit or stand behind him and see that big awkward scar. Some scars you can wear as a badge of honor. Some scars come with more stigma attached. Scott imagined people wondering "Geez, that guy had his head opened up. I wonder what's wrong with him."

"I'd like to try the surgery," Scott told me after doing some research. "It's not like it's brain surgery. Plus, it's outpatient with only a local anesthesia."

"Are you sure you want to go through any kind of surgery again?"

"I'd like to cover up some of my radiation bald spot, even for a few years before I go fully bald from old age. Assuming I live long enough to go bald from old age."

"Okay…I guess. It is your decision. But we better ask your doctors about it to see if they have any objections or concerns."

Scott told Dr. Arenson, who agreed the surgery was okay. "Self image after cancer is important," he agreed, "Even for men."

The procedure entailed cutting a long narrow strip of Scott's own scalp from low on the back of his head. It came from underneath where his hair was still growing strong, where the scar would go unseen like a hidden zipper. Each hair and intact follicle was separated into tiny plugs. Imagine using two scalpels like a fork and steak knife to separate hair follicles so that each resulting piece looked like a single bee stinger. The doctor would then pierce Scott's scalp full of slits in which, using tweezers, each follicle would be planted, one at a time. In theory, after a few days, each hair would take root and start to grow, resulting in a lush head of your very own hair. After a weekend at home, sleeping very carefully on a pillow so as not to disturb the new seedlings, and foregoing shampooing for maybe a week, poof—a crop of new hair with no one the wiser.

If only it were that simple. Some hair grew in. Most didn't, likely because of radiation damage to his scalp. But worse than that, where the IV with the sedative went into Scott's left forearm, his vein swelled up with painful phlebitis, or superficial blood clot. Scott had to see his family physician several times about that painful side effect and eventually consulted a vascular surgeon who offered to strip the vein. (Serendipity was the cure: using a power tool to sand paint from a door seemed to jiggle and disintegrate the clot. We have no medical proof that *that* is what worked.)

Since I couldn't tell anyone about the hair transplant, I cheated and in an otherwise honest email, I put in a prayer-request plug for Scott's hair. (Please forgive me, everyone, for deceiving you.)

If you wouldn't mind, for the sake of Scott's 1-year anniversary since his stem cell rescue, send an extra prayer and positive energy to him for his continued recovery and healing. And how about a boost to his hair that it keeps on growing like crazy to cover up the last remaining visible reminder of that long-gone tumor.

I must admit, the blood on Scott's scalp from his hair transplant procedure was way worse for me than the nice tidy staples and stitches of his brain surgeries. It drove me crazy to be back in the doctor's office again for Scott's vein in his arm, for something he elected to undergo (and knowing I approved in the first place). I wish he never had that damn surgery.

As if that weren't enough, we were blindsided by fate a few weeks later. We could not have been more surprised if an overzealous angel sporting a football helmet had appeared out of nowhere, charged across the room and—THWACK!—slammed into Scott, tackling him to the ground and knocking me out in the process, then jumped up shouting, "Ha! Gotcha! Get up! Get up! The game's not over yet!"

It happened at one of the vein-pain follow-ups with his family doctor when Scott felt a twitching sharp pain running between the top of his ear and the corner of his left eye. As Scott sat on the exam table, he mentioned it to the nurse, who looked more closely at Scott's face. We saw Doug's eyes widen.

"It's turning into a red streak as we speak," Doug said. "I bet you have herpes zoster, or shingles. Let me go get the doctor."

She didn't need much time to diagnosis that, sure enough, those were shingles appearing on the side of Scott's face. If after being blindsided you can summon any gratitude, it could be for a drug called Valtrex that shortens the duration and lessens the severity of shingles, if prescribed early enough. That's what she prescribed for Scott.

"What *are* shingles?" Scott asked, "And why me, why now?"

"Shingles is caused by the *varicella-zoster* virus, the same virus that causes chicken pox. After you've had chicken pox, it lies dormant in your body in certain nerve cells. Stress can bring out shingles, and they are common in the elderly. Interestingly, shingles are very common in patients after bone marrow transplants, like your stem cell rescue."

With that, Scott was back in patient mode, and I was back in caregiver and driver-to-appointments mode. What else can you do after being tackled but stand and dust yourself off? (Maybe throw a temper tantrum on the ground for a few minutes?)

Scott had to see a corneal specialist every day for awhile to make sure his cornea wasn't damaged by the shingles. He took steroid eye drops and had to wear dark glasses. Any light was painful. It was almost like quarantine all over again after Scott's photodynamic therapy.

Scott was lucky, however, that his shingles didn't manifest through the mass of nerves all over his torso, like so many people, because that causes unbearable pain.

When I told Wil that Daddy was sick again, Wil's reaction was more honest than my own. "Oh great, now Dad's gonna get all the attention again. Everything's about Dad, Dad, Dad."

Scott's next MRI was the last day of August. Scott and I were both depressed during the week leading up to it. To make it worse, Wil was dealing with a third-grade bully and his best friend at school who teamed up to tease Wil that his dad was a no-brainer. If life wasn't so raw, it might have been funny.

I was tired, worn out from the hard month. When I woke up the day before Scott's MRI, my mind was singing *Don't go breakin' my heart.* I took a walk by myself to Marcy Park, down the hill from our house, where I walked the loop around the soccer field, once, twice, three times, talking out loud, asking for help, for peace, for reminders to be in the present. I always knew when I was extra worried about an MRI because I made sure not to step on any cracks in the sidewalk.

I usually felt better as soon as we saw Scott's MRI, but only when we got good news. My email explained:

Scott's MRI 8/31
Dear Friends and Family,

Yesterday was Scott's MRI and dr. appointment and it has taken overnight to figure out how to write this email update. It's not bad news, but it's not clearly good news either. AMBIGUOUS is my word for the day. As we've said for the past year, there is "something" on the MRI that could be scar tissue, dead tissue, or possibly tumor. It is visible as a white area on the MRI called "enhancement." This time, the MRI film was developed with "brighter whites" so it is not clear whether that suspicious area is just brighter, or whether it's bigger. Ambiguous.

And so the neuro-radiologist and neurosurgeon will both take a close look at the scan and give their opinion. For us, it just means another 3-month "hall pass" to continue our lives until the next MRI verdict. If the scan had been clearly better or clearly unchanged, we probably would have moved the MRI's to every 4 months instead of 3 months. Intellectually and logically, we believe that Scott is doing better mentally/neurologically than he ever has since this all started. So the idea of tumor re-growth doesn't make sense.

SO, that's our news about the MRI. We're just feeling a little flat and disappointed, yet not really surprised. We would have preferred a nice surprise instead. The good news is that Scott's white cell and hemoglobin counts have improved, although his platelets have dropped (likely due to all the meds he's taking for the shingles). So his immune system is getting slightly stronger.

As for the shingles, you can't see any visible sign of them anymore on his face and the eye doc says his cornea is healing nicely. Unfortunately, the nerve pain in his eye is still very aggravating and Scott is extremely light sensitive. He's been in a dark cave for several weeks, so to speak (and you can imagine what light deprivation and constant aching does for a soul). We're trying more steroid eye drops and starting another anti-seizure drug called Neurontin, which might help and might also replace Scott's other seizure med, Dilantin. We'll see.

Wil goes off track from school next Friday and later in September we plan to spend a week in the mountains, in Steamboat Springs, thanks to a timeshare condo arranged by Scott's parents (THANKS!). We're also heading to Cincinnati in October for my sister's graduation from her master's degree program in Lay Ministry (way to go, Jenéne!). We're looking forward to a nice long weekend there.

That's all for now. If we hear more news regarding the MRI, we'll pass it along. Otherwise we'll just be in touch . . .

Love always,
Shelly

On the day of Scott's ambiguous MRI results, I found a yellow sticky note in my calendar that I stashed back in the winter, sticking it on a random future page when I could reconsider my needs. It was the phone number for a psychologist and licensed social worker named Meredith who specialized in grief counseling for cancer survivors. I booked an appointment. I felt like the MRI had pushed me back into a hole and I needed one more person pulling on a rope and cheering me on so that I would have the strength to climb out (and not run in the opposite direction when I did).

It was nice to talk with someone who had a fresh perspective ,who didn't know me yet, or Scott, and who knew in depth about life after cancer. Meredith used to coordinate the weekends retreats and workshops for Qualife, where Scott had been going to the men's cancer support group.

Her ideas about cancer survival helped me:

"In times of crisis," she said, "We circle the wagons and lean on each other. In times after crisis, we need to go back to our autonomy and individualism. Families and marriages are stronger and healthier when each person is an individual who contributes to the whole. But the search for your new identity after cancer has to be your own. Have you heard the story about the butterfly? If you help a butterfly out of its cocoon, its wings will be crippled. It's the struggle to emerge that creates wings strong enough to fly."

Here's something else Meredith explained, which I found useful:

"Anger, sorrow, and fear are hardwired emotions that God gave us for a purpose, which is to experience those emotions. Just like physical pain, feeling anger is an indication that something needs your attention. It's healthy (and better than okay) to let ourselves feel those emotions so we can address the issue and move through to a solution. If we don't, things will get worse."

As our meetings went on through September, Meredith gave me another tip for envisioning life after cancer. "Think about and say—say out loud—

what you want your life as a family to look like. Have family meetings to talk about it."

One day I wrote down my horoscope, wanting to capture its suggestion of hope. *It is time to break out of stagnant conditions and investigate new opportunities. Travel is very much part of this cycle. This can be a turning point. Be flexible, adapt, rather than make rigid plans.*

It seemed like the universe was giving me good advice from all angles. A friend gave me an angel card, which is like a fortune cookie sans cookie. The card said, *Trust life—the best is yet to be.*

Since Wil was off-track from first grade, being on A-track at Trailblazer Elementary, he and Scott took a three-day trip over the mountains with my mom. (I happily agreed to keep working and basked in the downtime being home all alone.) They stayed with my aunt and uncle, Chris and Greg, playing in their swimming pool for a few days while my mom visited her mom in the nursing home. On the drive home, past orchards and vineyards, while Wil busied himself in the backseat with books, Scott and Mom talked about someday living in such a place.

"After growing up around my grandpa's farm in Michigan," Scott said, "I wouldn't mind living somewhere like that again."

The next week, Scott, Wil, and I took a short family vacation to the mountains to Steamboat Springs. We took Wil horseback riding for the first time, and he was tickled to meet his horse, Willy. We rode a hot air balloon, a first for both Scott and Wil. We loved the eagle's eye view of the valley, the way the flame roared from the propane tank, how quiet it was (in between blasts) to float far above the ground, and the way we could look down on the steeples of pine trees below. We drove through the countryside looking at houses and ranches, fantasizing about leaving the city and living somewhere like this. We walked in and out of galleries and gift shops in the town of Steamboat Springs, one day having lunch at the drugstore deli counter. Scott and I smiled at each other as the waitress spoke to the local patrons, making their regular sandwiches, scooping ice cream for their kids, knowing them well enough to ask specific questions about their day.

"Wouldn't it be nice to live in a small town like this?" Scott asked.

"I never thought I'd want to leave Denver again, but now I'm thinking it might actually be nice to have a fresh start. It'd be nice to go somewhere new, do something different, meet all new people, stop being "the brain tumor family." I can take my business anywhere there is high-speed Internet and that's almost everywhere now. But do we want to go alone? Do you think we could convince our parents to leave Denver, too?"

"Maybe. Maybe we could have some land, several houses together, our family-compound idea."

"Yeah, except instead of waiting until we're all old and decrepit, needing to take care of each other, we could do it now when we're healthy. That would be a nice change of pace."

We drove home the next day, still a bit restless to keep traveling. We found an excited message from my mom on our voicemail.

"Hi, Shel. We're over here in Grand Junction visiting Gramma. We have a proposition for you. Is there any chance you can come meet us and stay over for a few days? Call me when you get this message."

Wil had a week left before school tracked back on, so we figured, Why not? I called Mom back,

"What's up?"

She sounded all high-pitched happy and bouncing around on her feet, which is not my mom's normal phone voice. She is usually warm, steady, and calm.

"Well, all these years we've been driving over to Grand Junction and fantasizing about living here someday on a small piece of land. One day this week we drove around Palisade, you know, the small town to the east with the orchards and vineyards—where we stopped that one time on I-70 to buy peaches?

"We were driving along this county road and stopped at the end, just before the road bends, to take pictures of the mountains, and we stopped right in front of a place with a for-sale sign. The people were out in the yard and there was a sign on the garage that said 'Honk for Fruit' so we drove in to talk with them.

"When I introduced myself, the man said, 'Rena? That's my grandmother's name' and I said, 'I was named after my grandmother, Rena.' Wasn't that a coincidence?

"Anyway, we talked awhile. It's a peach orchard, with apples, cherries, and pears, plus a few plums, apricots. and grapes. This couple has owned the orchard for almost thirty years, raised their family there. Two years ago their daughter-in-law was killed in an automobile accident and they spend most of their time in Denver now helping their son with his two boys, who are just three and five years old. The orchard is too much for them to take care of now, so they're ready to sell it.

"Here's a crazy idea, and it's still just a thought, but what would you think of moving to Palisade with us and learning the orchard business together? You'd have to come see it first, of course, and then think about it."

"That's so funny," I said. "We were just saying over lunch in Steamboat Springs this week how it would be nice to move to a small town like that, but only if we could get our parents to go, too. But geez, I wasn't serious."

And so began a serious conversation on whether this was a move we could make. Scott, Wil, and I drove west over the mountains, four hours from Denver, so we could look at the property together with my parents. In the 24 hours since our phone call, I had painted the most romantic picture in my mind of a quaint Victorian farmhouse with wrap-around porch and wicker couches, with a tree-swing, a red barn with cows and horses nearby. That was house down the road and around the corner. The real house and orchard for sale was the one with knee-high weeds, rusted heaps of unrecognizable metal under a lean-to roof, and a faded-yellow squat house with pale-purple shutters (that I couldn't even call periwinkle). The place was, well, run down and ugly. Inside, the kitchen was chock-full of tables, cupboards, washer and dryer, with green and orange-flowered wallpaper right out of the Seventies. The ceilings were not even eight feet high, and one of the two bedrooms had pink walls, red shag carpet and popcorn-textured ceilings with sparkles you couldn't even call stars. The September orchard itself was empty of fruit except for some apples and a few cling-peaches that had been left on the trees, hard, almost tasteless, and unmarketable. I tried hard to see the potential, but I wasn't impressed. It was dreary, droopy, dirty, and rural. Add to that the drizzle of rain that day.

When my uncle asked me over dinner what I thought of the place and the concept of moving, I burst into tears and ran from the table. In the guest bedroom I talked first with Mom, then with Scott, trying to stay positive but admitting my overwhelming fears of the move. All those weeds, all the renovation required. I don't know if I said this out loud, but I was thinking *I'm still tired from last year. I don't have the energy for something this big.*

The next morning, under blue skies and sunshine, the orchard (even the house) looked better. Everything looks better after a good rain. The orchard sparkled and, in cahoots with our souls, beckoned, whispering *Wouldn't it be lovely to wake up to this view every morning? You know you're ready for a change.*

Change here—with the trees, the birds, and the seasons. I promise it will be a price-less experiment…I mean, experience.

Like the doctors who gave Scott a fighting chance to survive, the orchard didn't promise an easy, quick fix. It offered an opportunity to take a risk for an uncertain outcome. It offered hope for a future that was far beyond the one we once planned that was no longer ours. It meant moving to the other side of the mountains to leave the past behind and find a new life. Do you want to hear about the whole decision-making process, or can I just tell you that after weighing all the pros and cons and possibilities, we agreed to take a leap of faith and say yes? Within a month, we were ready to say it out loud, without even waiting for Scott's next MRI. It felt right to make a move based on hope, not fear of the unknown. If cancer hadn't taught us that, it hadn't taught us anything.

The prospect of moving and starting a new life gave me the strangest sensation. It was part terror, part sadness, for sure. But something else was bubbling up from the depths, and it took me awhile to identify that long-lost feeling. I felt happy.

November 2000
Dear Friends and Family,

For the past few days, we've been celebrating Scott's 35th birthday and his 2-year anniversary since his brain tumor diagnosis. It feels great to be at this point, when all was so uncertain before. We remain very humbled though, to be so lucky with Scott's remission, as the past month has brought us to our friend David's funeral and news of tumor growth for another friend, Charlie. Please send some healing thoughts and prayers to their families, please.

We have been lucky to come a long way, even since August when Scott was still in pain from the shingles in his eye and from the blood clot in his arm, and we were deflated by the uncertainty of that month's MRI. He's feeling much better now. Our next MRI is November 29th. We're facing that with optimism, as Scott recently had another neuropsychological evaluation which shows he has improved neurologically in many areas AND because we are facing a big, new adventure in 2001:

My parents are buying a 6-acre fruit orchard in Palisade, Colorado, and asked us to go with them. The plan is for Scott and mom to work the orchard of peaches, apples, cherries, pears, grapes, and berries, and a big vegetable/herb garden, while my dad and I will continue our respective businesses of iron work/architecture and website design/writing. Palisade is a very small town by Grand Junction, on the western slope of the Rockies and about 40 miles from the Utah border. My aunt, uncle, cousins, and grandma live in Grand Junction, so we're very happy to live close to them. Wil is excited because there seem to be RVs in every yard, which fits his utopian version of a chicken in every pot.

So, mom and dad are going to sell their house, ideally "for sale by owner". If you know of anyone interested in a 1917 brick "Denver Square" just two blocks from Washington Park, please contact us.

Plans are for my mom and dad to move first, and then we'll follow sometime next spring. We're really excited at starting a brand new life. There has been an enormous amount of synchronicity leading to all of this, which confirms this is a perfect prearranged plan by the universe, however it turns out in detail. It will be extremely hard to leave our wonderful friends and neighbors here, as we couldn't have managed the last 2 years without them. But now we have a great place for everyone to come visit – to the land of peaches and vineyards (and RVs). :)

We will be in touch again after Scott's MRI on November 29th.

Hope all is well with all of you!!!!!

Love,
Shelly, Scott & Wil Vickroy

November 29, 2000
Hi everyone,

Here's a quick note to say that Scott's MRI today looked great! The questionable area of enhancement (the unknown white stuff) on the MRI was not there this time, or at least was much smaller. The doctor says he was nervous last time, but now he is not nervous at all and officially called it "no visible signs of disease." Also, Scott gets to taper off his seizure medication and be done with that. And we don't have to go back for the next MRI for 4 months (instead of our 3-month schedule). Scott gets to stop taking his Tamoxifen a year from now, and since Scott's health insurance is continuing to May (instead of my original prediction that he'd be on Medicare by now), it means that we'll only have to pay for six months of Tamoxifen instead of over a year's worth. All this adds up to SO MUCH RELIEF for us. We're taking the day off to celebrate by seeing the movie "Unbreakable."

We're looking forward to December, with Wil off track of school from this Friday until mid-January. He's turning 7 years old in a few weeks and has big plans to get a dog when we move. We are spending January 5-12 in Maui, Hawaii (thanks to the generosity of Scott's parents) and can't wait to ring in the New Year on a warm, sunny, beach.

So, happy holidays to everyone! We'll keep you posted on our upcoming move to the orchard next spring, and send out our annual year-in-review photo collage (or a website version) sometime soon.

Hope you all enjoy a wonderful holiday season, wherever you may be. We're think-ing of all of you and sending you our love.

Love always,
Scott, Shelly & Wil Vickroy

March 22, 2001
Dear Friends and Family,

Get those positive thoughts and prayers geared up. Scott's MRI is next Wednesday, March 28th at 8:00 a.m. Our follow-up appointment with Dr. Arenson is at 9:00, so we won't have to wait long at all for the results. We fully expect an even cleaner, clearer MRI since Scott has been feeling so great the past few months.

More excitement for next week is my parent's big move to Palisade on Friday, March 30th. After 30 years in the same house, you can imagine what this means not only in quantity of packing, but in the amount of emotions we'll be experienc-ing as we say goodbye to 360 S. Corona Street.

The house in Palisade is in the midst of renovations, drywall going back up and wood floors going in next week. My parents will not move in until closer to Easter, when my sister, Jenéne, comes from Cincinnati to celebrate the new move.

Our house here in Highlands Ranch has been on the market 3 weeks so far. We've cleaned, caulked and painted so much there isn't anything more we can do except wait for the right buyer to come along. We're confident that the perfect family will show up at the right time -- whenever that is -- to buy our house. Originally I had hoped for Wil to start school in Palisade before summer vacation so he could meet some friends, but it's looking like he'll finish the year here -- which is just fine with everyone.

As with all the challenges we've faced since Scott's brain tumor, we've learned that once we have done everything in our power to do, the rest is up to God and the Universe for the finishing touches. We're just focusing on the idea to "let it be" and trust in the big picture!

Of course, we're always looking for signs that we're on the right track, so here's what our latest fortune cookies had to say:

"Your efforts are budding. Results will appear soon."

"The hard times will begin to fade. Joy will take their place."

"Your blessing is no more than being safe and sound for the whole life-time."

And so, we'll be in touch next Wednesday after the MRI and catch up with all our other news. Thanks, as always, for sending us your love and support!!

Love,
Shelly, Scott and Wil Vickroy

April 25, 2001
Dear Friends and Family,

I just looked in shock at my calendar today to realize that our move is exactly one month away!!! We will be packing up and heading over the mountains to Palisade on May 25th, the Friday before Memorial Day. We have sold our house (contract pending; we're confident it will go through) and will close on Wednesday, May 23rd. Date of possession is Friday at noon. YIKES! and YEE-HAW!!

Wil's school year isn't over until May 30th, but after some soul-searching I've decided that it's best to just move and be there, rather than move and drive back to Denver for 5 more days of Life in Limbo. The dates were vital to the buyers, so we're stuck with that. It also happens to be the busiest moving weekend of the year, so we're doing the best we can to locate a U-Haul truck and to book the same awesome guys who helped load Mom & Dad's house.

The ironic thing about these dates is that they coincide to the day 5 years ago when we moved here to Desert Willow Way! And also the same week when I moved to Tennessee back in 1990. I guess that it's just in our destiny to move on Memorial Day weekend. But hopefully, we won't be moving again for a good, LONG time.

Other news for the Vickroy's includes a bout of chicken pox for Wil the past five days. It was such a surprise, since he had the vaccine as a toddler. The docs say only 1 percent of people vaccinated still get chicken pox, but I've read on the Internet that the rate is more like 25 percent. Luckily, Wil's case has been very mild with not much itching. Cabin fever has been the worst of it. That, and the scare with my next-door friend, Diane, pregnant with twins and on bedrest who never had chicken pox (turns out her vaccine a few years ago did not confer immunity for her, either!). Because she spent the afternoon with Wil on the day before his pox poked out, she had to get a globulin immune-boosting shot to protect her and the babies. Please think immune-protecting thoughts for them!! (The twins should arrive late in May, making it hard for us to think of moving then.)

Scott managed to miss the chicken pox quarantine due to a trip to Michigan, but for a sad reason. His Uncle Eddie was diagnosed with kidney cancer and isn't doing well at all. I am so glad that Scott was able to be there with him this week. I know it was a bittersweet visit. Scott is flying home tonight. Please send Uncle Eddie and the whole family some prayers!

Well, we had a great Easter weekend in Palisade. Jenéne came from Cincinnati, and Scott's parents drove over for Easter dinner at the Haifley's (my aunt & uncle's). We spent two days of hard labor, working in the orchard picking up tree limbs and trimmings. We learned to drive the tractor, too! I must say, we made the prettiest piles of wood I've ever seen -- with apple blossoms still clinging and blooming on the cut branches. We really saw the difference between peach, cherry and apple wood, and marveled at how much more we will learn in the coming season.

I'm still battling with Rocky Mountain HMO to accept my insurance application. Even today they're still wondering if I have a legitimate corporation to purchase group of one insurance. The hassle has been so frustrating. I've had to also convince them that I am moving to Mesa County and should qualify for Mesa County rates ($80 less a month). I'm keeping my fingers crossed that it all works out today! Please send some encouraging thoughts to the underwriter! :)

Mom & Dad have still not moved into their house in Palisade, but hope to by this weekend. They're waiting for the final certificate of occupation and a few minor touchups. They're exhausted, I think, but hanging in there. It will be good to finally crawl into their own bed and eat off their own dishes.

That's about all for now. We're having a garage sale on Friday, May 11th (nearly everything goes!) and then we'll start packing. Scott is planning several trips to Palisade to help with the orchard and set up the computer network at the house. We have lots to do in 4 weeks!

Hope you're all doing great! Will keep you posted on our move.

Love always,
Shelly, Scott & chicken pox'd Wil

Wednesday, May 2, 2001
To: HRMOTHERSANDMORE

Dear Friends

Many of you have known me since the very first year we formed our chapter of Formerly Employed Mothers at the Leading Edge (FEMALE) which has now become Mothers & More, some only know me through my email updates about my husband Scott's successful brain tumor battle. Well, this message is to say goodbye and thank you for all the years of support and friendship. We've sold our house and are moving to Palisade (near Grand Junction) on Friday, May 25th, off to the land of orchards and vineyards to start a new life.

It's with tears on my keyboard that I say goodbye to you all with this message. Before I go, I wanted to tell you what this group has meant to me.

At the very first chapter meeting back in June 1997, I looked around the room and saw the faces of women who I wanted to know, whose friendship I knew would make a big difference in my life. After being in Denver a full year, having quit my job when we moved here with a 2-year old son, I had yet to meet kindred spirits who shared my truths about motherhood and womanhood. At that first meeting, there you were! Being in on the chapter's birth and watching her grow from 30 to well over 100 members was a great source of pride and fulfillment for me. Like a happy workaholic, I spent many satisfying hours working on chapter subcommittees, the first chapter website, and other chapter and national business during the time I was our chapter's 2nd leader. I truly loved the months where I knew every member's name (and email address) and where I could be the first person to smile and welcome unfamiliar faces at the door. And then in November '98 Scott was diagnosed with a brain tumor and my life as I knew it changed forever.

Thank goodness and THANK YOU for stepping up to catch me. Anne Streech was there within days to relieve me of the chapter leader "crate" and a team of women and friends stepped in to continue leading the chapter. Meals kept pouring in throughout the next 9 months of Scott's treatment, and friends made sure to check in on my frame of mind during that time.

But just as my life took that unexpected turn, I also found myself on the outside of the chapter I loved so well -- by my choice and my circumstances. As much as I missed the camaraderie of Mothers & More, it also became a constant reminder of the life that was no longer in my present or my future. Wives with healthy, working husbands; mothers with new babies or happy pregnant tummies; women with time, energy and available hours for playgroups and book groups and gourmet dinners. It became painful and awkward to step into that circle where I only saw my losses. I was in a stage of grieving that I couldn't share out loud because, no matter how empathetic, you just had to be in the same boat to understand. I know I'm not the only one who went through devastating losses, grief and changes -- and you may not understand how I can look at it that way when my husband is still alive and is free of his brain tumor. I hope that someday you'll read a book of mine and it will become more clear -- until I write it, it won't fully be clear to me either.

Now, with this new opportunity to move into a new life and have a fresh start, I am saying a fond farewell to many parts of my life and opening the door to unknown joys that I trust await me on the Western Slope. It is part of my own recovery to take this leap of faith that "the best is yet to be." I just wanted you all to know that FEMALE and Mothers & More was "the best of what was" for the time I lived in Highlands Ranch. I have never known such a vast and giving group of beautifully strong, intelligent and loving women who could create such deep friendship out of the shared experience called motherhood. I hope that each and every one of you has found at least one lasting friendship, a true kindred spirit, from your membership in this chapter.

Just because I'm moving to the Western Slope doesn't mean I'm disappearing forever. I plan to come back for business possibly monthly, and when the fruit crops are ripe this summer, we'll be back with truckloads of peaches and apples. If anyone is interested, we can arrange rendezvous with the fruit. We'll be growing peaches, apples, Bing cherries, pears, raspberries, boysenberries and some veggies & herbs. So, I will find a way to let you know about that (like a website, prob-ably)! And you're welcome to visit us on the orchard any time of year! Or you might just need to arrange a moms-only 12-vineyard wine-tasting weekend! :)

I'm going to be at the Broadway Starbuck's coffee on Tuesday, May 15th at 10 a.m. if anyone wants to stop in for coffee and a hug goodbye. Or you can find me at our huge moving sale on Friday, May 11th from 8 to 3:00. We're selling almost half of our household.

Love and hugs to all of you,
Shelly :)

I'm gonna miss the way you used to
holler for help before you found your courage.
—Dorothy's farewell to the Cowardly Lion

42

Moving Over Mountains

Our crescent moon was in the sky the morning we moved over the mountains to an orchard in the desert. I felt like the moon was waving goodbye, the same way our neighbors waved goodbye with tears running down their faces, filling the gutters, and cresting in a tidal wave of grief half way down the block. They stood in a circle in our driveway for our last moments on Desert Willow Way: Bob, Pam, Kelton and Judy, Warner and Andrea, Traci and Regis, Chris, Nancy, Rachel and Julia, Eric and Caro, Fred, Kathy, Rachel and Andrea, Scoot, Drew, Noah, and Diane holding brand-new baby Sam. Caro sent us off with a beautiful quilt she sewed of houses and flowers and orchards. She put a Xeroxed-to-fabric photo of our house in the center, and everyone signed their names in indelible markers. We could sleep under that quilt to recover their love.

Each friend waited in turn for a hug, hugging so tight it was hard to let go. We were like Dorothy saying goodbye to the Tin Man, Lion, and Scarecrow. Instead of by hot-air balloon or by clicking magic red slippers, we left in a U-Haul. Scott drove away first, Wil's tearful face pressed to the window. I followed in the minivan with our two cats wailing from their plastic carrier cages. Everyone was bawling.

Oh no, what have we done? I thought, needing windshield wipers for my eyes. *How could we leave this wonderful life, our wonderful friends?* In our five years on the street we shared so many heartaches, so many dinners and birthdays and New Years together. We were as one family with plans to live next door and next door and across the cul-de-sac and down the street from each other until our children were grown and had kids of their own. We were *that* sure of our guaranteed tomorrows and our places side by side.

But on the day we signed the sales contract on our house, it seemed as if we signed the bottom line on our soul-contract with the neighbors as well. Contract Fulfilled, the stamp would say on such a document.

"All obligations have been met to a satisfactory level, exceeded in fact," the soul advisor would say, handing the paper back to us for our records. "If you wish to continue this association, you can sign a new contract for Everlasting Friendship. While it doesn't require the same level of daily commitment, the bonds of your heartstrings will remain strong with intermittent yet dedicated upkeep."

I knew our contract was complete, that although our time on the street had ended, our friendships would endure. As with my friends, I said goodbye to every room of our house, pulling in all the energy of our time there so that I took all the love with me—the same way I was taking cuttings from my strawberries and lilac bushes, too. I knew I was ready for whatever came next, that I would return a month later with the first crop of fruit. I was ready to say goodbye, but that didn't make driving away any easier.

When I was three and my family moved from the yellow trailer in my grandparent's big yard, I watched as Dad and Granddad loaded my bunkbed mattress into the pickup truck. I turned to my mom and hugged her knees, crying in little-kid lisp, "I'll nevah evah be happy again." We were moving a mere thirty miles from Lakewood to Boulder to live in the apartments at Student Family Housing while my dad finished college on the G.I. Bill. My childhood mind couldn't imagine how change could be good. My adult mind knew better this time.

Ten miles from home which was no longer our home, a song came on from *The Road to El Dorado* soundtrack CD, reminding me that friends never say goodbye. I bawled even harder, but this time with thanks—for true friends who helped us survive a phase of our life we could now leave in the past.

On cue, the next song perked me up, and I sang along, "Look out new world here we come...we are just the team to live where others merely dream." I knew we were blazing a new trail over the Great Divide, part of a sumptuous grand design (to paraphrase Elton John's lyrics). I had faith that the beauty of that design would be revealed, but only in the same slow way we would learn how to grow cherries, berries, peaches, pears, apples, and grapes.

I drove thirteen miles and parked at Scott's parent's home. That's as far as we had to go on the first day. It felt like a thousand miles. In the morning before we left, Scott's mom showed me their family album with photos of their going-away party when they left Michigan for Colorado. Scott was twelve. "I guess it's in the Vickroy genes to move," she said. "At least Palisade is closer to Denver than Michigan."

I spent most of the drive over the mountains singing along to various CDs. The cats had stopped crying, except for when I drove around curves. By the time I pulled off I-70 into Palisade, I was singing *Alleluia* as alto to Julie Andrews' soprano on the *Sound of Music* CD. Scott and his dad followed in the slower U-Haul. Wil rode with Grammy Binny in her SUV.

My parents stood on the patio as we pulled into the gravel driveway at the orchard. Hung on the garage over the "Honk for Fruit" sign was a big plastic banner proclaiming "Happy Birthday!" I laughed.

"Welcome home," my mom and dad yelled with open arms.

"Thanks, it's good to be here."

Part Three:
Full Moon Faith

If Part One could be considered Treatment, and Part Two called Recovery, then Part Three of our story is all about Healing. What is healing? Not cure. That's a quasi-medical term for the body, while healing happens in your soul. Healing is to find wholeness again, and that cannot happen in an instant, with one step, three wishes, or a year of good sleep. Healing happens slowly, in concert with grief, reflection, integration, awakening. Healing has to do with letting go of losses and learning to trust life, love, and laughter again.

For cancer survivors, and that includes caregivers, healing involves creating The New Normal and accepting how different that is than before. It means defining a new sense of The Future. It means facing the threat of recurrence. It means regaining strength not only in your body but in your psyche, in case, just in case and inevitably, you are faced with hard times again, cancer or not. Healing means—as it always did—having faith in uncertainty, but hopefully for a longer unforeseeable length. It means learning to grieve while you're grateful. Healing in the long-run means surpassing survival and daring to embrace life, reset priorities, redefine who you are, and reclaim your purpose in life.

For us, it took time to forge a new future.

As my writing friend Betty once offered many years later, "We think healing is about returning to the person we used to be. But really, healing is about becoming someone new. We might not recognize ourselves when we get there."

ॐ

Live in each season as it passes;
breathe the air, drink the drink, taste the fruit.
—Henry David Thoreau

43

Orchard Life

Cherries, berries, peaches, pears, apples, grapes. Say it fast: cherries, berries, peaches, pears, apples, grapes. This is the order in which the crops came in, the order I listed them on the website I designed to market the fruit from St. Francis Farm, and, ironically, the best order for rolling the words off your tongue. I've learned from the orchard, from cancer and life, that when we say "ironic" we might as well say, "It's a God thing." Inexplicable yet somehow perfect, appropriate, and probably predestined.

I learned a lot from living on the orchard. I wasn't supposed to even be working in the orchard. The deal was, I would keep up with my website business because we needed the money and the group-of-one health insurance, and I would take Wil to swimming lessons at the Palisade town pool. We would all share the grocery shopping, cooking, and cleaning. I would pitch in when needed, helping out on irrigation day, picking fruit, spraying weeds, hoeing weeds (hating weeds), driving to Denver on alternate weekends to sell bushels of fruit, watering the half-acre garden and patio pots when it was Mom and Dad's turn in Denver. It was more work than any of us expected. That is an understatement. We were so tired we rarely stayed up much past roasting marshmallows after dinner on the grill. When we did see the Milky Way, the Big Dipper was right over the orchard as if watering, too.

Learning was hard work. The fruit kept us focused on learning the ropes one crop at a time. Cherries, berries, peaches, pears, apples, grapes.

Cherries. I won the prize (no tangible prize) as the fastest, best picker of cherries, the one who could fill up her bucket (a three-gallon plastic bucket curved to fit across your chest, harnessed over your shoulders) with the best quality cherries, the fewest bird-pecked, and able to retain the most cherries on stems. Someone who came to buy fruit told us in a disdainful tone that sweet cherries should be picked with the stem on so they would keep longer. Before that summer, I didn't know anything about cherries other than the Bings at Safeway and the acidic Montmorency pie cherries from my childhood backyard that we picked stem-off. Now I know better.

I learned to twist and pick, twist and pick. I learned it was just as well to pick without looking, to rely on my sense of touch, judging the best cherries by how sticky or slick each cherry was. A sticky cherry would be one where a bird sampled the fruit like a piece of Valentine's chocolate tasted and put back in the box. Smooth cherries, often found three to a clump just like on vintage tablecloth fabric, would be ripe for picking. We picked the first batch too soon, still a bit tart, not yet fully dark and sweet. Compared to pie cherries, they were incredible.

I learned to climb high on the ladder to where I could see over the twelve rows of peach trees, clear over to the pears and apples on the west side of the orchard. The row of eighteen cherry trees, on the east side, was first to feel the morning sun, but also the chill canyon wind. The sun burned the back of my knees as I perched on the rungs.

Twist and pick, look for bird pecks and poop. Lightly drop to the bucket, be careful not to bruise. Twist and pick. Picking cherries was a religious experience, I would exclaim in surprise, though I couldn't say why, I just felt it. Each red cherry grew from a blossom, survived late frosts, was kissed by bees, warmed by the sun, protected from sparrows, robins and crows, watered every few weeks, then emerged through the miracle of ripening, a bit more each day, to perfection.

Bing, Van, Lambert, Hedelfingen, Stella—you pick those sweet cherries when they're purplish-black, because that's when they're the sweetest, perfect for eating by the handful. The sweet, white Ranier cherries you pick when they blush peachy-pink. You wouldn't bake a pie with sweet cherries (unless you pick them early when they're sour, or reduce the sugar and add lemon for tartness). For a pie, you want the sour pie cherries that ripen later in the month. We didn't grow sour cherry trees on St. Francis Farm; for those, you have to go down the road or up to East Orchard Mesa where a woman once told me she won't pick pie cherries until someone comes to buy them, otherwise they're too much trouble.

The cherry trees were dying a slow death of raspleaf disease caused by nematodes in the soil. All the cherry trees in the valley are affected, an oldtimer told us, by this "curly-leaf" disease. You can tell because you'll notice a branch of leaves that are not just wilted but look almost shredded and curled back into themselves. The parasitic nematodes puncture and suck on the roots. A tree can survive for years with Curly Leaf, offering full branches of cherries that taste just as good as can be. As proof, our trees looked like clusters of grapes on the vine, thick as your arm, that first summer. No cure for the nematodes, we were told. You just prune what you can in the spring, let the tree grow, and produce as long as they can, 'til the disease takes over. Then you cut down the tree, pull up the stump, and replant something else. That's just the way it is, the oldtimers said.

From the cherries, I learned that you need strong legs for the ladder and both patience and speed for picking, that your arms do grow stronger, that you might as well plan on losing a lot to the birds because loud noises, plastic owls, and shirts on coat hangers flapping in trees do little to discourage their hunger, and that you have to accept that someday the cherry trees will die. That summer, from nuances still too subtle to share, I learned why life is a bowl of cherries.

Berries. I didn't pick many berries that summer or since. The heat took its toll on that short-lived crop. Mom spent countless days trimming back canes, shoring up wires, training the vines to grow, wearing thick leather gloves up to her elbows, picking in silicone gloves til the plastic was punctured. I never knew berries lived among so many thorns, or that the thorns would be so spiderweb fine and sliver sharp. Blackberries, raspberries, dewberries, boysenberries. I learned that horticulturist Rudolph Boysen created that hybrid berry in 1923 by crossing a raspberry, blackberry, and loganberry. I also learned that nothing tastes better on hot buttermilk waffles than fresh boysenberries and whipped cream.

Mom showed me once the best way to "go on a treasure hunt" is to use a forked hand-trowel to hold up the vines, looking for the ripest berries underneath, in the dark. How they ripened beneath all those leaves, away from the sunlight, I don't understand. Seems to me, it's a bit like searching your soul for meaning, having to look in the dark for the sweetest fruit, living with the stains on your fingers, licking them clean.

Peaches. Ah, peaches. The perfect fruit, so I thought when I first met our 330 trees. To walk down the rows of the Early Red Havens those mornings in July was to revisit the Jolly Rancher factory and inhale the candy itself. No, it was better than that. To find the first ripe peach of the season, a peach so heavy and ripe it would fall off the branch if you breathed too close to its face, was to find bliss. That first peach when it fell, we called a windfall, and that's when I first knew the true treasure of the word. Kathy Matsey came visiting from Denver the weekend we found the first peach, and we shared it for breakfast, everyone in the family taking a slice. To this day, we agree, there has never been a peach sweeter. Close, but not quite. Was it sweet because it was our first, or was it perfect for real? I will always wonder and never know.

Early Red Haven, Red Haven, Red Globe, Washington, Blake, Suncrest, Redskin, Monroe, and Gleason. Did you know that Elberta peaches, the ones people ask for with nostalgic snobbery as if nothing less will do, are not a specific peach but a variety of late-season peaches. We learned you could tell those folks the Gleasons were Elbertas and they would be happy.

Picking peaches, tree ripe, entailed filling up twenty-pound boxes in two careful layers so you didn't touch a peach more than twice, sneezing and scratching from the peach fuzz (as bad as installing attic insulation, Scott swore), stacking full boxes behind the tractor, moving them to the cooler as soon as possible. We had to know just when to pick; too soon and the hard fruit would be no better than the bins harvested green for the grocery stores, too ripe and it would bruise on the way to market, too late and the fruit would be wasted. Everyone we asked had a different method for telling when a peach was ready to pick: by feel when you can press your thumb in; when it smells like peach sugar; when the crease down the side of the peach plumps and flattens; or my favorite, by tasting another peach on the branch. The sacrificial peach. We called it our breakfast peach.

We'd set one peach aside, saying "I'll have this one for breakfast with my cereal." At first we would rationalize keeping the breakfast peach, pretending it wasn't perfect, saying the skin was torn, it was a bruised, too ripe to pack, had leaf rub, or a dent from where it swelled into the branch. We knew some buyer would scoff at its lack of beauty and call it a "second." But we knew this breakfast peach was one we deserved to eat and enjoy, not give away, not sell, not pack in a box. Some peaches are meant to be eaten right off the tree, unwashed, ignoring the pesticide residue just this once. Sometimes a peach is so perfectly ripe you can pick it and stand there, peeling away the skin in one or two pieces, then you take a large bite, sucking and slurping the juice, not caring how much drips from your chin to your shirt because it's just a sweaty, dirty picking t-shirt anyway.

That's what I learned from the peaches. You can spend all summer wishing to relive the taste of that first perfect peach, or you can devour a new peach every day ripe off the tree because you deserve it.

Pears. I don't get pears. I like picking them, though, because they won't bruise and they don't make me sneeze. It's ironic semantics that you pick pears when they're hard, so it's easy. Pears are easy to pick, which I figure is how Nature rewards your careful picking of peaches all summer, letting the next something be easy. Palisade pears are ready to pick in September, over-lapping the late peaches. To pick a pear, you lift it up toward the branch and the sturdy stem snaps, just like that.

One day driving past a fruit stand, one where generations have been growing fruit one after the other and are still all together, we stopped in to ask, "How do you know when pears are ready to pick?" The old man orchardist, perhaps seeing a sucker, told me he looked at the sugar spots, and he held up a pear close so I could see what he meant. "When those spots multiply so that they're touching, that's when you know the pear is ready." I believed him, but everyone else (to this day) thinks he was teasing. "The other method," he said, "Is to buy an instrument that measures the pressure in the fruit, which indicates the sugar level." We had only one row of pears, so nobody felt like spending the money on the pressure sensor. Instead, Mom selected a day and said it was time to pick pears.

Someone else told us that pears should be kept in the cooler for six weeks after picking so as to let the sugar set. I didn't eat a single pear that year. You can't eat them ripe off the tree. Like I said, I don't get pears.

One year somebody came into the driveway and asked to pick pears to make wine. They didn't mind the windfalls, or the overripes, or how ugly the Asian pears looked. I don't remember if they ever brought us a bottle of the finished product.

What I liked best of the pears was a picture I took. We were mostly too tired to take photos of each other that summer. But that pear picture I love. It shows Scott in his boots, with a picking bucket on his waist full of pears, standing in mud. You can't see his face, just a top-down view of the pears to his Levi's to his boots to the mud. It reminds me that one row of the orchard was easy, and he was there.

Bartletts. Red Bartletts. Moonglows. Did you know Red Bartletts are red from pear-hood? (What do you call an inch-long baby pear?) They don't ripen and turn red. They're red from the start. I didn't know that before.

What I learned from the pears is that sometimes you should just let life be easy.

Apples. I loved the apple trees. Loved them to tears. We had heirloom apples, an official term meaning nearly extinct, of complex, unique genetics, apples with flavors that surpass (beyond poetry) the bland, waxy, and hybridized breeds bought in bulk as unblemished but boring. In 1892 around 735 apple varieties were available from commercial nurseries; today there are fewer than fifty. Our apple trees were the great-grandparents of the orchard, over thirty years old, sturdy and stocky, offering their bountiful fruit for our first season as if with their last beautiful breath. You can't find apples like this in a new orchard. Nine rows by twenty of apple trees, grouped somewhat together by name but some planted here, some planted there when through the years dead trees were replaced: Northern Spy, Ginger Gold, Grimes Golden, McIntosh, Granny Smith, Winesap, Gravenstein, Rome Beauty, Cortland, Yellow Delicious, Jonathon, Late Jonathon, and Old Fashioned Red Delicious.

To fully appreciate heirloom apples, I recommend reading *Botany of Desire: A Plant's-Eye View of the World*, by Michael Pollan. You might become an activist, an advocate of apples after that, refusing to buy the imposters from agribusiness or New Zealand or China, more willing to spend your cash on hand-hewn heirlooms, despite a few worms. To truly know apples is to taste them right off the tree, crunchy, juicy, and sweet.

I first fell in love with the apple trees over Easter when they had been pruned and we learned to drive the Ferguson tractor so we could gather the prunings. Branches and branches lay over the floor of the orchard, waiting for us to stack them for drying and burning. Covered in pink blossoms still kissing bees, those branches on the ground were the prettiest firewood I'd ever seen. My heart ached for each blossom that would never be fruit.

I fell deeper in love with the apples on every irrigation day, standing with my hoe, exhausted from smashing dirt clods and scraping weeds, listening to the water trickle down the row, seeing the sunlight skate in the ripples. The grid of trees are planted and pruned, we were told, so that birds could fly a diagonal path through the orchard and the tractor could till each row north to south, east to west. If you looked at one tree, straight on, the rest of the row lined up, disappeared. The leaves were so dense on the apple trees that I felt alone with the orchard even though Scott, Dad, and Mom might be hoeing mere rows away. The Granny Smiths watched over Wil, busy floating Action Man in the runoff with his new friend, Marshall, from the orchard across the road. On those days I met the old-soul energy of apple trees that invites orioles and hummingbirds to nest, moths to alight, worms to feast, wind to blow, tears to flow.

By autumn, when we were exhausted from the first season, needing to be at our desks to earn money, and my mom broke her foot in the uneven orchard-row dirt, we had to be done. We couldn't pick all the Rome Beauties from fifty-six trees and they fell to the ground in a blanket of red. Poor trees, to have offered such bounty, rebuked. We couldn't find buyers who would pay what it cost to grow, spray, harvest, and market the apples. It was easier, but sad, to let the wind and dirt have them. It felt wrong to give them away to persnickety people who expected the same price as two decades ago. But when a woman walked by one day, asking if she could have some for her pigs, we said yes. Lucky pigs.

What I learned from the apples is more than immense. My heart aches with the fullness of gratitude for having lived on the orchard that summer so I would know the bittersweet intimate details of apples. It may take another book, or may go with me to my grave, but the apples and the orchard will always be a part of me.

Grapes. Good old grapes. Did you know Concord grapes taste exactly like Kool-Aid?

I wish I could tell you we found our new calling in life with the orchard, in the same way I wish I could say life after cancer was easy. I don't want to disappoint you. I wanted to tell you only the good, like a reprieve and a prayer. I could tell you too much of the bad. The truth is, life on the orchard was both. Like life. Like cancer. Like love. Both good and bad.

The short version is that—despite all its beauty and the value of learning so much on so many levels—Scott, Wil, and I left the orchard after the first summer for reasons too many to mention. There are reasons we don't live with our parents when we grow up, or parents with their grown children. There are reasons people get degrees in horticulture or become master gardeners. There are reasons most people who own orchards have other careers, or that when people retire to live on an orchard, a for-sale sign often appears after a year. There are reasons most orchards contain one fruit, not six or seven. There are reasons, good reasons, why Americans mostly stopped living on farms. It takes more work and commitment than you can imagine if you're used to buying your food already grown, picked, sorted, and washed. I will never balk at the price of cherries, berries, peaches, pears, apples, or grapes ever again.

The orchard might have been the reason we moved, but we had to find a new reason to stay.

I don't regret our orchard summer. My soul is stronger for walking the rows, for tasting the fruit, for learning how many steps are required to keep each tree alive, for being aware of the seasons like never before. It was worth doing once. But I'd never do it again.

Life can only be understood backwards;
but it must be lived forwards.
—Søren Kierkegaard

44
Making a House into Home

We found our own house in town, two miles from the orchard and not far from a park where the Colorado River flowed through. The house had been empty all summer, one contingency contract had falllen through, so it felt like the universe had put the house on lay-away for us until we were ready. The day we toured the house with our realtor, we saw an empty wooden quilt bracket hanging high on the dining room wall. "That stays with the house," our realtor said.

"Scott, we have to buy this house. It already has a place to hang our quilt from our old neighbors."

"Well, it's not perfect. But it'll do."

Not long after moving in, I painted a red wall in our living room.

From: Shelly
Subject: Merry Christmas 2001 and Happy New Year 2002

Dear Friends and Family

After moving to Palisade in May 2001, we had a nonstop season on the orchard with my parents, Rena and Jeff. It was cherries-berries-peaches-pears-apples-grapes. We've learned about tractors, irrigation, weed control, pesticides, picking properly, marketing strategies, box availability, and recipe possibilities. It was fun, exhausting, overwhelming, interesting, challenging, and truly an adventure. And we're so relieved to be done for the season.

In August, we decided to buy our own house in Palisade rather than build an addition to the farmhouse. We found a nice house on a quiet suburban-style street, not the Victorian we thought we'd find but a house with all the items on our wish list, including an awesome view of the Grand Mesa, walking distance to school, and kids on the block. Scott got his Internet satellite system, his own office and a big garage in the deal, Wil got a 2nd story room of his choice and a dog house and kennel for the eventual addition to our family (someday when Wil agrees to daily scoop-patrol in the yard). And I have a sunny office, an east-facing kitchen, shade trees and a shady backyard in the afternoon. We already finished a kitchen remodel and the addition of wood floors instead of linoleum. It's exciting to create our own space, and be able to afford it with the lower cost of housing in this town. We're just two miles from the orchard, and Wil still gets to ride the bus there some days after school.

Wil is enjoying 2nd grade at Taylor Elementary, where he's very impressed that they've had more than five fire drills already. He gets to close the classroom door and turn out the lights on the way out during the drills. Wil mostly likes living in Palisade, but he sorely misses his friends in Highlands Ranch. The orchard wasn't exactly his kind of lifestyle, he'll tell you, mostly because it wasn't on Desert Willow Way with 20 other kids to play with. But he did meet a kindred spirit on 35.6 Road (the orchard), named Marshall, who we've enjoyed having around. And for the first time, we have a boy his age on our new street.

Scott worked hard all summer at the orchard, driving the tractor, picking fruit, and growing squash, corn and cucumbers. The hard work was good for his muscles and gave him renewed confidence in his abilities. In September, he introduced himself to a few professors of computer science at Mesa State College in Grand Junction. He offered to help them with a programming project, for the sake of getting his feet wet and relearning some skills. It's good for him; he'll always be a computer programmer at heart.

I've been busy catching up with my website business, after taking most of the summer off to help pick and market fruit. My summer website project was for the orchard – visit it if you haven't already at st-francisfarm.com and click on the family link to see photos. I don't have any local clients yet, but plan to expand my business this winter. I haven't had a spare minute for my book writing, but hope that can happen this winter, too. One of my favorite new "to do's" is volunteering at Wil's school every Thursday afternoon during "writing time," something I've always wanted to do.

We celebrated Scott's 36th birthday on November 6th. It's a great milestone for us. Scott had a clean MRI in August and again in early December. Ever since moving to Palisade, we've hoped to make a fresh start and downplay Scott's brain tumor. Yet even here on the Western Slope, we have been contacted by several brain tumor patients and continued to share our story and offer our support. No matter where we go, we will always be part of that special community of brain tumor survivors – and happy, humble and honored to be able to continue that role.

In other news, we went to Palm Desert over Thanksgiving to spend the holiday with Scott's parents there, with a night in Las Vegas on the way home. One highlight of the trip was completing books 1 and 2 of Harry Potter and seeing the movie (Wil's new passion) and reading chapter books aloud is a nice family treat. In 2002, we'll be happily settling into our new home and just going about our days as normal. That in itself is a real pleasure.

And so, that's the news from the Vickroy Family. We hope this message finds you all happy, healthy and safe. The tragic events in America certainly remind us to count our blessings, and we count each of you as blessings to us. Happy 2002!!!

Take care and Love always,
Shelly, Scott & Wil

My inner chipper Pollyanna wrote that email, ever convinced that the best way to manifest happiness was to say it was so, make a note when it was, and catch up to the whole picture later. With that goal in mind, my Pollyanna Glad Game was more like the board game Life. When we played at Christmas, Wil focused on having as many kids as possible, Scott on a high-paying career, and I picked at artist's cottage by the beach. And as when I was a kid, it was hard to keep playing when the game didn't go my way. Long-term survival and the game of Life entails some jumps forward, some moves back.

God is a comedian playing to an
audience that is afraid to laugh.
—*Christopher Moore*

45
Fire Fighting Mode

I t's easy to feel like you're cursed.

Leaping awake at the screech of smoke detectors at 4:00 a.m., the whole-house wiring makes the sound ricochet, ripple through the house. It is June 2001, less than a month since we moved to the orchard to escape and recover from cancer fire fighting mode. Wil runs down the stairs like a shot, before I can sit up in bed to cover my ears. Our bedroom is on the main floor, under his. My parents are in their bedroom upstairs, and I hear them moving around.

"What's happening?" Wil cries.

"I don't know," I reply, reaching to pull him on the bed with a hug. After 30 seconds it stops. Silence. We wait. Nothing. No smoke. "Wouldn't it keep going if there was really a fire," I ask Scott, who is already turning back on the pillow, groaning in frustration.

Fifteen minutes later, the smoke alarms go off again. Each time, we wait for a minute to see if the sound will continue. Again it screeches at 4:30, 4:40 and 5:00. At 5:30 I say, "This is stupid! Smoke alarms go off for a reason. We can't just ignore it!"

So Scott and my dad walk around the house, poking in closets, looking in the utility room accessed by an outside door. I'm thinking one of our computers has a short in the wiring. I start packing my bags to head for a hotel with Wil and the cats, dang the rest of them if they're not concerned. The men find nothing to explain the smoke detector's false alarms. No smoke, no smell, no evidence. Grudgingly I go back to bed.

When I was a teenager and sitting on my back porch one day, I heard the smoke alarms going off in the bungalow next door. Mr. Brooks was older than ninety that year (and lived to be ninety-nine and nine months). I did odd jobs for Mr. Brooks and drove him on errands. When I heard his smoke alarms buzzing, I yelled to my mom "Call the fire department!" and I ran to his front door, smelling smoke through the screen. I went in. Smoke filled the house, but like Mr. Magoo, Mr. Brooks couldn't see it or smell it. He stood on a wooden chair in the front hallway, in bare feet, bashing the smoke alarm on the ceiling with the heel of his brown oxford shoe.

"Shirley," (he called me Shirley), "This damned smoke alarm is broken."

"No, it's not, Mr. Brooks. Something's on fire."

I helped him down off the chair and took him outside. The firemen arrived and discovered a big cast iron pot on the extra stove in his basement. Mr. Brooks had been dyeing his socks and underwear brown and the water had boiled clean away. The fire was from the clothes roasting, scorching, and turning to ashes. Nothing was harmed, but we had to repaint a few walls.

That's why we have smoke alarms.

Wil hated sleeping at the orchard that summer in the upstairs room with only seven-foot ceilings, his bed beneath the smoke detector with its ominous green eye blinking and winking, every few minutes blinking red. (Apparently it blinks red to let you know it is working.)

Two weeks later, it happens again. This time my parents are out of town, it's us three at 5:30 in the morning wondering what the hell is happening. Later that day Scott's dad, who happens to be driving through town on his way to California, gives us a clue. It might be fruit flies, he surmised, attracted to the single light on the ceiling at night, that red eye of the smoke detector.

"Vacuum them out," he suggests. We do, as well as replace the batteries with the recommended Duracell (not the generic store brand) and for the rest of the summer we survive without the dawn alarms, except for some sporadic chirping once in awhile.

Wil is further terrorized (and me, indirectly) by the thought of house fires in July when he visits Aunt Jin in Cincinnati. He tells us about it on the phone, "I was in the shower and Aunt Jin runs in saying, 'Get out of the shower, the house down the street is on fire and we have to get out.' So I jumped into my clothes and helped get the cats and we ran across the street to Gary and Cindy's. I helped take care of Bart and Radar, too, you know, their dogs. And we watched the house burn down to the ground. There was a fire in the kitchen, but nobody was home. It's a good thing the little old lady doesn't live there anymore. One of the neighbors heard the smoke alarms going off."

The house was two doors to the left of Jenéne's and about 100 years old, a Victorian on a very steep San Francisco-like street, with a kitchen renovation underway. Wil watched as the firemen did their work, not saving the house, but saving the neighborhood.

At the end of the summer, we moved into our own house in Palisade, a young house on one of the few suburban-looking streets in town. At our final pre-closing inspection, we noticed the smoke alarms chirping and chalked it up to old batteries since the house had been empty for months, and the high ceilings hard to reach without a ladder. We replaced the batteries on the day we moved in.

Wil's first night in his new room under a ten-foot ceiling he sighed with relief. "I like this new house. The smoke alarms are way high up on the ceiling." Next morning he reported how well he had slept.

Two days later, we wake to that same damn noise at 4:30 a.m. for just half a minute. More gnats? Bad alarms? Blown batteries, it turned out, but why? How, after thirty-six years and so many homes, did we manage to live in two houses with the same problem in the same summer? What bad luck was this? What in the world was the universe trying to tell us? Was some ghost playing tricks on us?

Six months later, it happens again. With recent new batteries, it couldn't be that, so Scott replaced all the smoke alarms in the house, except two because the bulk box from Home Depot wasn't quite enough and he always meant to buy more.

Months later, it happens again. That time we saw that the battery itself had popped at the seam. I wondered if it had something to do with human error upon installation of the battery. (Of course, I blamed Scott.)

Next summer it happens again. I trust the batteries. I say to myself *It's the gnats, those pesky fruit flies that came with the box of ripe peaches. They're at it again. They went looking for light instead of squeezing out though the kitchen window screen.* The next night, I leave on the light of the refrigerator icemaker, telling the gnats if they need a nightlight they can flitter by that one. That works.

I remember times in the past when my sense of panic was instant. Panic is real, but how valid the panic? That's relative.

Laying in bed in the dark, countless times before early morning flights, I wake in a panic that I've overslept and will miss the plane. Waking every hour. Never oversleeping. Never missing the plane. Just irrational worry.

Laying in bed in the dark, in our first house in Oak Ridge, Tennessee. It's 1:30 a.m. on December 18, 1993. I'm in labor. You'd think in a panic, but instead soothed by the words to the song in my head, *Here comes the sun.* ..

And I say, it's all right. Wil on his way. A message from the universe, as lyrics, replacing my dread.

Laying in bed in the dark, listening for Wil's baby breath sent over the crackling radio waves of the room monitor. I'm sure he has stopped breathing. I hear him. He hasn't. A new mother's worry. Heightened awareness of ultimate responsibility for my son, fear of SIDs, and just in love with the sound of his life.

Laying in bed in the dark, five years later in Highlands Ranch, listening to Scott's breathing every night since his brain tumor surgery, jumping sometimes at the sudden twitching of his feet like a dog chasing squirrels in a dream. Then silence and stillness. Panic over life and death, seizure or sleep. My ears always open for five-year-old Wil creeping into our room, sleeping on the floor by my side of the bed, too scared to sleep alone. Me, just too scared to sleep.

Two more post-orchard years go by without the alarms. Scott's MRI's stay clear those two years as well. But my panic still sits at the surface some nights. If I accidentally remember the memory of the smoke alarm going off without warning or reason, I can feel it, instant panic. When that happens, I lie in bed with my hands folded over my heart, trying to release the pain in my chest. I'm trying to stop the energy from leaking out of my heart. It is so easy to recognize that total sense of dread, but not so easy to make it go away.

My fears play out in possible scenarios of a real house fire, and I don't know if it's because I'm scared of the smoke alarms, a real fire, or tumor recurrence.

I am mad at the smoke alarms who are behaving badly, playing tricks, crying wolf. I worry, *What if I don't take the alarm seriously and next time it goes off for real?*

Clearly, I'm worried more about Scott's brain than the smoke alarms.

Sometimes, still, several years and fresh batteries and safe MRI's later, I wake from a single-scene nightmare in which I hear one screech of the smoke alarm, sometimes with one warning dog bark. I sit up, half way convinced, and poke Scott, "Did you hear that? Was that the smoke alarm?"

Clearly, since the alarm isn't still reeling through the house, we are safe. Scott goes back to sleep, and I try.

No, no, no! I say in my head. *You are safe. Wil is safe. Scott is alive...We've replaced all the batteries and the alarms. We have a safety ladder in Wil's room and he knows how to use it (but is it buried in the closet under shoes and toys?). There aren't any gnats. Just sleep. Sleep.*

Usually, I can put out the fire of panic and drop off to sleep.

We've done all that we can. It's time to let go and relax. Whatever happens now is beyond my control.

This is why we have smoke alarms…and another MRI every six months.

In cancer fire fighting mode you live on adrenaline, on the high of self-awareness that comes with facing death and choosing life and feeling surrounded by synchronicity that speaks to the true nature of God. You're surrounded by support from loving friends and family, acquaintances who suddenly seem so close, and strangers willing to help out by saying your name in their prayers and at church. You're amazed by the people who give you money, or bring meals, or go so far as to donate blood, even platelets, to help save a life.

And then that life is saved. The crisis ends. There's no more adrenaline, just fatigue. *Go back to your lives, citizens.* The support network dissipates, like a spider's web spent by the long night's efforts, bits drifting away in the morning breeze, some strands still clinging to the rafters, with dewdrops catching the light of the morning sun.

Big spiders. Now, *they* can cause panic. Scream. Swat. Splat. Panic ends. In Brisbane, Australia, after my mom's cancer when my parents lived a year there on a teacher's exchange, they told stories of big, really big spiders on the walls over the bed or in the shower. "You wouldn't believe the size," my dad said, holding up hands like he was clasping a softball. "But by the end of our year, we'd see them at night and just go back to sleep. No worries."

Sometimes I almost miss the high of cancer fire fighting mode. Of being reminded that life is short, joy is vital, and friendships and love matter most. But you can't live life in fire fighting mode. (I don't know how fire fighters do it.) For a while after cancer, you are stuck in survival mode (or is it survivor's mode), just eating and sleeping and breathing through the months, then years, of recovery. Slowly, it seems, survival mode is replaced with a fresh, somewhat raw, awakening. You climb up a few rungs on Maslow's Hierarchy of Needs.

After the fire is out and the smoldering smoke finally gone, you have to rebuild your web once a day, using patterns that work, adding new strands as needed, doing just enough to strengthen your soul.

If I lay down at night feeling taut in my heart, let it be over fullness and gratitude that I'm listening to deep, roaring snores from Scott on the pillow next to mine, from Wil down the hall, from the dog at our feet…and from trusting that all the gnats are rising to greet the full moon, not swoon over smoke alarms.

Happiness is not a station you arrive at,
but a manner of traveling.
—*Margaret Lee Runbeck*

46
Witness Protection Program

I was so tired of being the Brain Tumor Family. I was tired of everyone asking me, "How's Scott? How's Wil? How are you?" — in that order. One great benefit of moving to the other side of the mountains to an orchard in the irrigated desert was the gift of anonymity. I didn't care what I looked like when I drove to the hardware store to buy tall rubber boots for slogging through tractor-tilled mud or to purchase plastic picking baskets with shoulder harnesses. I didn't need to wear mascara to convince anyone I wasn't tired. My ponytail stayed under a ball cap and I didn't mind letting a few gray hairs grow out until I could find a new salon. I wasn't in lipstick-and-minivan suburbia anymore, and it was such a relief. For awhile.

As Scott and I worked hard with my parents learning how to grow, fertilize, pick, and market our cherries and peaches, we didn't have much time or energy to make new friends. We traversed the mountains almost every weekend back to Denver, selling fruit to our old friends who envied our new lifestyle while they continued living the lifestyle we had abandoned. I pretended our former house was an invisible black hole on the cul-de-sac when we parked in our neighbor's driveway for our come-and-get-them peach rendezvous. During pear, grape, and apple season, we were moving into our own house, enrolling Wil in second grade, and replacing carpet with wood floor, old kitchen cupboards with new.

It was *after* all that, when the pace slowed down and we found ourselves in the dark days of winter, when I realized that we had relocated to some Twilight-Zone Witness Protection Program for cancer survivors and Grand Valley newcomers. It was as if we had seen too much, knew too much, and chose to assume a new identity to protect ourselves from the dangers of Living an Authentic Life. We had decided against sharing our brain tumor story, preferring instead to say we were helping out with my parent's orchard and Scott was helping me with my website business. I soon realized, however, that people weren't buying it.

For instance, "So what do you do, Scott?" the plumber once asked when he came to plug up the raging leak in the powder room after Scott failed to properly solder the copper fittings of the new pedestal sink. "I know it isn't plumbing."

"Oh, not much. I help Shelly out with her business," Scott said without further facts. Jerry assumed Scott was independently wealthy, perhaps making it big in the dot-com boom (the opposite of true for our investment portfolio).

I resisted rolling my eyes or blurting out more. Later I said to Scott, "You need a better line than that. You could say you're on a sabbatical or you took early retirement, or...or...or something. It sounds like you're lying."

"So what? Should I tell them I've had a chunk of brain removed and now I'm disabled? That'll really scare them off. That's not a conversation starter."

"Well, maybe not that. I know...you could say you're living off a rich uncle's trust fund. You don't have to tell them it's Uncle Sam. Don't you just wish you could say, 'I am a cancer survivor. Killed myself off and came back to life with my own stem cells. Lost part of my brain but I'm doing just fine, thank you very much. What do you do for fun?' "

"Nah, just let 'em wonder," Scott said.

It was a long year. The next autumn, Scott (despite his master's degree) decided to take a class at Mesa State College, Biology 301. He wanted to see if his brain could still learn. When he'd gone through college for his first two degrees, he was solely focused on computer science and this time wanted to broaden his knowledge. He found that he could learn again, but only in short spurts. By the end of the semester, the test-taking was much more difficult and studying took much longer than he expected. He also learned that it was nice for awhile to be able to say he was a student.

One day mid-semester Scott stood outside the lecture hall revealing to another student that he once had a brain tumor. Scott told him about the very first symptoms, how his right hand didn't move when he told it to move, how he felt dizzy and couldn't make a plan to fill a glass of water. In the midst of the telling, as if in the telling itself, Scott grew dizzy. He told me about it that night.

"It was so weird," he said. "It's like I was reliving the symptoms. Or that my symptoms are back."

"Do you think we should call Dr. Arenson, or tell your doctor here?" I asked. I started to panic, despite knowing his MRI was all clear a month earlier in October. When his tumor first appeared in October '98, his symptoms were so very subtle but real. I didn't want to ignore what could be real this time as well.

"Maybe. I don't think it's my tumor again. But maybe it's better to find out for sure."

So we called our new family doctor, who agreed to see us that day. From our appointment with her, we walked across the parking lot to St. Mary's Hospital to have an MRI. I was impressed by the speed of her response; I was grateful but scared. Then we had to wait for a return call with bad news, telling us we had to drive over to Denver to see Dr. Arenson. At that point, I didn't consider that the news might be good. I have no idea where my inner Pollyanna went.

Instead of waiting by the phone, Scott went back to campus for his biology class. He said he'd call me if he heard back from the doctor, or he'd see me at dinnertime. I couldn't stay home by the phone because I had to drive Wil to an after-school acting class. I sat outside in the minivan, trying to write in my journal to ease my panic. In my head, though, I was planning Scott's funeral. The worst part was wondering how we could cope, in fire fighting mode again, without a network of friends.

I couldn't wait until I dinnertime. I called Scott on my cell phone. He was home by then.

"Well, was there a message? Did you hear any news?" I was afraid to hear his reply.

"Oh, yeah. I forgot to call you. She called back to say the MRI is all clear. Nothing to worry about after all."

I could have killed him.

By springtime, I was starving to make friends who knew who I was, what I'd been through, how I got to be where I was, to find friends who would be willing to help...just in case. I was tired of being an acquaintance. It's hard to establish new and deep friendships. People are friendly but they're busy with their own lives and orchards and families. It's not their fault. I have a feeling that, like horses who sense fear in new riders, people sense when you're not fully open. If they don't know you from Adam, why should they trust you?

The universe decided to intervene and make it easy on me. It was the end of Wil's third grade year in school and the last parent/teacher conference night of the year. Wil led us to his classroom, showed us his portfolio, took us to the library for the Scholastic Book Fair. We were in the school parking lot unlocking our car when we realized we forgot to see one of Wil's teachers.

"Oh no. We better go back in," I said, even though we were hungry for dinner. We walked back toward the school's side door. The doors opened and out came a family of four, a very tall father, two girls, and a petite brownish-red-haired woman who looked vaguely familiar. She and I both squinted and slowed. We looked at each other, then both of us said, "I know you, don't I?"

"Carrie?" I ventured a guess and identified myself. "Shelly. From CSU. Carrie?"

"Oh my goodness! Shelly? What are you doing here?"

"I live here. We moved to Palisade about two years ago. We moved over here from Denver at the same time as my parents, when they bought an orchard. What about you? Oh, this is my husband, Scott, and our son, Wil. He's finishing third grade."

"This is my husband, Mike. And this is Jolie; she's in second grade. And this is Callie, who's in preschool. We moved here two weeks ago from Wyoming. We transferred with the Forest Service. I can't believe it." Carrie put her arm on mine after we smiled and shook hands all around. "Mike, I know Shelly from college. We lived in the same dorm our first year."

"What a small world," Mike said with a deep voice and a broad smile. "Don't tell me. Your parents live on St. Francis Farm, right?"

I gasped. "How did you know that?"

He gasped. "You mean I'm right? I was just joking? When we were trying to decide whether to move to Grand Junction and then whether to live in Palisade, we looked online for local websites. We found the St. Francis Farm website and I was looking around at all the pictures. I showed Carrie and said, 'See how pretty it is here.' I showed her the family photos on the website."

And Carrie interjected, "And I said, 'Oh, wouldn't it be nice to be friends with that family.' I didn't look closely, of course. Oh my gosh! I never dreamed I would know anyone. I can't believe it!"

"I can't believe it either. I designed that website. Yeah, that's us in those pictures. Holy cow!" I said, stunned at the synchronicity. I was feeling the same hint of destiny as when my next-door neighbor in Highlands Ranch turned out to be my old friend, Diane. At least Carrie's husband wasn't also named Scott. Something strange and wonderful was happening and I didn't know what to say. It was almost too much. Carrie and I had almost ten years to catch up on. And besides, Conference Night was almost over and we had to go back inside.

"Well," I said, stalling, as if pinching myself to see if I was awake. "Um, well, let's get together soon, after school is out." I dug in my purse for my business card so she would have my phone number and address. "Here you go. Call me after you get settled, and we can get together."

Almost a month passed before we saw each other again. Carrie called and I invited her family to come for dinner. We hadn't had friends over for dinner in years. It had been our favorite thing to do our first years in High-lands Ranch with our next-door neighbors. It was so exciting, and scary, to think we might have come-over-for-dinner friends again. It felt too good to be true.

I picked up two large take-and-bake pizzas from Papa Murphy's, way too much for only four grown-ups and three kid appetites, but I didn't want to have too little. We all sat around the kitchen table and I didn't know whether we should say grace or not. I was out of practice for all those intri-cate getting-to-know-you niceties. We skipped grace, made a quick toast with our ice tea and lemonade, and couldn't finish all the pizza. The kids went outside while Scott and Mike did a slow tour of our small downstairs; I heard them stop to admire Scott's widescreen TV and hear our new joke, "Sold a house, bought a TV." Mike was a good conversationalist. Scott was keeping up his end of it, too.

Carrie and I stood in the kitchen, putting glasses and plates in the dish-washer, updating each other on old college friends (her roommate, Judy, caught the bouquet at my wedding). Carrie is gifted at skipping small talk to get straight to the real stuff, like "Is your life now all that you hoped for in college?"

How do you answer that one? I skirted it with something like, "Oh, I don't know. What about you?" And we talked a bit more, but she kept com-ing back to the real question.

"So what brought you here?" she asked.

I hesitated, trying to gauge whether I was ready to spill the beans. I did the duck-and-dodge first.

"We were ready to get out of the city. When my parents found the or-chard and invited us to come, too, we thought 'Why not?' I can take my business anywhere with the Internet." That was all true but she wanted more.

"But how could you just pick up and leave? What does Scott do?"

I still wasn't sure so I tried another tack. "Oh, he was ready for something different. The idea was for him to work with my mom on the orchard while my dad and I kept our own businesses going. The people who sold them the orchard said it was a two-person job. All four of us worked on the orchard that first summer, though. It was such hard work."

"So you're not doing that anymore, you said." Carrie countered, clearly wanting to understand and grappling with her own sense of boundaries to keep asking. She went for it. "I don't get it. What does Scott do now?"

I wanted to be friends with Carrie. I wanted to be done pretending and tell the truth. She was so sweet and kind, just like in college. I felt I could trust her with the truth and she would hold it gently. So I decided to spill my guts.

"Okay, here's the situation. Scott had a brain tumor a few years ago — cancer — and he doesn't work anymore. So we moved here to cut our expenses in half and build a new life."

Poor Carrie. Her eyes filled up with tears as she realized how big the secret had been. I know part of her felt terrible for dragging it out of me. The other part of her was pure compassion. That's the part I fell in love with. A friend at last. Someone to share my secrets.

"Here, let's go upstairs where we can talk. I'll explain," I said, handing her a Kleenex from the box on the counter and pulling her down our short hallway and up the stairs. To anyone else, it would look like a house tour continuing.

We sat on the end of my bed as I filled her in on a few details. Not everything, but enough so that she knew a bit more.

"It's been hard to decide how much to tell people," I finished. "But I wanted you to know."

"Oh, Shelly. I can't believe what you've been through," she said, patting my leg and wiping her eyes. "But here you are. And here we are. It's amazing we ran into each other. This is going to be great."

Our friendship was cemented, and it just kept getting better. We both liked to garden. We both loved FiestaWare dishes, both the old and the new (we both have the original pale-yellow salad bowl). Our kids got along great. Her house behind the big hedge by the road was halfway between mine and my parent's. I'd been driving by it all this time.

Carrie soon met a woman who lived around the corner from her and generously offered her friendship to me like sharing a box of chocolates. When Carrie moved into her house, Laurie was driving by when she saw

Carrie and her girls in the yard. Laurie stopped her car and jumped out saying, "You have daughters!" Laurie lived on Meadowlark Farm with horses
and chickens and an old hedge of roses, which I noticed every time I drove
down that road, as if something were pointing out places where my future
friends lived. Laurie's older daughter was in Wil's class, and she and her
husband were people I smiled at during class field trips or volunteer afternoons.

Our friendship became a threesome, and then larger still because Laurie
knew Mel and Nancy, who lived on the next stretch of road, who also had
daughters in Wil's class at school. They lived in houses, as with Laurie's,
that I had noticed for years, one on Bliss Drive (I envied that street name)
and the Victorian house on G.4 Road with the grape-motif gingerbread trim
and tree house. I swear something was showing me where to find friends,
but it took Carrie to bring us together. And time. It was time, and I was
ready to leave my introvert-self at home and become my true self with new
friends. After that I could rewind and go back to the women I met the first
summer, like Jody and Val, and let our friendships develop beyond waving
hi over the heads of our kids.

As another year went by, coincidence convinced me it was time to leave
the Witness Protection Program forever. One day Laurie called to say that
Nancy's mother, who lived in Wisconsin, had been diagnosed with a brain
tumor. Maybe I could call Nancy, she suggested. So I did, and she said it
made a difference to talk with someone who knew about brain tumors. It
gave her hope.

During those same years, we spoke on the phone to a local woman
whose husband had just been diagnosed with a fast-growing brain tumor.
She turned out to be the cousin of my cousin's father-in-law. We never met
in person, but she said it was nice to know someone else in the same boat.

One August at Scott's regular six-month check-up, we sat in the MRI
waiting room in Denver and introduced ourselves to another young couple,
as it turned out, who lived in Grand Junction. The wife, Karole, had a brain
tumor and saw our same doctors. We exchanged phone numbers and they
came to our house to talk about a month later. We talked for hours, connecting like old friends, and promised to see each other again after her surgery.
She called me once to say her surgery had not gone well. I was so sad to
hear a few months later when she died, and I mailed a note to her husband.

Confirmation continued when new neighbors moved in across the street.
I brought them warm brownies and was secretly pleased their names were

Jane and John, just like the kids down the street where I grew up. In making introductions that night in their foyer, not even thinking, I blurted out that Scott didn't work because he was recovering from a brain tumor. Jane's eye's opened wide and she said, "My father died of a brain tumor when I was a little girl." She and I would have been friends anyway, but I also believe it was synchronicity all over again. Jane said more than once through the years how nice it was to see someone going on with their life, someone who had survived. When Jane and John had to move, their realtor was Karole's husband. It amazes me how life loops around and revisits us.

I believe that friends are people whose lives are meant to intersect our own "for a reason, a season, or a lifetime." If Scott and I had not been willing to tell the truth of our story, we would not have been able to help share what we learned or pass along hope. It was the easier route to let Scott's story on our family website be the only path to finding us, answering emails and phone calls from web-surfing brain tumor people. Sharing our story with Carrie opened me to a new life of friendships. Sharing with Nancy made me realize it was time to come out of the closet. Each step of sharing after that has taught me that we don't have to wear our brain tumor survivorship on our sleeves or post a sign in our yard. Neither should we stay silent.

The summer after I reconnected with Carrie, Scott proudly walked the Survivor's Lap at Grand Junction's annual Relay for Life. While there, he saw a woman who works at our local bank. They were both wearing the t-shirts that said, "I'm Still Here." To see each other as survivors made our town seem a bit more like home.

When the soul is exhausted,
no beautiful flowers can grow from it.
— *Mira Kirshenbaum*

47
Learning to Play

Creativity saved my life.

I called on my grandmothers' souls, an Irish saint, and my inner artist to save me. They showed me the way. I didn't know I was saving my life at the time.

The Irish say that when a soul is lost, you can call on Saint Brighid who will ask the fairies to help lay out a thread for the soul to follow back home. She is the Lady of Smithcraft, Healing, and Poetry who weaves together the mental, emotional, and psychic threads that make life worthwhile. She integrates mind, heart, and soul.

When my mother and grandmother taught me to sew at eight-years-old, it may have been because my legs had grown long enough to reach the electric sewing-machine pedal on the floor and my fingers had grown long enough to guide the fabric under the needle with my right hand, while pulling gently from the back with my left. My thoughts were old enough to envision a finished skirt from flat pieces of gingham, a zipper, and thread. My first skirt I made from a white sheet, because that was for practice. I wore it to school, proud as could be.

The Christmas I was nine, my grandmother surprised my sister and me with two dolls surrounded by a full wardrobe of finery, with matching wool girl-size coats. My doll was blond and we had green coats. Jenéne's doll was brunette and their coats were red. We imagined ourselves in one of our favorite fairy tales about the two sisters, Snow White and Rose Red (not *that* Snow White). Our grandmother made magic with her Singer.

For Easter, school dances, and proms, my mom and I made dresses. I picked out the fabric and pattern, and learned that to match the fabric you should use thread one shade darker. We put a leaf in the dining room table to have room to fold and smooth the yards of periwinkle satin, without caring whether the pins scratched the surface. She taught me to pin tissue-paper patterns in a layout more efficient than the instructions so as to have extra fabric leftover. We cut with my mom's left-handed pinking shears so the fabric wouldn't fray. All this on the mahogany dining room table with brass feet that had been my grandmother's and now is mine. When we were done, the Kirby wound a multi-colored record of our project.

When I was in my last year of college, for my birthday, my mom gave me a Singer of my very own. I made skirts to wear to my first real job as a technical writer. I almost made my wedding dress, but then didn't. When I was pregnant with Wil, I sewed blue striped curtains and re-upholstered the gliding rocking chair to match, as well as made crib bumpers and a soft cotton quilt. When he was little, we sewed clothes for his bunnies and Rugrats. Wil watched when I wrestled white organza and taffeta into two flower girl dresses, and he danced with those dresses in his mini tuxedo at Aunt Amie's wedding.

When I was facing the uncertain outcome of Scott's second surgery, I bought myself a new Elna and sewed curtains of my own design that I see now as the tree of life appliquéd. The diversion and designing of those tree curtains kept me sane throughout those months, as if I was reinforcing my soul with straight pins and zig-zag.

When my grandmother was too old to sit at her sewing machine, too arthritic to sew anymore, she gave me her boxes and boxes and boxes of silk, wool, polyester, polished cotton, organza, and ribbons, seam-binding tape, and an assortment of thimbles, one silver with turquoise beads, one hand sewn of leather for Granddad's thumb for when he patched his truck upholstery, and scissors all sizes, and arcane but essential gadgets, and seam rippers, and plastic shoeboxes of thread. Silk button thread on short wooden spools. Cotton/polyester thread on white plastic spools. Every color you needed to stitch any fabric you desired.

My grandmother was a fabric junkie. So am I. She gave me the ancient weaver's gene, but we called it loving to sew.

That was my dad's mom, who because her first grandson was born from her first daughter, she became known to the rest of us grandkids as MomMom. Her friends called her Gretchen.

My mom's mom, Gramma Liz, was the oldest daughter of the oldest son who came from Ireland to work in the coal mines so his next youngest brother could keep the family farm in Roscommon. She gave me the saints and the fairies, a teapot for tea parties, and her recipe for apple cake that is best with Granny Smith apples and walnuts. She always said, "Go outside and play."

I used to know what I loved, and then I forgot. There was a time, despite our forward-backward steps toward Healing, that the only way to describe it was dark. Dark times. Dark like mid-winter. Dark like mid-forest. Dark like thunderstorms with enough rain to rain forty days and forty nights. Dark, dark, dark, dark.

One particular night, after a cranky dark dinner, Wil asked me a question instead of saying his prayers, "What is your greatest fear?"

"Losing you."

"Mine is having an unhappy family."

"Oh, that's a good one."

My son is the most empathetic, enlightened old-soul that I know. Seasoned traveler that he is, Wil can mimic, with perfect inflection, the flight attendant's speech saying in case of emergency, put on your own oxygen mask first and then help the occupant in the seat next to you. He didn't say it right out, but that's what he meant. I was his flight attendant and he relied on me for safety. Wil also relied on me to be light-hearted enough to play and connect my inner child to his only-child self. You can't play shadow puppets without a bright light.

My dad always said, "You'll ruin your eyes if you try to read-write-draw-sew in the dark." He was right.

In addition to visits from friends for afternoon tea, we did have moments of light, like candles on cakes, like dappled light through the leaves, like late-day sun that gives you a rainbow, but just for a moment, and then the sunsets. But it wasn't enough. The rest of the time felt lifeless and flat. Like all the crayons had melted and the only ones left were burnt orange and raw umber.

One January after our birthday (we're Irish twins, one year apart), my sister delivered a message to me, as if Gramma had sent it herself (but she died the October before). In Jenéne's dream, among other things, Gramma told her, "I'm sad about Shelly. She's not living her life."

When Jenéne told me, I burst into tears. "It must be true if it makes me cry." I was laughing, but gasping at the same time. I sat with those words for days, wondering what does it mean to Live Your Life, *living* your life, really living *your* life? Having something to love? To laugh about? To look forward to?

At a bookstore one day, and this happens a lot, I noticed a book wanting to jump off the shelf. (There's a reason for eye-catching book spine design.) The book was *The Gift of a Year* by Mira Kirshenbaum. So I bought it. You might like it. It gave me permission and roadmap to carve time out of my days full of normal commitments to make time for something I'd love. Don't think of this gift to yourself as a disposable treat. To identify and pursue your heart's desire is the path to saving your life. The question to answer is "what is my heart's desire?" and her book helps us find answers.

My mom knew I was struggling to find light in the dark, so she suggested another book that once worked for her as a flashlight, then spotlight, then sunlight, *The Artist's Way* by Julia Cameron. The book has two subtitles that say, "A course in discovering and recovering your creative self" and "A spiritual path to creativity." You might like that one, too. It gave me permission to take my inner artist on a date once a week to find inspiration or color or something surprising, and asked me to fast-write three pages in my journal every morning to capture my dreams. With it, I accomplished a lot more than that.

As I worked through Mira Kirshenbaum's and Julia Cameron's chapters of suggestions and insights and side quotes, I noticed my inner artist starting to chatter. And then she wouldn't shut up. She woke up my inner everyone-else's and I realized they'd all been asleep, or banished. In fact, I remembered, once on a very dark day, telling my inner Pollyanna to shut the fuck up. Ever since, she'd barely attempted to breathe. I finally said sorry and welcomed her back. Thank goodness! It wasn't until I started to wake up myself that I realized how much I had stymied and stifled my inner resources.

My inner executive, it seemed, was the only one who I had allowed in my new house up until then. I was relying too heavily on her for my business, inflating our combined sense of urgency, intensity, and responsibility. I told my inner executive it was okay for her to take a vacation. I appreciated all she had done to help me keep my head above water, now I was okay on my own. Work would be waiting when she got back, but I thought maybe she needed a well-earned trip to Tahiti. I think she had Nike treads on her butt when I kicked her out the front door. *Whew! Got rid of that party pooper*, my inner artist yelled to my inner seamstress, brushing her hands like they'd been covered with dust. *Now let's have some fun!*

My inner artist could not contain her enthusiasm. She insisted we get out the crayons and paper and fabric and thread, promising we had fun projects to start. She insisted we pull the blinds on the windows all the way open, and the sun couldn't wait to get in. She even made me turn off the computer during playtime. Can you imagine the way she was hopping from foot to foot in excitement, rubbing her palms together? She turned the music up loud and insisted we dance. Then she insisted on shopping.

My inner hippie flower-child insisted on a new wardrobe of play clothes. She said I was done wearing black and helped me find (on a sales rack at REI) a pink batik t-shirt with long, slightly flared sleeves. She said pink is a good color for you/me. She also pointed out pink Shasta daisies, and mini white daisies with yellow centers, and other multi-color daisy things that we bought at Mount Garfield Nursery and planted outside the window of my office, I mean, studio. Then, she told me to start looking around for a used VW New Beetle in lime green and to ditch the boring soccer-mom minivan. We ordered a greatest hits CD by Simon and Garfunkel so we could look for fun and feel groovy.

My inner preschooler insisted on color, so not only did we buy a new box of 64 crayons, but two gallons of paint. I had tried living with professional, grown-up beige walls in my office, only to realize I was surrounded by mushroom soup that matched the PC's plastic case. I wonder how I ever designed good websites with those walls looking on. So in one fast afternoon I painted two walls Ocean Dream blue, two walls Muscat Green (thanks, Sherwin Williams and Martha Stewart). My inner perfectionist tried to get me to touch up the splotches at the ceiling, but I told her not to worry, I was cultivating imperfection instead. I asked her to please leave the room.

My inner artist, in cahoots with the others, insisted on something to form with our hands, and so we became intimate with the inventory of Hobby Lobby, Joanne Fabrics, and Michaels. I saw a smorgasbord of raw materials and I was starving. So I fed myself, just a bit at first, then I went back for seconds. I combined my new treasures with those from my grandmother's boxes, her creative source, and the methods she taught me. I found new ways of my own.

Some people have Starbucks. Creativity is my caffeine, a grande mocha full-caf plus double shot of espresso. Creativity caused me to lie awake on my pillow brainstorming what else I could do with that fabric, those beads, and that ribbon. *So be it*, I thought. *Let me be addicted.*

"You're having way too much fun," Scott would say as he passed by the dining room where I was bent over my sewing machine, using its 20-watt light bulb to help me cut leftover threads from a seam.

"Nuh-uh. I'm having *exactly* the right amount of fun."

Scott didn't really mind because he liked what he saw, me coming to life. I rationalized and affirmed the dollars I spent as worth every penny because what I bought was art therapy, which it was. As L'Oreal says about hair color, it's okay to splurge, because I'm worth it.

I could tell you exactly what I bought, what I made, but that isn't the point. The point is the process: to begin to create and then to beget even more creativity, like spontaneous combustion. Like Eureka! I learned that the point was to get out of my head and into my heart, which I find especially ironic considering it was Scott's brain in his head that caused me to need the strength in my heart.

Creativity was my lifeboat. It not only kept me afloat, but it gave me the buoyancy to lift my arms and my face to the surface, frog kicking, breast stroking my way to the shore. Creativity was swinging from a rope like Tarzan's transformed Jane, letting go, falling, feet first in a pond, squealing and yelling just to be loud, not caring how stupid you look soaking wet in a swimsuit. Skinny dip, if you dare.

As my creativity swelled from a ripple into a wave, I wanted to body surf, hoot and holler, and dive back in the ocean for more. Creativity let me float between waves and talk with the whales and hear them talk back. For the first time in a long time, I was feeling carefree.

Other women taught me to find a thread for my soul so I could follow it home. Your solution would look different than mine, so here's how to find your own thread, your own answers. What are your forbidden joys? What did you love to do as a child, or before cancer caregiving made you feel seriously old? What hobbies have you locked in a closet, buried under boxes of tax forms and medical records, clothes that don't fit, magazines you never make time to read? If you could take any class now, perhaps one an unenlightened school counselor discouraged you from pursuing, what would it be? If you had a gift certificate to the store of your dreams, in whatever dollar amount you deemed perfect, what would you buy for yourself? What makes your heart sing? What turns on your lights?

I found that while most of the darkness had lifted, the darkness always came back (as it does once a day, as intended). Instead of darkness falling with nightmares, however, my nights were lit with a full moon or star shine or porch lights or bonfires of pruned apple wood at the orchard. At that point in my healing, in my creative recovery, I didn't know if I'd ever write My Book, whether I'd ever get started. And that was okay. I was learning to breathe again. I needed more time to play. But I *was* on my way.

I held a conversation with God one night that went, "Thank you, God, for making me creative."

"Oh no, thank *you*, Shelly, for being creative."

"Oh, no-no-no, thank *you*," I said, but God had the last word.

"We make a good team."

"What is life's greatest burden?" asked the child. "
To have nothing to carry," replied the old man.
—a fortune cookie

48

Scott's World

On a flight back from Chicago in January 2004, having visited my sister for our birthday, I was reading *Sophie's World*, a Norwegian novel that is also a history of philosophy. I didn't have my pen out, so I was turning down corners of pages to mark good thoughts to ponder later. Without giving away the secret to Sophie's story, I can say that without warning the book flipped my brain inside out. I felt dizzy and wanted to cry. I began to question reality. My own reality.

What if Scott *did* die from his brain tumor, back in 1999 or sometime since then? What if I have been living a delusion so real that I believe he still exists? What if nobody else has seen him or interacted with him, but only know of him by the stories I have told? What if? Holy shit!

I was sitting there on the plane, the paperback face down on the seat tray. I looked out the window, twisted the wedding ring on my left hand, and really wondered?

How crazy am I? Am I crazier to consider this flip of reality, or did I just awaken from craziness that might have lasted for years?

I put up the seat tray and reached under the seat for my backpack. I pulled out my pen and my journal and started to write. I had to sort this out on paper, immediately, to see the faults or the truth in my logic. My pen couldn't keep up with my mind.

What if...what if I never let go of the "Scott who died" —as in the "previous Scott" (or maybe neither has he). Have I ignored or discounted the new one, the Scott who lives?

What if Scott is not living his own life, but letting me live it for him? As in the way I seem to be keeping all his relationships alive by being the one to make phone calls, send emails, write Christmas cards, buy presents. Have I become so overprotective, or perfectionist, or disabling, because I think it's my duty as his caregiver or wife? Have I lost belief in his abilities to carry on? Or do I do those things because I always did those things when I was the stay-home mom and he worked full time, before I became the caregiver? Does he even need me to be a caregiver anymore?

To what extent has he allowed me to intercept his father-son relationship with Wil? Has it become easier for me to be both parents? Has it become too hard for Scott to pay attention to Wil? Or have I been protecting Wil from Scott's role as parent because Scott tends to think it is more about discipline than playing? Such as this weekend whenever I called home, Wil always sounded so lonely, saying he missed me, because Scott was in the garage, or on the computer, or up late watching a rated-R movie that Wil couldn't watch.

So could Scott really be dead instead? Has he not interacted with Wil because he isn't alive? Have I left Wil alone? Is my mom taking care of Wil, like she usually does, and she's just saying she'll make sure to feed both my boys?

Should I ask Carrie if she ever met Scott in person? What if she told me no, that she's only heard stories and seen photographs?

Of *course* Scott is alive. I should ask him to sign and date the oak side table he made me for Christmas as proof. Ironically, and now I am going crazy, he made it from oak that he's had for five years. Did he make it five years ago and I'm kidding myself that it's new? What if, before he died, he made all sorts of presents and asked my parents to give me one every year so that I would always remember him? But what about the sawdust in the garage?

Would my parents really let me believe this delusion for so many years? Would my doctors tell her it was safer to let me have my illusion, delusion? God, am I really that crazy?

It's conceivable. It's inconceivable. Either I'm nuts or I'm just waking up from years of being crazy. Here are all the reasons this could be true that Scott could be dead:

1. Scott's wedding ring has been sitting on my desk in a cup for over a year. He took it off (at least that's what I think) because he said he was too skinny to wear it and he was afraid it would fall off and he'd lose it. Since it is gold lined with titanium, it couldn't be sized. He said I could just keep it safe until he got fat enough to wear it again.

2. Scott's MRI's haven't changed in almost five years. Maybe the doctors are in on it, too, and they're showing me the same MRI every six months. After all, I sit in the MRI room all by myself. I walk though the

hospital with Scott following me, along those black and blue tiles that point the way to Radiology and back to the elevators. I do all the talking, it seems, with the doctors. I seem to answer questions for Scott instead of letting him talk. Like that last time we ran into the neurosurgeon in the elevator. He seemed so surprised to see us (me?). He asked "How are you doing?" not, Hi Scott, how are you doing? And Scott waited so long to say anything, I just answered for him, "We're good. We just had a six-month MRI and are on the way to see Dr. Arenson." And the surgeon looked at me funny, which he would do if I were pretending Scott was there, too, or perhaps because Scott hadn't spoken (and maybe he wondered if Scott was not doing so well and his speech was affected?).

3. Who taught Wil to ski? It wasn't me. But I dropped him off at Powderhorn and he came back later. Maybe he had group lessons?

4. Every November 6th I tell the same story, of how Scott was diagnosed just days before his birthday and every birthday since then we have another big party, toasting to another year of survival. But it's always me making the toast, never Scott. Is everybody in on it, and we're just pretending to remember Scott on his birthday as if he's still there? Who blows out the candles?

5. I've been having such dry eyes lately and my vision has gotten so blurry. What if it's because my body is fighting so hard to see the truth, and I'm just now able to see it? God, is even my body and the desert-dry air conspiring against me in this delusion?

6. We're still getting Scott's Social Security check every month, but through direct deposit, so he never has to endorse the check. Is that actually my widow's benefit? Should the amount still be that much?

7. Scott's clothes are still in the closet, and I still wash them. I find his jeans on the floor every day and it's not like they're dirty but I wash them anyway.

8. Whose whiskers are in the second sink in our bathroom? I'm sure they're not mine. Have I been shaving my legs on the counter with his electric razor again? God, am I that crazy?

9. What about Scott's silver Ford F150 parked in the driveway? I'm always complaining that he hardly ever drives it. He tells me it's because it gets lousy gas mileage and anyway, where would he go? He's been letting me do the driving since the day he was diagnosed. We bought him that truck because of the automatic transmission. But it has barely

more miles on it than two years ago when we bought it. I even had to co-sign on the loan, even when I didn't want to, because he said I was the one who would be responsible for paying it off in the end. Geez, were the car salesmen in on this delusion as well?

10.   Whenever we have visitors, even from Scott's friends who come all the way over the mountains to visit us, it seems like I do all the talking. I never thought I was that talkative before? Is everyone going along with this hoax? How crazy am I?

11.   Who has been fixing the computers in our house? Now I know that couldn't be me.

I wrote all this down in my journal until the Boeing landed in Denver. I packed away my journal and walked to baggage claim, too afraid to get out my cell phone and call Scott at home, because by then I wasn't sure if he answered whether I would know it was a real human being, not just a ghost or some hoax of a message machine. Besides, my voice was on the answering machine recording, not Scott's.

I walked from baggage claim, pulling my black suitcase, shaking my head. I've either got an extreme imagination, or I'm just waking up. This is so weird.

I kept up the queries in my head as I started the engine of the minivan, paid the fee for long-term parking, pulled onto I-70 for the four hour drive home back over the mountains. At one point, crazy with thinking, I pulled my journal out of my backpack and set it on the passenger seat (where Scott always sits) and clicked on my pen. I wrote notes while I was driving, not willing to pull over but unwilling to let the thoughts wait. The handwriting on the page is all over the place. Perhaps that was my mind, not my driving.

Did I make him disappear? When? Can I bring him back? Can I get back to reality? What can I do to make him reappear? Live, just live!

How crazy is that?

Very crazy.

Halfway home, my delusion went out the window, evaporating at 10,666 feet when I drove over Vail Pass. I was feeling sane by the time I pulled into the driveway at home, with one last skeptic pause.

Relief welcomed me. Scott and Wil came out of the house, waving and happy to see me. Wil held my hand while Scott carried my suitcase inside. If he was a ghost, could he do that?

I looked Scott in the eyes, connecting with his blue irises behind his glasses, and I reached for a hug. A real hug. He hugged me back.

"Hi honey, I'm home," I said.

"Good," Scott said. "We missed you."

Wil pulled me out of Scott's arms and into the kitchen. "Look, Mom. We wrote you birthday poems with your magnetic poetry. Come see."

On the side of my fridge were rectangles of words from the Magnetic Poetry Kit plus the words we had printed and stuck to magnets ourselves (like our names, plus groovy, crescent, sew, spleen, and crap, because the kits don't know all the necessary words and jokes a family needs). Some poetry refuses explanation.

I will always love Shelly

devour champagne as if it were
squirming decaying spleen crap

chocolate
kisses
sewing
cute animals
laughing
velvet
porcelain
perfume
peace
and
crescent moons
perhaps Scott and Wil

Once I saw Scott alive, I had to address whether he was really living his life, without me as concierge, director, or ventriloquist. It wasn't my job, exactly, but I wanted to find a way to nudge him into action, short of telling him how I spent six hours imagining that he was a ghost (*why didn't I tell him?*). The first step was to redefine my role as wife and friend versus caregiver. I wanted out of the caregiving job.

The next week Scott had an appointment with the local neurologist. The appointment was to further sleuth out why Scott could not fall asleep easily and then would wake up and couldn't go back to sleep (which had plagued him since his first operation). For over a year, the neurologist had been tweaking the brand and dosage of Scott's anti-seizure medicine while trying to balance the side effect of worsened insomnia.

"So you've been taking the medicine early enough, at dinnertime, like we talked about last time?"

"Yes, mostly," said Scott. "It doesn't seem to matter when I take it, early or late. I still can't fall asleep."

"Well, if taking the pills before dinner was going to make a difference, we would have seen the results for your sleeping by now," he said. "I'm sure I'm a good enough judge of your character, Shelly, to know you were reminding Scott to take his drugs at dinnertime."

At first I didn't say anything, feeling guilty—like it was my fault Scott wasn't sleeping, like it was my fault that maybe he didn't always remember to take his pills before dinner, like it was my fault that I wasn't even paying attention to Scott's pill practices at every dinnertime for six months.

The doctor repeated his joke, slightly altered, at the end of the appointment, something like "So you'll stay on top of him with his meds for the next six months?"

"I stopped being that kind of caregiver years ago," I said, probably glaring. What I meant was, *It's no longer my job, so back off.*

The doctor looked at me funny, as if I were about to go postal. I can say now that it wasn't unreasonable of him to expect my help…he didn't know the extent of Scott's memory problems or the extent of my role in Scott's daily maintenance. The doctor chose the correct response. "Oh…kay."

As Scott and I walked out of the office and down the steps to the parking lot, I asked Scott, "Should I have been responsible for you taking your meds these past months? Being so responsible for your survival and drugs that first year nearly wiped me out."

"No, you're not," Scott said with a firm grip on my arm, not just to steady me on the stairs. "I don't want you to feel that way again. You are not responsible for my survival."

"Until I have to be," I said, half aloud. But I nodded. "Thanks. I needed that."

I reaffirmed for myself that it wasn't my job any more to keep track of Scott's medicine. Scott was more than able to sort his pills into his twice-daily boxes, to reorder his prescriptions when they ran out. It was liberating for me not to worry, and even more so to be absolved of my guilt.

That event seemed to open the door to more steps in my personal goal to coax Scott back to life, to his own life, and release him from my...care? ...protection? ...concern? It wasn't the first time Scott tried to find a new purpose in life. Years earlier Scott tried Habitat for Humanity, but it wasn't a good fit. They didn't need another guy with a hammer and his inner carpenter was frustrated at their methods. Scott offered his computer programming services for free to Mesa State College, as a way to test his ability to keep learning, but they didn't understand why a guy would do something for free, and that didn't pan out.

Scott was depressed at so many doors slamming shut, but he refused to try anti-depressants when Dr. Arenson suggested it might help him surface enough to be able and willing to talk

One night we saw *A Beautiful Mind*, which struck too close to home, especially the scene where the once-genius husband sits in the kitchen unable to participate in life and the wife asks him to start by simply taking out the trash like people do. "What *do* people do?" he asked, not understanding how people without high IQs manage to exist without the thrill of a career that challenges their mind beyond normal limits. During that scene I couldn't even look over at Scott to see how he was reacting. In the dark car driving home, though, we agreed it was the closest we'd seen to an accurate reflection of our life.

I insisted against his wishes that Scott go talk with a local neuropsychologist who I hoped would be able to sort out the cancer grief from his brain deficits, but all she said was "Pick up the Yellow Pages, Scott. Plenty of places could use you."

I saw an article in the *Grand Junction Sentinel* of places to take kids on the weekend. One caught my eye: the Western Colorado Math and Science Center. It was a place of hands-on exhibits for kids, more than a museum but an Exploratorium.

"Scott, check this out," I said, clipping the newspaper article and sending it over the breakfast table. "Why don't you take Wil and go visit this place on Saturday and see what it's about. It sounds like the Science and Energy Museum in Oak Ridge. I know the school takes field trips there. It's supposed to be great."

"Okay, that sounds kind of interesting."

"This reminds me of another article I saw awhile back about this high school kid from Grand Junction who invented a sign-language interpretation glove. It was attached to a digital screen so that somebody could read what you were saying, like when ordering at Burger King. This kid won first prize in an international competition for his invention and lots of scholarship money. His mentor is the man who started the Math and Science Center."

"Cool. I'd like to meet that guy."

On a Saturday morning, I stayed home when Scott and Wil went to the Math and Science Center, which is housed in part of an elementary school. The school district donated the space, although it wasn't in charge of running the center. The large room was awash in colorful tables of science equipment that seemed more like toys and signs inviting kids to explore some concept in physics or biology or magnetism or sound waves. Scott paid the two dollar entry fee, putting the bills into a large glass jar at the entrance, signing his name in the guest book.

A petite white-haired man walked across the room with a smile. "Welcome. I'm John McConnell. Where are you folks from?"

"Oh, just from Palisade. This is quite the place you have here," Scott said, extending his hand to shake.

"It sure is. Take a look around. Have you been here before, young fellow?" he asked Wil.

Wil shook his head no, being shy and standing almost behind Scott.

"Let's go see that big magnifying glass," Scott said to Wil.

That first encounter turned into another. Scott went back alone another day to ask John if the center needed volunteers. "I was thinking it would be fun to learn more about electricity and oscilloscopes. Maybe I could volunteer some time in exchange for some lessons."

"We can always use volunteers," John said, "But you're welcome to come here and learn whatever you want anytime. That's what we're here for."

Scott's learning time turned into volunteer time, first with one afternoon a week, then sometimes three days, sometimes four. Within months Scott was talking with John, full of ideas for a database that would schedule the school field trips. Scott talked like a new man at the dinner table at night, telling about the other volunteers he met, "They're a bunch of really smart guys. They're mostly retired engineers and physicists who worked at places like Los Alamos, the Jet Propulsion Lab, and the National Labs."

As time went on, Scott helped build exhibits, network the computers, and act as a tour guide and general question-answering guy for people who came to visit the center. He enjoyed John's camaraderie, lunches at

Conchita's Restaurant, being surrounded by people who loved learning and teaching.

Thus began a beautiful friendship. Scott had somewhere to go where he had something interesting to do with someone who earnestly needed what Scott had to offer—his time, his brain, his passion, and his humor. Scott was happy again and coming alive.

Do you take this man as your lawful husband
to have and to hold, from this day forward,
for better or for worse, for richer or for poorer,
in sickness and in health, to love and to cherish
as long as you both shall live?

49
I Do

On the morning of our wedding, I awoke alone in my childhood bedroom, where you'd think I would be waking up happy. But I awoke from a nightmare of pink-orange-red flames and then saw those flames matched in the sunrise out my window. Moments before in my dream I was walking away from a burning jetliner, holding Scott's hand. Silhouetted people were running and screaming in the background, but I was calm with my hand in Scott's, squeezing fingers for comfort. Steadfast, he led me away from the crash, resolutely toward safety. At first I wondered if it meant our marriage would be a disaster, or if it meant we would someday survive a plane crash, or if we should cancel our honeymoon flight to Cape Cod the next morning. I sifted through the panic dissipating from my dream. I could not find a shred of doubt about marrying Scott. If the dream had been meant to dissuade me, I decided, I would not have seen myself holding his hand.

That afternoon, at ten minutes til two, tuxedoed Scott observed how the priest was more nervous than he was. While the groomsmen were waiting those final moments before stepping onto the altar to watch me walk up the aisle, the young Jesuit priest joked about maybe needing to drink some sacramental wine to calm his nerves. Scott didn't need any wine.

Forty minutes later we said our I do's. Then we each said, "I take this ring as a sign of my love and faithfulness in the name of the Father, the Son, and the Holy Spirit."

Because of the way my wedding band gold wraps around the diamond solitaire like a puzzle, I thought Scott slid my ring on backward. So I whispered to him and made him turn it around. Then I saw it was right the first time and he turned it around once again. We laughed. Then we kissed.

I had our wedding date engraved on the inside of Scott's band so he'd never forget. As the years went on, he forgot the date was engraved there, but he never forgot the date.

Close to our first anniversary, when we were still blissful, naïve, and renting a condo on High Point Lane, one of Scott's friends at work was diagnosed with breast cancer. The day he heard the news, Scott gave me a dozen red roses, a pint of Ben & Jerry's Cherry Garcia, and a card on which he wrote, "I know you know I love you, but do you really know how much?" I do, I told him.

It's no secret that a marriage must change when a baby makes your couple to a trio. You don't split up your love, dole it out, and decide who gets how much. Love multiplies, as do hours in the day allotted for laundry, diapers, and dishes. You just agree to sleep less. When we were both working parents we shared everything in equal parts, and the points balanced out.

It surprised me then that marriage changes when you stop being a dual-income couple with one kid, wanting more kids, and the wife decides to quit working and the budget gets tighter. Where we once shared household duties right down the middle, it changed when I became a stay-at-home mom and he worked full time, halving our income while doubling our mortgage and confusing our duties. We seemed to start tracking points, like who vacuumed last, who had to drive when we went to our parent's house for Sunday dinner, who should take out the trash, who deserved a back rub more, and who knew better what to do with the grass clippings: mulch, bag, or bury.

Scott's brain tumor signaled its very first symptom a week after our eighth anniversary. Ironic, isn't it, that the universe asked us to remember our wedding vows just about then? Scott's tumor reignited the memory of my pre-wedding plane crash dream, and I tried to focus on the part where Scott held my hand as we both walked away from the flames.

So what changes when cancer arrives in your marriage? For the nine months of Scott's brain tumor treatment, I must say our marriage, on most days, grew stronger and wiser. We were a team. We were in it together. I did the driving, I gladly gave him back rubs and foot rubs. Our neighbors took care of our lawn, and somehow the carpet got vacuumed. Every day we said "I love you." We took turns crying and comforting. I was proud, amazed, and impressed by Scott's courage. Our marriage strengthened during Scott's cancer because, I believe, we never stopped talking or telling the truth. We were on the same page, and we weren't keeping score.

It's true that we found ourselves wearing new roles, he as patient, me as caregiver. You do it because you must, but also because you promised "in sickness and in health."

However, the vows had an escape clause, so to speak. "I prepared myself for the possibility that you might leave, you know, if the situation became unbearable," Scott told me years later, and I remembered how he even gave me permission before the first surgery in case he woke up as a mean, horrible person. "Leaving should always be an option. If it was killing you to stay, I would much rather that you left. There comes a point when you have to save your own life or go after your own happiness. Things change. And you shouldn't have to stay if you cannot be happy."

When he said that, he looked at me one second extra to make sure I understood his permission did not come with an expiration date.

Does everyone's marriage get harder in the years after cancer? If so, why is *that* kept a secret? If I knew to expect it, I might have been able to circumvent some of it. Or could I? Is caregiver burnout inevitable, and is that why marriage gets rough?

It's hard to admit that part of caregiver burnout is anger and blame. You're ready to kick him off the pedestal everyone put him on and realize he's still just a man. He's thinking the same thing. You wake up and look in the mirror, shocked to find wrinkles you never noticed before. Literally, overnight wrinkles, gray hair!

If I could sum up seven years of wishful thinking and blame, I would skip to the part where one of us said, "I guess what I'm really mad about is that I miss my old life."

"I know. I do, too."

And that's how we find ourselves back together again, on the same page, in the same boat, on the same team, understanding the root of the problem. *All the king's horses and all the king's men, couldn't put Humpty together again,* but marriage might mend. There are some things, like a brain after a tumor, that cannot be put back together, not the same as before. Not without deficits. Not without changes. If you have enough time, the swelling subsides, more healing occurs, and you dare to imagine the formation of new neural pathways. Or at least you find better ways of coping with what isn't the same as before. Part of long-term recovery is allowing time to make new connections. I once thought of making a poster from a photograph of Easter eggs with a caption that said, "If you're going to put all your eggs in one basket, make sure they're hardboiled."

While Scott's was too loose, I noticed my wedding ring was too tight. It took six weeks to send it to Helzberg's to have it resized. I felt guilty not wearing a ring, but I noticed my ring finger stopped being dented and hurting. At some point you have to resize not only your rings but your marriage.

At some point it's good to rewrite and renew your marriage vows, call them Marriage Vows for Real Life. Keep what works and clarify as much as you need. For instance: *For better or worse, for richer or poorer, in sickness and in health. In laughter and joy. Through fear and worry, grief and fury. Through cancer and caregiving, if that's where life takes us. Despite morning breath and body smells, belly flab, and wrinkles. On vacations or Mondays, every day wake up choosing to love. Remember we each do the best that we can. Help each other find hope. Encourage to laugh. Honor by listening. Forgive. Foresworn. Forever. Amen.*

P.S. Don't forget Cherish.

At what point in long-term cancer survival do you stop being patient and caregiver and return to being plain old husband and wife? It is subtle, like the day you don't order his prescriptions and he refills his pill box all on his own, that day and thereafter. Or the annual physical exam you don't attend because it's not about cancer and he doesn't need you to take any notes. Or the day he takes out the trash, mows the lawn, cleans the toilets (some days never come). Or the day you realize his selective memory is not a brain tumor thing, it's a guy thing.

Your role swings back on the pendulum if he tells you about a headache one day, then when it is resolved as a normal everyday headache, not a tumor, your pendulum of caregiver swings back to spouse.

Becoming married again might mean finally feeling sexy instead of too tired. It might be planning next year's anniversary vacation, instead of wondering whether you can count on him to still be alive in six months. It might mean celebrating a birthday like a regular birthday instead of a major milestone.

One thing that never went back to normal, to the way it was before cancer, was that Scott couldn't go back to work and I was the one who had a career.

"So that's the one thing you would change if you could?" I once asked Scott.

"Yes. Definitely."

I thought about it a moment, filtering through all our life's losses and changes.

"Me, too."

You can accept when life changes, you can try to embrace life and love it like never before. But to be honest, you may never stop missing some parts of your past. The question is, do you spend too much energy missing yesterday's loss and instead miss out on the present?

One day I realized I wanted points. I wanted points for all that I'd gone through. I thought I deserved points for everything I had lost, plus my sacrifices, plus my sorrows and angers, plus all the heroic things I had done that I never would have done if I hadn't been forced by choice and circumstance. I even wanted my points to add up higher than Scott's, or at least end up in a tie.

So here's my idea. Let's say you get points. Take as many as you think you deserve. Go all out. Give yourself points for every tear that you cried, every night you lay awake too scared to sleep, every mess you had to clean up, every bad dream, every time you didn't get to do something normal and fun because you had to be at the hospital instead. Count every minute or day or year of your time you deem worthy of points. Add them all up. You get to decide how many points to assign for each item.

Have your "patient" do it, too. How many points for each surgery? Each day of radiation? Each chemo drip? Each transfusion? Each vomiting binge? Each hair that was lost? Each day of life you fear was deducted from the total expected? You, caregiver, get to count each of those items—you were there, too.

So have you added them up? Does it feel good to see all those points? To say this is how much it hurt, how much I gave up, how much you owe me? I want recognition!

So here's what you do next. Print yourself a nice diploma saying you have graduated from the Caregiver's Program, *summa cum laude*. Frame it, sign it, and hang it on your wall.

Pretend you're at the Oscars, in a stunning dress and jewels, accepting your award for best actress in a drama. Give a long-winded speech, thanking everyone including The Academy, but especially the writers, the directors, the costume designers, the supporting cast, the snack prep team, your leading man, and of course, your family for their unflagging devotion, love, and support.

Or take yourself to a booth in your mind—like at Chucky Cheese, the county fair, or Las Vegas—where you exchange your points for a prize. Show with a flourish your self-tallied points and say, "See? Look what I did? What do I win?"

The person in charge of awards will give you a smile and do a Vanna-like wave to display the prizes at hand. What's on the prize shelf? Shelves full of stuffed pink unicorns, fake trophies, wind-up flying pigs, high-bouncing balls, lava lamps, t-shirts, real cubic zirconium, keys to a car, a ten-day vacation to Fiji? What prize is enough?

"Now that's a lot of points. Congratulations," the prize-keeper might say, "Well done. Thank you for playing. But didn't you know? Life is the prize. Do you want to keep playing?"

God wants to give you the frosting bowl to lick
and also the beaters.
—*Mary Jo Cartledgehayes*

50
In Seven Years
To Make a Long Story Short

Anniversaries shared among strangers.
September symptoms. October weddings, November diagnosis and
    death.
Young couples and malignant brain tumors.
Parallel lives spanning the continent. Stories and hope connected by
    Internet.
Clinical trials considered. Stem cell rescue after high-dose chemo.
Mike goes first. Rough but rapid recovery.
    Kathy tells Shelly. Shelly tells Scott.
Encouraged, Scott takes his turn. Rough but rapid recovery.
Mike goes again. Savage clinical trial. Twice is too much.
    Pneumonia takes over.
Mike dies. Scott lives. Tumor disappears.

Years pass.
Kathy survives and finds love again, a love that knows loss.
Marries David, who lost his first wife, Kimberley Ann,
    to a brain tumor, after surviving six years.
Kathy and Shelly share emails, support other strangers
    by creating tumorfree.com.
Young wives, caregivers, survivors of one husband's death,
    one husband's survival.

Friendship expands from email to phone calls to in-person hugs.
Standing knee deep in the ocean at Seaside, connecting.
Touring the Empire State Building, Ellis Island and Monet
    in the city, connecting.

Tasting wine from the barrel and soaking up scenery
    in Colorado canyons, connecting.
Applauding the sun as it sinks in the ocean,
    a foursome united, connected.

Years pass. Seven so far.
Survival lengthens. Friendship strengthens.
Autumn evokes anniversaries of marriages, diagnoses and deaths,
Scott reports a clean MRI, brain tumor still missing.
    Statistics defied another six months.
(Is it true that in seven years every cell in our body has died,
    been replaced, leaving us entirely new?)

Same day, 2,000 miles away,
Kathy and David deliver good news of their own.
Grace Anne. Seven pounds. Six ounces. 'Cute as a button.'
New life. Hallelujah!
Happiness shared among friends.

Someone who cannot move and live a normal life because he is
pinned under a boulder has more time to think about his hopes
than someone who is not trapped in this way.
—*Václav Havel*

51
Pain Tolerance

It was our seventh Christmas since Scott's brain tumor. Wil was twelve and finding his way through sixth grade at East Middle School in the Challenge Program. Wil was doing just fine. We measured our years by his passions from chickens to video photography to cell phones, and by marking his height on the door trim as he surpassed five feet two and his feet grew larger than mine.

I measured progress by my roses, lilacs, crab apples, and willow in my yard, the lineal feet of filled journals on my shelf, and one more wall painted something other than white. I smiled when I saw how our family photos had progressed from snapshots of me stretching my arms as if to protect both Scott and Wil, to pictures of Scott standing tall, beaming health, draping his arms around us.

Scott measured his progress by his latest computer, by how far he could run, and by how many times he went skiing. He submitted to a new vaccinations, which he'd been meaning to do for six years since his high-dose chemotherapy and stem cell rescue wiped out his bone marrow and any immunity from his childhood vaccines. It was progress that he thought he'd live long enough to benefit from updated vaccines. On his birthday, he traded in his gas-guzzling Ford F-150 for a small Kia Sportage, which came with a 10-year, 100,000 mile warranty, and he said he didn't mind that the truck's warranty was better than his own.

I measured Scott's progress by whether he whistled while he worked and how often he laughed. We were all making progress.

By our seventh Christmas, following a clean MRI in October, our fifteenth wedding anniversary, Scott's fortieth birthday, I thought we were home free. I thought it marked progress that we were not traveling anywhere for Christmas, content to have it at home even if that meant alone while our parents went elsewhere, not fearing it could be the last. I thought it huge progress that I didn't care about Scott's flu, which kept us home from church on Christmas Eve. It was such a relief for him to be sick with something that wasn't a brain tumor.

The thing about reaching such milestones after cancer is that sometimes instead of feeling lucky and home free, you feel like your warranty is about to expire. If you start looking for signs to confirm your suspicions, you'll find them—if you choose to filter your vision that way.

Scott told me about a few weird right-sided symptoms that plagued him all month, and I chose to ignore them. I pretended it was progress that I could live without worry. After all, he was winning Sudoku, sixth level. But I kept my eye on him when he wasn't looking.

The holidays seemed to be going quite well, when I started to feel a tight panic invading my chest. Panic. Despite Scott's latest weird symptoms, I didn't really think that was it. Despite learning that the extended warranty company had gone bankrupt, and my used VW Beetle no longer had coverage, I didn't think that was it. I did notice an irrational decision to stop putting miles on my Bug, park it in the garage, and drive Scott's new Kia instead. After all, it would be good for ten years.

I didn't think I was worried about Julie, even though her latest test results show her tumor markers rising. I wasn't too worried because she was happy with her new full-time job. She was living her life.

One day, however, I received an email from my friend since seventh grade, Amy. She and I had been best friends, locker partners, college roommates. We were butter and toast, Laverne and Shirley. We took care of each other, as best friends do growing up. Amy went backpacking through Europe the semester my mom went through ovarian cancer. When Amy came back, I left my roommates to move in with her. I met Scott the next month, and the next year we all lived together. By 2006, we hadn't lived in the same state together in a very long time. She was happily married with four kids in Connecticut and a fulfilling career. The second Christmas after Scott's tumor, she included us in her 1999 Christmas card, saying we'd been through a lot, send us prayers. Her December 2005 email just to me said she had breast cancer.

I didn't know what to say. I wanted to tell her all the secrets to cancer survival so she could skip straight to the end where you find courage and peace, no matter what. What I knew is that she had to go through her own journey. I was afraid to say the wrong thing. I wanted to tell her if Scott and

Julie could do it, so could she. But I didn't want to be glib. I meant healing, not cure, without guarantees.

Amy began her chemotherapy in mid-January. She said to send her good vibes. So I did, with this Magnetic Poetry poem. If I could have been there in person, I would have.

listen here woman
you are my life long sacred sister

do ask god why
but trust this secret will speak not in words

learn to use wild breath
make sad voice a deep embrace
the hard magic works slowly
come linger & explore it

we smile & laugh
we live with worry
needing less hard crap
but soon we know how to heal

understanding profound question
you ask for more grace
& let us bring you flowers
celebrate as though hearts were opening
bellowing there can always be joy

then when dark night is over
and one morning the clouds melt away
wake up and picture only the good things
perhaps you would lie down in cool grass with me
and look for translucent stars above in the steel blue sky

I say
may soft peace surround these women
two brilliant daughters born of this universe
remembering to dance

free will

love change

Around the same time, I heard bad news from Gail, a friend from my writing class. We spent two semesters sharing our stories, she knew all about my first drafts writing about cancer caregiving and had cheered me on when the words start to flow. She told me her husband was just diagnosed with throat cancer. She said knowing me gave her courage, that if I could get through it, so could she.

After so many years of replying to emails from newly diagnosed brain tumor patients, I thought I knew what to say. But when I found myself facing two friends who were facing new cancers, the stakes seemed higher. I questioned all that I knew and the best way to say it.

The panic in my chest grew tighter. Scott started telling me more of his symptoms. I started coughing, but only at night, not running a fever. I chalked up the cough to a virus, the panic to fright, the tight pain in my chest as my heart breaking for friends. I didn't take myself to the doctor, and I didn't get better. And still I didn't get better. I got worse.

Finally, a friend who is a physician's assistant said to me, "I think you have pertussis." He meant whooping cough. I went to the doctor, too late. Pertussis could not be confirmed so they called it bronchitis, and the antibiotics, two rounds of them, finally helped. My lungs remained sore, like a knife was twisting in my chest. It turns out the panic in my chest was my lungs, that a panic sensation is also a symptom of asthma-like attacks. It turns out that whooping cough is making a comeback as a silent epidemic because our vaccinations as children have worn off. I should have seen a doctor about it much sooner.

"Remind me to take myself to the doctor next time I'm sick," I told Scott, mad at him for not insisting I go and madder at myself for not making myself a priority.

"I was wondering why you didn't go to the doctor," Wil said.

"I know. It was stupid. I would have taken you right away. Why couldn't I take care of myself? I should have. That wasn't a very good example, was it? Next time I will do better."

All that's to say that my body was crashing, my defenses were down. Worries for Scott, and Amy, and Gail and her husband were in my thoughts every hour. Plus, I didn't like being sick.

Ironically, as Garrison Keillor once said on his radio show, "The good thing about being a writer is that no matter how bad life gets, you always have something to write about."

Every time I started feeling better, it happened to be on a Thursday, which happened to be the night of my writing class, so I could go. Women Writing for (a) Change was another God thing that saved my life. I was in my third semester and I was feeling prolific, perhaps enhanced by the pertussis that gave me bedridden time to read Parker Palmer, Jean Shinoda Bolen, Mary Pipher, and others, and facing life and death all over again with my friends, not to mention Scott's symptoms. Insight and inspiration dripped out my fingers. Words arose from deep within or beyond myself, straight from my soul or much higher. As sick as I was in my body, my soul felt strong and wise, at least more days than not.

Yet I questioned my wisdom. I wondered if I knew, really knew, what to say to my friends. I wondered if I remembered what it feels like when your husband is first diagnosed. Gail said she kept coming back to one question, "Why?" I remember that question. It took time to find my own answers. I wished I could sum it up on a page, I thought, because my book isn't done.

This poem came out for Gail one morning, sticky brief thoughts snapped to my fridge via Magnetic Poetry, my soul-saving device. By then I had the Starter Kit—Part Two, the Healing Words kit, and a kit that came with my 2006 calendar. I liked to use all the words. I liked finding that laugh, live, and celebrate came in each kit, with multiple whys.

Question Blessings

come here, friend
give question blessing
ask openly if
you will heal from this treatment
no question

say, I am present
feel deep desire for balance
angel, spirit my being through fire
bear the long cycle
between hard day & possible peace

begin women's work
sacred journey from chaos
birthing wisdom in between
why not let go of time
fly beneath night sky
the star shine is deep inner god
play with clouds
look beneath dark smoke
like piercing a needle through marble
use courage to challenge self and endure storm
o learn all over again and trust strong soul

pray why
meditate why
but we were so happy
you bellow
when we suffer'd you would sing to me
his voice doubtful now
this man is haunted
with weary understanding
his sad breath too aware
to see relief there

remember, strong & young
let him make a hard wish
ask him for a kiss
he was never more safe with eternity
surrender mind & melt steel heart
perhaps our men are almost there

we growl ferociously
wanting to keep our sons from weight of season
yet two boys must see how to transform dark night
trust in their brilliant fathers who do it
only then would believe it
like secret hard truth
and could grow up whole

look how these days I can
bring more clean flowing water
drink from well of worry
nourish dreams
accept time
we will get by

rest would do me good
speak self-love
you give compassion
encourage hope create joy
but remember you are fragile
ask for care too

it takes time grace energy
to heal heart
have faith

soon wake from hard dream
believe you could live without knowing
then live like you were born yesterday
see gratitude as only path

celebrate
though maybe only after
pick his present
one birthday gift
delicious cake
laugh
then eat another popsicle

The thing about writing is that when you think you're writing for someone else, it turns out you're writing because it's what you need to know. My
poems surprised me that way. When I began thinking our grace period was
about to expire, the poems spoke as if to prepare me.

May I be safe,
May I be healthy,
May I be happy,
May I be fully at ease.
—Ancient loving-kindness meditation

52

Taming Lions

I woke up that morning at the end of February and rolled onto Scott's shoulder. The alarm clock said 6:14 and I thought, *Whew, ten minutes to snuggle.* I savored a second, and then I thought, *Huh. Oh, yeah. This is what it feels like to remember that time is precious.*

When you remember that, you bother to snuggle each morning, even if just for a minute. And you say "I love you" when he leaves the house to take your son to school. And you realize that life is still good and things are okay if you still trust him to drive, trust him with your son's life, with yours. And then when they're gone, instead of going back to bed to sneak an extra hour of sleep, you sit at the kitchen table, write in your journal, and have a good cry. That's what my morning was like.

That is, the Tuesday morning after an appointment with Scott's primary physician, Dr. B, a young guy who had not dealt with Scott's brain tumor before, or should I say *yet*. Let me back up.

Here's how it goes, when Scott gets a symptom and tries to discern whether it's something to worry about or if it's just the new normal. He'll walk into the room, hem and haw, stand there a minute and say, "I should tell you something in case I drop dead later today."

That gets my attention. Then he'll continue with details. On that Monday night it sounded like this:

"Something weird just happened. I got out of the car at the pharmacy and I couldn't grab the handle very well. It was like these two fingers were sticky," and he gripped the pinky and ring finger on his right hand with his left.

Here we go again, I think. *Right hand, left brain. Brain thing.*

"Does it feel numb?" I asked. "Is it still feeling like that? How long did it last?"

"A few minutes. It's just kinda tingly now." He held out his hands and the right one was shaking, but not the left. My heart clutched.

"Hmmm. Shit."

And so I picked up a 4-by-6 blue spiral notebook that had been sitting under my desktop calendar. I bought it after Christmas to carry in my purse in case I had a spontaneous thought to write down, to capture my creativity, and move ahead with my book. I said, "Well, let's write down the symptoms, keep a diary sort of, so that when you go to a doctor you can tell him specifics. I've already called Dr. Arenson's office to move up your MRI to spring break instead of April. But maybe you should see your primary doctor or the neurologist right away? What do you think?"

That was our conversation on Monday night. The next day he called the primary care doctor's office and made an appointment for Thursday. Over lunch in our kitchen that day, he agreed I should go with him, which I had not done for a few years. I tucked the spiral notebook in my purse before we left. When I pulled it out again in the exam room at the doctor's office, I thought it significant progress to downsize my spiral to one that fits in my purse. Seven years earlier I took a new five-subject notebook with me. *I wonder where I put that notebook?* I thought, and clicked the ballpoint pen to start writing.

The young brunette nurse brought us into the room. "What are we seeing you for today?"

Scott hesitated, deciding how much to say. "Neurological issues," and he sat on the crunchy paper on the exam table. She fell silent while taking Scott's temperature, 98 even, and blood pressure, 120 over 80. I thought *That's not enough detail* and said, "Scott's in remission from a brain tumor, grade three. He's been having right-sided symptoms again."

The nurse looked up with a jolt and said, as she opened the door, "Okay, the doctor will be here in a few minutes."

"Well that shut her up," Scott laughed after she left And I remember how we laughed in the neurosurgeon's office the day his staples were removed after his first surgery, and how the neurosurgeon said how he had heard us laughing down the hallway, how that never happened in his office before.

"Okay, Mr. Vickroy," I joked, "Tell me what you've been experiencing." And changing my tone, I said, "Tell me now so I make sure we don't forget to mention it when he comes in."

I make a damn good interviewer, I thought. *I know how to probe to make sure he gives the specifics that might make the difference in diagnosing these tremors, twitches, and tics.*

Dr. B walked in and said hello to Scott, not even introducing himself to me or glancing my way. *Lose a point, doctor,* I assessed. *Let's see how you handle the rest of this appointment.* I know that sounds bitchy, but listen, this is important, and I set the bar high. I nudged Scott along through the process of describing his symptoms since early December—the sunburn-like sensitivity on top of his skin, along the outer right side of his arm, torso and leg; the way his foot thinks the sock is scratchy like it had been dried in a ball when in fact it's clean and soft as the sock on the left; the tic beneath his lip on the right that comes and goes; how sometimes his eyelid feels sticky and Scott uses his fingers to open it wider.

"Tell him how it started, back in early December," I urged.

"Well, it started after some serious physical exertion," he began, shooting me a glance like *Geez.*

And I shot back exasperation and said, "Tell him what kind of exertion," and it's not to be rude or mean, but because I think it matters, and doesn't he remember that nothing is sacred when you're trying to diagnose whether the tumor is back. It could be significant, so why give the wrong impression that it was incredible sex or heroic lifting or marathon running. "It was pooping!"

Dr. B laughed and commiserated with Scott, "Do you ever feel like you have a second mother in the room?"

Ooh, there goes another point, doctor, and I say—I'm sure with a pout, "Hey, it's my job as his medical advocate," and I'm pretty sure the doctor understood what I was saying was *Don't mess with me, doc.*

"What I meant was you remind me of mothers with teenage boys who keep nudging to get them to talk," he said with a smile, trying to win back his point. And I thought *Yep, it's like I'm the mother again of a grown-up kid. Shit. Here we go again.*

And so we kept talking and asking questions, and I gave Dr B a few extra points when he explains that what Scott is experiencing is not a stroke or a bleed, because that would have happened suddenly, severely, and would not have subsided. Clearly, this is a brain thing and we all know it. We just don't know whether this is something more seizure-like or more like a tumor recurrence. I asked him whether he thinks it's okay to wait three weeks, until March, for the MRI or if sooner is better. I detect pissiness in Scott's voice when he said, "What does it matter if I find out tomorrow or three weeks from now?"

And Dr. B earned a few more points when he said, "This is where I'd get into trouble if I ignored it," and I agreed, mumbling partly aloud about how many tumors go undiagnosed for too long by doctors who blow off the symptoms.

"I hate to even say this," Dr. B cringed, then set his shoulders to speak. "Let's just say hypothetically that if the tumor is back, and it's growing quickly, then three weeks could make a difference."

That's true, I said to myself. We all know the likelihood that when the tumor comes back it will return as a higher-grade tumor and weeks do make a difference. Shit. Shit. Shit. But true. And Scott knows it. And he agreed, begrudgingly. I didn't stop to think then if his hesitance was because he didn't intend to have treatment, or if he just wasn't ready to give in to the possibility that the tumor was back.

We went back and forth talking, deciding whether it made sense to book an MRI in Grand Junction or drive to Denver, back to Swedish Hospital where our neuro-radiologist works, where all of Scott's scans were already in the system and could be compared, apples to apples. We had an MRI here at St. Mary's once, in 2002, and I remember that it mattered to have the MRI performed by the same equipment or team, something about matching up slices to see if there was change.

And so in the end we agreed to call Dr. Arenson's office ourselves, talk to him about whether to schedule it here and send it digitally to be read in Denver, or to just drive to Denver next week, or to wait until March. We left the exam room and headed down the hallway,

"I'd be surprised if he wanted to wait," Dr. B said. Scott and I were ambivalent; we just shrugged and walked on. It was okay that Dr. B was being cautious. It was a good thing.

I knew both Scott and I were thinking about Schrödinger's cat. To see the next MRI—whatever was there—would be to reopen the box. Did we want to do that tomorrow or three weeks away? It seemed to me that this time the box contained not a cat, but a lion, and I thought I could hear it growling. I felt myself gearing up to do battle, just in case it was a lion.

I was wearing my new cowgirl boots that day, the soft brown suede Ariats I bought myself for my birthday, as if I somehow knew I would soon need shit-kickers to summon my inner cowgirl. And I was wearing my new favorite pink sweater from Mom, another birthday present made of yarn that looks like homemade pink frosting, you know, where the butter is still a bit cold so the red food coloring doesn't quite mix all the way with the powdered sugar, leaving it speckled.

In the Kia on the drive home, heading east on I-70 to Palisade, afternoon sun creating dazzling shadows on the treeless Bookcliffs, fresh snow on Grand Mesa, I recognized the moment, me driving, him back in the passenger's seat. New mountains this time, but otherwise very familiar.

"Funny how easily I slide right back into the caregiver slot," I said, patting his thigh, then wanting to hit him hard on his chest for putting me back in this role. "It's so easy to be the medical advocate again, asking questions, taking notes, being bitchy if I have to."

He just looked at me and then out the window. "I know."

I considered what I just said and was surprised to realize I was feeling both scared and strong. *Wow, I know how to do this. I can do this. I'm going to be okay. If I have to battle that lion, I think I can do it.* At first I thought that hardness in my chest was panic. I poked around to see if my inner bricklayer had thrown up a wall for my protection. *No, that isn't it,* I realized. It's more like a Kevlar vest sensation, bullet-proof. *Or maybe my superhero costume just materialized under my sweater. Wow, that's it. My superpowers! They're back!*

So I woke up the next morning and rolled onto Scott's shoulder, feeling stronger than yesterday and thinking *This is what it feels like to remember that time is precious.* Not in a panic. Not yet. Over my breakfast of Froot Loops I had a good cry, then laughed at the thought of eating a bowl full of chakra colors. I journaled awhile. I picked out some Magnetic Poetry words, eyes closed, and slapped them on the side of the fridge, asking my soul for help arranging the random words into a message of hope. Then I took a shower and put on my comfortable jeans with part-cashmere pink hoodie and my pink quartz necklace with the charm that says "Laugh." My next thought? Now it's time to get to work. Thank God it's Friday.

Pickup Poetry

worry
but nourish gratitude
this man would hope
accept it like translucent dark time

we shine
celebrate our son
then do live
ask for faith too

encourage
but flow
safe breath
chaos
why more?

Can all spirituality and any experience of the reality of God
be reduced to a fleeting rush of electrochemical blips and flashes,
racing along the neural pathways of the brain?
—*Andrew Newberg, M.D.*

53

Profession of Faith

The Monday morning before driving to Denver for Scott's MRI, I was at my computer trying to catch up on several client website projects. I wanted to be able to clear my plate before leaving town. I was just starting my second To Do of the day, marked my timesheet to start, when the phone rang.

"Hello. How are you doing?" the young man's tentative phone-voice said, sounding so kind, and I wondered if this was the nicest telemarketer I've ever met.

"I'm good, thanks. Who's this?" I answered, with more cold skepticism than I meant.

"I found your website. My name is Kevin," and I knew I was speaking to someone with brain tumor questions. "I have a brain tumor, and I wonder if I could ask you a few questions. Do you have time to talk?"

"Yes, of course," I said and pulled over a notepad to write down his name, feeling instant connection and not just because one of our best friends is a Kevin. He wanted to know more about our experience getting a second opinion from M. D. Anderson. He was almost three weeks out from his second surgery for a low-grade astrocytoma, back again after a silent two years since his first surgery, having had no immediate follow-up treatment. Tingling sensations on one hand and leg were the only symptoms he had, and I thought, *Sounds like a parietal lobe tumor like Scott's.* I was right. I asked him if he had new symptoms this time, or if the tumor just reappeared on his regular check-up MRI. Except for some tingling, there were no other clues—that's exactly what happened.

As I listened to him talk, and I answered with what seemed like mostly clear-headed facts and encouragement, part of my mind was talking to God, *What are you up to? How ironic is this to send me a phone call from a guy whose symptoms are just like Scott's, in mirror imagery, whose tumor is back, and day after tomorrow we're going to find out if Scott's tumor is back. If it's anything like this Kevin's, it sure could be back. This is so weird.*

Then this nice young Kevin asks me, after we've already agreed on the value of ignorant bliss, "So how do you deal with the statistics? I mean, I couldn't help reading about them online this morning."

"Well, we've always said that statistics are just numbers, but you are a person, an individual. You can look at them as a way to light a fire under you, to make decisions about your treatment based on information instead of on fear." I went on to describe how Scott's first neurosurgeon gave him two to five years, and how now Scott's at seven. How so many people out there beat the statistics. I blathered on until I didn't know what else to say, and then he affirmed he had heard me.

"I like what you said about lighting a fire. It gave me chills."

Whew, I said something right, I thought like a mental back-pat and brow-wipe. *Thank goodness.*

We talked on, about living your life, letting people help you and love you, finding your inner samurai, that maybe it's more about your process than it is about the outcome, that cancer sucks and it sucks every day, but it's possible to find moments of love and courage that will amaze you. Before we hung up, I told him we'd be happy if he ever wanted to call back, talk to Scott, or just keep us posted by email.

"Thanks for talking to me," he said.

"It's totally my pleasure, getting to help other people." I said, "It's the reason we're here."

When I hung up the phone I thought to myself, *Maybe the universe sent me this phone call from this Kevin and his astrocytoma because it's important for me to share the wisdom I've gained, to pay it forward. Maybe if I believe all this today, and I've sworn it out loud like an oath (which by definition means cussing allowed), then on Wednesday morning after we see if a tumor is on Scott's MRI, I can remind myself that I do know the truth.*

It's not about the outcome. Death is not a failure. Cure and healing are two different things. Survival is about how you live every day, not just breathing and hearing your heartbeat, but really living your life. That is what matters. It's about *surpassing* survival.

We live our life in semesters between each MRI. If this one is clean, there's always the next. I can let worry and fear overwhelm me, or I can just live my life every day. I can let the potential tumor recurrence ruin my life with some statistical deadline, or I can let it light a fire under me to not take time or life or love for granted, but to live every day. You and I have the same exact choice, cancer or not.

It's so hard to remember this.

Hence, this life of yours which you are living
is not merely a piece of the entire existence,
but is in a certain sense the whole...
—*Erwin Schrödinger*

54
Schrödinger's Lion

A week later on the last day of February, Scott and I drove to Denver for his MRI, which would be the next morning, Ash Wednesday. Wil stayed home with my parents. He didn't know this MRI was a month ahead of schedule. He didn't need to know how scared we were. If the MRI turned out to be bad news, that would be soon enough to tell our son. Ignorant bliss.

Scott drove us over the mountains to Denver. It seemed defiant for him to drive, daring the gods to send him a seizure.

I was in charge of the soundtrack. Only Scott's CDs were in the Kia. I hadn't packed any of my own. It seemed defiant for me to not bring the music that kept me alive way back then when Scott was first diagnosed. That didn't keep me from over-analyzing the lyrics I was left with, looking as always for a sign. The group called Train came on first, calling all angels. *Oh great, how does Train know how much I need to know that things are gonna look up? I do feel us drowning in a sea spilled from a cup.*

The lyrics got worse from there, a sad album overall, so I opened the center console and started looking for a different CD. We were far between mountain towns, so radio wasn't an option. I was looking down when CRACK! I jumped despite my seatbelt. A piece of gravel had hit the windshield like gunshot. In front of my eyes cracked a star the size of a quarter.

"Damned Halliburton," I said, cursing the big red truck in front of us as if blaming it for all brain tumors, bad things, and war. Then I burst into tears, my courage cracked worse than the windshield.

Scott patted my leg, but laughed, too. "It's okay. It's going to be okay."

I have an out-of-print book called *The Body is the Barometer of the Soul* by an Australian healer, Annette Noontil. Her final chapter, written in all seriousness yet sounding like a joke, talks about your car being the barometer of your soul, too. Any part that breaks down in the vehicle you drive corresponds to a condition in your body. The body likes metaphors for making us pay attention. I always thought it ironic that our Honda Civic was dented in the left rear passenger door, just like the location of Scott's tumor. A cracked windshield, so said that book, meant you were afraid to see into your future.

I am NOT afraid of my future, I shouted inside my thoughts. That damned windshield. It was not a bad omen, just bad luck. It didn't mean anything. That crack mocked me for two hundred more miles.

We stayed with Scott's dad in Denver. Scott's mom was in Palm Desert enjoying a warmer winter, just like she was gone when we first learned of Scott's tumor. The coincidence scared me. We went to bed early, wiped out from the drive and our pre-MRI angst.

My final dream before waking tried calming my nerves. I dreamed of opening a box and finding a purring orange-striped kitten. I was too nervous to interpret the dream or eat any breakfast. So was Scott.

At the hospital in the MRI waiting room, Scott emptied his pockets into my hands, keys, coins, watch, and wallet, and I put all that in my purse. I miss my routine of putting his ring on my thumb.

It's always strange to wait for Scott during his MRIs. Since November 2, 1998, I sat alone in that MRI waiting room about two dozen times. Always the same room, the morning news on the television that hangs from the ceiling, sometimes alone, sometimes smiling at others who wait for their turn, always wondering if their MRI will be of their brain (sometimes it's obvious). Sometimes I write in my journal. Sometimes I read a worn magazine. Sometimes I bring my own book and sit there pretending to read, but I'm always too nervous to think. Sometimes...sometimes I can only wait. I listen to the clattering thrum of the MRI behind the wall. And then Scott returns, holding out one hand for his keys, holding his other arm stiff because it still contains the IV needle. He learned to keep the IV in so as not to be poked twice. Dr. Arenson always orders blood work on MRI day to check Scott's immune system recovery: white cells, red cells, platelets, and more.

We walk from Radiology following the blue tiles, down the surgery hall to the black tiles, around the corner and down the long hall to the glass walkway that connects Swedish to the medical plaza where Dr. Arenson has his office. We wait in his waiting room. The fish tank is gone. A small stone water fountain tries to make up for the loss.

Cynthia comes for us, holding Scott's chart. She is Dr. Arenson's longest survivor, a year ahead of Scott, surviving a grade-four glioblastoma multiforme, against the odds. Cynthia was a nurse at Swedish when her tumor appeared. Like Scott, she had photodynamic therapy with her surgery, plus radiation and the same aggressive chemotherapy (minus the high-dose chemo and stem cell rescue). Cynthia credits Dr. Arenson's team and the Lord for saving her life. She never worked again but Dr. Arenson lets her volunteer in his office three days a week. We're always relieved to see her there, as if her long-term survival is tied to our own.

After Cynthia checks Scott's weight and blood pressure, she shows us to Exam Room One. We have a window overlooking the sunny gardens below, still bare and asleep in March. One time Dr. Arenson took a Polaroid of us in that room, for his "wall of fame," and in the snapshot a bright light appeared over our shoulders. It was probably the flashbulb's reflection in the window, but I like to think it was our guardian angel. I wonder if our guardian angel comes to every appointment.

"How are you doing?" Cynthia asks, keeping us company until Dr. Arenson is ready to look at the MRI with us.

Holding back tears, I admit, "Actually, we're pretty nervous this time. Scott's been having some symptoms."

Cynthia rolls her stool closer and holds out her hands to both of us. "Can we pray?"

We nod, unable to speak lest tears turn to sobs.

"Dear Father, be with Scott and Shelly this morning as they see the MRI. We ask that you give them strength…and that this MRI be okay. If it's not, we can fix it. In Jesus' name we pray. Amen."

She squeezes our hands, smiles, and leaves. I blow my nose on some Kleenex from the box on the windowsill and wash my hands at the exam sink. I pull myself together. Scott sits there, folding and unfolding his hands, eyes closed, doing his samurai deep breathing.

Then Dr. Arenson comes to the door and says, "Ready to see the MRI?"

"Ready as I'll ever be," Scott says.

We walk down the hall to a room with no windows, painted a deep warm brown with artwork on the walls. One photo I know was taken by one of Dr. Arenson's patients, before he died. The photo is of a desert cavern with sunlight shining in from above.

Scott and I sit together on a bench, like an antique carriage seat or a church pew, facing the monitor where Dr. Arenson was pulling up that morning's MRI scans side by side with the previous scans from October. In our early brain tumor years, we viewed twenty-inch films clipped to a lightboard on the wall. Now we can take home our own copy on a CD from the hospital's radiology file room. Dr. Arenson curses the keyboard, as always, then scrolls through files with the mouse, moving through images that take our view deeper into Scott's brain. He scrolls each layer more slowly until he has a perfect match, side by side, of Scott's brain, before and today.

For a moment, Dr. Arenson says nothing. Scott leans forward, almost squinting to make sure he is seeing what he saw. The scans are damn near identical to the ones from last time. Dr. Arenson says, "See, nothing there."

Scott and I sat silent, snapping back into our bodies as if our souls had been near the ceiling ready to flee if the news had been bad. It's hard to believe that this MRI, this Schrödinger's box, held neither a lion, a cat nor a kitten. It was empty.

After a moment of skeptical relief, I said, "Then what has been causing Scott's symptoms? Could it be increased seizure activity?"

Dr. Arenson shook his head and with a slight smile, not at all condescending, just wise, said, "It's Damocles Syndrome."

"Yes," I nodded, thinking *Oh, of course.* It was the survivor's syndrome I read about a few months ago in a study of long-term cancer survivors. Scott didn't know about it, so Dr. Arenson explained.

"*The Damocles Syndrome* is a book written years ago by a man named Koocher about survivors of childhood cancer, how they never feel completely cured, always expecting the cancer to come back."

My inner know-it-all interrupted and said, "Damocles was the Greek-myth guy at the feast, sitting under a sword that could fall any moment and kill him."

Scott said, "Oh, yeah. I call that my AA syndrome, like once an alcoholic always an alcoholic. Once a brain tumor patient, always a brain tumor patient."

Dr. Arenson nodded and bent his head to write a few notes in Scott's chart. "I'm glad you're okay. This is good news. It's been a hard, hard time."

"You mean losing patients?" I asked, sensing his broader meaning and knowing Scott's survival meant as much to Dr. Arenson as it did to us.

"Yes, lots of patients lately. Lots of our favorites. We didn't need you to be another one," he said, pointing Scott's way with his pen, his head still inclined toward the chart.

I wanted to ask for names I might recognize, but it didn't seem right.

"So, we'll schedule your next MRI in six months," he said.

"Or eight, if you'd rather," Scott said, an arbitrary extension of time.

"No. I tell all my patients that they should have an MRI every six months for the rest of their life, or until I retire and another doctor replaces me with a different philosophy. But that will be ten years from now. I'll be 71. Assuming my own health holds out, and you just never know. That's twenty more scans together, Scott."

"We know some good vineyard land when you're ready to retire," I joked, fully serious. I knew of his dream to grow wine grapes someday.

"Sounds good. I'd like to grow Rieslings or Viogner or some kind of grape that would need lots of TLC. I don't like California whites," he laughed.

By then our official appointment was over, and Dr. Arenson abruptly walked out of the room without a backward glance, leaving Scott with the IV from the MRI still in his arm. We walked back to the exam room where the nurse, Mary, was ready to draw blood and then remove Scott's IV, working slow and gentle to loosen the tape with a cotton ball soaked in magic solution. As she worked we chatted, telling about Wil, asking about her daughter. Mary had been our oncology nurse since the very beginning when Wil was in preschool and her daughter a preteen. Mary left with the tubes of blood and came back soon with a printout of Scott's complete blood count. His platelets showed 131, which was up from 108 five months earlier, though still in the low range.

"What am I doing right?" Scott asked, curious about the increase.

"Living the good life," she answered. "Recovering."

Before we left Dr. Arenson's office that day, we stopped in the hall to hug the social worker and Cynthia, who said, "How was it?"

"All clear," I said, grinning.

With her hug she uttered, "Praise Jesus."

Scott's neuropsychologist happened to walk in the office just then. He handed a thin book to Dr. Arenson and I heard him say, "It's poetry," as if continuing their earlier conversation. The book was *Facts about the Moon: Poems by Dorianne Laux*, which I took as my own good luck sign.

That's why I love this team, I thought. *They're poets in disguise.*

I later Googled some poems by Dorianne Laux and loved finding these lines from "Music in the Morning":

... but I know it's only luck
that delivered him here, luck and a love
that had nothing to do with me. Except
that this is what we sometimes get
if we live long enough. If we are patient
with our lives.

After our appointment, Scott kissed me good in the elevator and we walked to the car holding hands. Scott called his dad on the cell phone to share his good news and then called my folks so they could tell Wil after school. I drove us to the Pancake House at Orchard Road and University, and when we passed Mission Hills Church at the intersection I thought about Reverend Clyde McDowell who ministered there and who was the first brain tumor patient we met on our journey, he and his wife, Lee. We never had an MRI day when we didn't think of the brain tumor patients we once knew.

I ordered Eggs Benedict and Scott had scrambled eggs, sausage patties, buttermilk pancakes, and coffee. While waiting for pancakes, I posed a question.

"So, now that your MRI is all clear, are you going to live life any differently, extravagantly?

"Do you mean is the sky more blue, the trees greener, the clouds puffier? I hope I see that every day, not just today. And I already bought my new computer. I suppose that's as much as I've spent on myself in six years."

He wasn't counting his big-screen TV when we moved to Palisade, or the new Kia Sportage he bought for his most recent birthday. To Scott, he who dies with the best computer wins.

"Fair enough," I said. "I'm starving."

On our drive home over the mountains that afternoon, while still within radio range of Denver, a song on KBCO continued our pancakes conversation. Tracy Chapman asked us whether, if we knew that we would die today, see the face of God and love, would we change?

Scott was paying attention, too. I squeezed his leg, he squeezed my hand back, and we laughed.

Do you change out of fear, or gratitude? Or do you need to change at all?

Before we left town for the MRI, I told a friend that if it was clear, I would celebrate by booking our family on a cruise, even though I couldn't afford it. I don't know if that was a decadent plan, or bargaining for Scott's survival. It's like telling God, *Okay, if it turns out he's safe, I promise to live life more fully.*

After we knew Scott's MRI was clear, his brain safe from a tumor recurrence for now, I had another decadent thought. *Maybe it is time to replace the water heater in our house, before it breaks.*

What is more decadent? To take a trip as if you had six months to live, or to buy a water heater you plan to use for ten years?

Maybe neither. Maybe both.

Maybe it's enough to celebrate with a nice dinner and wine.

If you make your choice with fear,
your path ahead will not be clear.
But if with Love is how you choose,
in the end you cannot lose.

55
Damocles' Feast and My Dragon

I have never seen such a big crescent moon. As it fell toward the western horizon, it glowed huge as a harvest moon, showing the upper white border of its true circle.

"Look at the moon," I pointed, as Scott and I stepped out our front door and walked to the Kia. We were on our way to the Red Rose Café for a celebration date to toast Scott's clean MRI, while Wil was still at my parents' house.

That crescent was the most beautiful moon ever. It was and always will be our lucky moon, and it brought luck that day. The previous Friday morning at seven I saw it through the branches of our willow tree, Jupiter above to the east, the sun still asleep behind Grand Mesa's bulk. When I saw the waning crescent moon two weeks ago, I noted it there. Not just any moon, but our crescent coping moon. *The moon will always be with you*, it said of itself.

Five days later, I thought we were alone in the dark phase of the moon and I wondered with pre-MRI superstition what it meant to go to the MRI without our standard morning crescent.

I only thought we were alone. The moon rises forty minutes later every day. It rose unbeknownst to me that day on the prairie east of Denver and followed us home over the mountains, invisible in the cloud-ridden sky. It wasn't until evening that we saw the moon's thin bottom lip blowing us a kiss through the cottonwood branches.

From our booth in the Red Rose Café, Scott saw it again through the plate glass window, more huge than before.

"Look at it now," he said, and I turned around in the booth to see. I turned back with a toast.

"Here's to a clean bill of health," I said, clinking my Mount Garfield Estates Fumé Blanc against the glass of Scott's Palisade Red, the kitchen-sink combo of wines that is the cheapest of the local reds and our favorite. Mount Garfield Estates planted their vines the same summer we moved to Palisade, in the same section south down the road from my parents' orchard.

We feasted that night, starting with house salad for Scott and soup d'jour for me, Manhattan clam chowder with chunky vegetables and spicy black pepper.

"You'd like this," I said, holding my spoon toward him, then thought maybe not since most things tomato still remind Scott of the tomato-paste smell of his stem cell rescue. But maybe after seven years his taste buds had adjusted.

"I'll take your word for it," he declined.

Next we had calamari, crispy deep-fried, drizzled with fresh lemon juice, and a big bowl of homemade marinara. It was the best calamari I ever tasted. For dinner we each had a Vietnamese rice noodle bowl (the owner of the Red Rose Café is Italian, his wife Vietnamese). My bowl had grilled shrimp and egg roll, Scott's had grilled chicken.

Scott ordered a second glass of wine and we sprang for dessert, chocolate mousse cheesecake, one plate, two forks.

Louis Armstrong filled the air with his jazz, and the tables began to fill with other local diners.

"I forgot how much I liked this place—these bright yellow walls, all the pictures, the old oak floors, high ceilings, the music. How long has it been?"

"Probably a year and a half," Scott answered. "Remember that extra long lunch when we waited and waited. The food was good, but it took forever."

"We should come back more often—for early dinners when we have plenty of time, like tonight, or some night just for dessert at the bar."

Scott nodded agreement and took another bite of cheesecake. I'm glad the waiter didn't ask what we were celebrating. To say "no brain tumor today" would not have done our mood justice.

Only Scott and I knew, as we feasted, that a sharp samurai sword hung in the air over our table, over Scott's head, his Sword of Damocles. From where I sat, I could see it quite plainly. Is that the caregiver's curse—to notice that sword on a thread more often, more clearly than the patient himself? It was time to step out from under that sword. With a sword in our hands, not over our heads, we can slay dragons.

The day after Scott's MRI and our feast, my cough came back with a vengeance, as if relief over Scott's MRI left a hole in my chest and bronchitis swooped in. I stayed in bed, taking care of myself, eating Girl Scout cookies (Samoas), drinking hot tea, alternating naps with writing in my journal.

It reminded me of seven years before when Scott came home from the hospital after his stem cell rescue—how my body knew it was finally safe to be sick once Scott was out of the proverbial woods. Back then I spent four days in bed with strep throat, too ill to move. On the fourth night I emerged from my bed and wandered downstairs, needing fresh air and starry skies. Wil was in bed, Scott was watching TV. I sat on the back deck, sipping hot tea, wrapped in a fleece blanket despite the warm summer night.

I asked the stars for inspiration for a story version of heartstrings, a way to convey what I had learned from our nine months of being loved, supported, and connected to friends near and far while Scott faced his brain tumor battle. In my emails, I used to call his battle slaying the dragon because that's what he dreamed after his first surgery. Looking up, I saw inspiration unfold. A shooting star, then another, dropped from the sky toward the porch.

Was it cosmic significance that the previous day, August 11, 1999, presented the last solar eclipse of the century and that night on my porch I was witnessing the peak of the annual Perseid meteor shower with 50 to 150 shooting stars per hour? Good timing or God thing?

I ran inside for a fresh spiral notebook and then went back outside in the dark with a pen. I wrote for an hour in the glow of kitchen light and suburban backyard glow. As I wrote I felt more awake and alert than I had for weeks, maybe months.

Once Upon a Heartstring

Once upon a time and not so far away, there lived a boy with his mother and father in a small, peaceful village. On one side of the village was a strong, forested mountain range, providing a beautiful backdrop on which they leaned in comfort. On the second side were checkerboard fields full of vegetables. On the third side were rows and rows of fruitful orchards and grapevines. The fourth side of the village was open—open to the wind and the rain and the road that went out to the rest of the world.

Happy, safe, and well fed, the people of the village were content, their lives full of joy, until the dragon came. Winter winds brought a mean and terrible dragon that ravaged the village and farms. The fields were charred from the dragon's fiery breath and poisoned by his venomous spit. Though now it was springtime, the earth was still in shock. Very few leaves peeked out from the trees and not many flowers chose to bloom. Too many villagers died fighting the ruthless dragon, leaving children without mothers and families without fathers.

The boy's father was wounded by the cruel dragon, his head slashed by the dragon's terrible claws. The scar had not yet healed since the poison still simmered in the wound. The father lay in bed, unable to think and too weak to move about. The mother tended the father's wound, unwilling to leave his side until she could be sure of his recovery.

The boy did all he could to help his family, cooking meals, milking the cow, and helping his neighbors as well. He was growing strong and tall, but nobody noticed in their worry for the sick.

The village healer had done all she could to mend the wounds the dragon had left behind. The herbs from the alpine forest were proving helpful against the dragon's poison, but the recovery was long and slow. Now only patience and time would transform the wounds into healed scars.

Without more strong hands to mend and tend the fields, what food would the villagers have to nourish them through the next winter? Several of the boy's neighbors met one day in the village square to discuss what should be done.

"We must go to the next village over the hill and ask for help," the old baker pleaded.

"We must find the dragon and slay it, before he comes back to harm us again," roared the blacksmith.

"We cannot afford to lose a single pair of strong hands, not now," said a woman in the crowd. "We must all stay together and help each other water, weed, and harvest the crops."

On and on they talked, wondering what to do with so many people still sick from the dragon's marks. The boy tried to speak, but nobody wanted to listen to a child, even if he was growing stronger and taller every day. Despite all their talking, the grown-ups couldn't decide what to do. So nothing was done . . . until one day the boy himself decided to go for help. He didn't know how just yet, but he believed he could find a way to help the village and make sure the dragon never returned.

After making his decision, the boy visited his teacher to say farewell. They spoke awhile and then the teacher gave him this advice. "You will face danger, fear, and loneliness on your journey. But each time you will discover a way to conquer the danger, face the fear, and overcome your loneliness —and find Truth. Remember this rhyme my own teacher once gave to me:

"If you make your choice with fear, your path ahead will not be clear. But if with Love is how you choose, in the end you cannot lose."

The boy tucked away these words in his mind, not sure of their meaning yet but grateful for a final lesson from his teacher.

"Remember our heartstrings," the teacher spoke in parting. All the villagers were in the habit of saying so as a fond way to part with friends, patting their chest over their hearts before waving goodbye. To the boy it was a nice saying but mere words. He had never given it any more thought.

The boy spent a few days saying goodbye to all his friends and family in the village, amazed at all the well wishers. Although he cried tears of sorrow at the partings, his heart was full of strength and joy upon realizing how many people sent their love with him.

The next morning as the sun began to rise, the young boy said his final goodbyes. He said goodbye to his father, still weak and sick in bed, who gave him a sword for protection. He said goodbye to his mother, with tears on her cheeks, who gave him a new cloak to keep him warm. And he said goodbye to his grandparents, smiling with pride at his bravery, who gave him a basket of bread, cheese, and apples.

With these parting gifts and the embraces of all who loved him, the boy started his journey to find and slay the dragon. "Remember our heartstrings," they called out to him, waving farewell.

And so the boy began his journey, setting out on the road that led to the world beyond his village. Along the way, the boy passed through other villages showing signs of damage from the dragon. From the top of a very tall hill, the boy could see all the dragon had ravaged—trees broken, fields burned, ponds sucked dry, and not a speck of growing green in sight.

He met only a few travelers along the road, and asked if they knew of the dragon. On the other side of a broad river is a rocky mountain range, they answered, where the dragon is said to live in a cave on the peak. To get there, the boy must retrace the path of destruction.

That August night in 1999, I couldn't imagine the details to write the middle. I knew he'd have several adventures and tests, since that's how fairy tales go. *The middle doesn't matter now,* I thought at the time, *I can flesh it out later, but I know how I want the story to end.*

On the night before he faced the dragon, the boy sat under the cloudy sky. The crickets were chirping in the meadow and a gusty breeze whistled through the trees. It seemed even Nature felt unsettled this night. The boy looked inward and upward, then began talking with the Great Creator.

"Along this journey, I have faced many fears. I see how much love follows me wherever I go, helping me in ways I never expected. I thank you for that. But tomorrow I face the dragon that all but killed my father, and I am afraid. What if the dragon wounds me, too? What if the dragon kills me? What will happen to my parents and grandparents, my friend, my neighbors? What if I can't fight the dragon? I am afraid the dragon will win and I will never see my loved ones again. I am afraid!"

The night grew very silent. The cicadas stopped chirping, the brook stopped still, and even the wind stopped rustling the leaves of the trees. The clouds parted then and all the stars in the heavens began to sparkle and shimmer more brilliantly than ever before.

Streaks of lightning flashed in the distance. Slowly at first, then more rapidly, out from the stars sprang heartstrings — arching, curving, and spilling to the earth in all colors imaginable, even colors the boy had never seen before.

All night long he watched the skies as the stars and their heartstrings floated, twirled, and splashed to the earth. The cicadas began singing again, as well as the brook and the wind in the leaves, until the whole world seemed in harmony, as if the very earth was falling in love.

In his heart, the boy felt the Truth. He then knew that the whole world is connected by heartstrings and the strongest heartstring emerges from within and reaches above, filled with love, courage, and peace from the Great Creator.

The boy no longer feared meeting the dragon tomorrow. The boy now knew that even the dragon's fiery breath couldn't sever the heartstrings that the boy carried inside. With a happy sigh of relief, he lay down to sleep, with this whisper to the sky "Thank you, Great Creator. I have faith that no matter what happens, all will be well, as it is meant to be."

The next morning the boy awoke with a smile on his face and much courage in his heart. He smoothed over the ground where he had spent the night, ready to face the dragon.

Still thinking of all who he loved and all who loved him, the boy strode out of the woods and into the clearing, which lay at the foot of the last cliff he must climb. And climb he did.

Up in his cave, the dragon stirred from his sleep, hearing the scuttle of rocks below and the flutter of startled sparrows flying away. The dragon crept out of the cave and in stealth looked over the edge of his cliff. He gazed below in astonishment.

Below was a boy, not so big if he'd been all alone. But this boy was surrounded by ribbons and strings of every color and hue, trailing from his chest, sailing behind him, rippling out like a cloak as far as the dragon's very long-sighted eyes could see. And biggest of all was a huge silver strand that reached all the way to Heaven itself.

"What kind of warrior is this, summoning and sending such strong magic?" thought the dragon. "Not a warrior I care to combat!" And with that realization, the dragon knew he could not win a battle with the boy so wholly protected by heartstrings. The dragon launched from the cliff to the sky, spreading his wings in flight.

The gust of wind from the dragon's leap flattened the boy against the cliff. He looked up and saw the dragon's broad wings and long tail disappearing over the mountain top.

See, I knew how I wanted the story to go. I just had to write it.

When I shared the first draft of my fairy tale with a few friends, with a disclaimer about the unwritten middle, their reaction was nearly universal.

"Why couldn't the boy just make friends with the dragon? Why do you have to leave it so ambiguous, with the dragon still out there?"

"Because. It's not that kind of dragon. This dragon is cancer. You can't just make friends with it. You're not guaranteed a happy ending. You never know when or if it will come back, just like the dragon. The boy has to go on with his life, not knowing. He has to be strong either way."

"Hmmm. Okay," was their answer. My friends knew not to push me. It was *my* story, after all. The stubborn writer in me refused to go further with the story, stumped about what adventures to describe for the middle, unable to allow a neat ending with the dragon befriending the boy. It didn't ring true, not for me. What I forgot is that fairy tales, by definition, must have happy endings because that's what children need to believe. What if I wasn't writing a tale for children, but for my inner caregiver who needed her own adult truth?

I could not write the middle back then. Like the boy's father who still had to recover from his wounds, our whole family began a new journey to recover from cancer and the effects of Scott's treatment. We moved over the mountains, we grew fruit in the desert, we endured a long drought, and re-landscaped our life. It was time to move on, lurking dragon or not.

At last, I knew. All these years, I was living The Middle, moving from angst to adventure, so on and so forth, step by step, year by year, always fearing the future with each MRI. With Scott's latest MRI I knew we had come to a crossroad. It was time to choose life over fear, to surpass mere survival and begin fully living. It was time to finally embrace living our life beyond cancer and leave the fears of recurrence behind. It was time to make peace with the dragon, or at least make peace with the dragon's escape.

As we entered our eighth year of survival, I finished the ending.

He could hardly believe the dragon was gone. And so the boy wondered what to do next, where to go, whether to consider his quest a success or a failure. Was the dragon not his to slay after all? The boy could not know until later, when he was a father himself, that it was his powerful cloak of courage and heartstrings that chased the dragon into the sky, out of sight.

The young man, no longer a boy, sat on a rock and welcomed the sunrise. From his vantage point on that mountain peak, he looked in every direction, north-south-east-west, and every point in between. He saw rivers that ran from their source to the sea, and he pondered which one to follow. He saw the way home, back where he'd been. His options were endless. He knew he could sit on his rock the whole morning, being warmed by the sun. But eventually his legs would grow numb, his stomach would growl, and his heart and his mind would grow restless.

"Maybe I need not know my destination. I need only to pick a path and start walking. One day I will return to my home, though I cannot say when. I do know at this moment it is a beautiful morning, a good day to travel, so I must be on my way."

Life is all about the journey, fraught with peril and rewarding adventure. As all heroes know, it's about daring to be brave so that later, by the fire with your friends, you have a tale to tell.

So what happened next? I started craving white walls (in particular, Swiss Coffee by Behr), a blank canvas for life, seeking new inspiration. And what else besides that? Simply this:

To live happily every afternoon.

THE END
(Of the Middle)

Truth is an eternal conversation about things that matter,
conducted with passion and discipline. Truth cannot possibly be found in
the conclusions of the conversation, because the conclusions keep changing.
—Parker J. Palmer

About the Author

Shelly L. Francis grew up in Colorado reading fairy tales and stories of strong women—and writing her own—and is glad her first book is one to help others engage their own strengths. She was a delegate to the Lance Armstrong Foundation LIVE**STRONG**® Summit in 2006, where she pledged to publish this memoir as her personal action plan to raise awareness and effect change around the needs of cancer survivors.

As *Damocles' Wife* goes off to the printer in 2012, Wil is graduating high school and going off to college. Scott is traveling around the world, tumor free. And Shelly is packing her proverbial knapsack with fresh music, her camera, journal, art supplies, and dark chocolate, to set off on a new path, 'carefree' in a normal sort of way.

"All of us are written upon by the challenges we faced, but with many more unwritten pages ahead," says Shelly. "We are each living the next new 'book' in our life—beyond just new chapters."

You can reach Shelly with questions, comments, or to share your own caregiving and long-term cancer survival stories by sending email to shelly@CaregiverHope.com. For resources, visit CaregiverHope.com.

"If the only prayer you say in your life
is thank you, that would suffice."
—*Meister Eckhart*

Many Thanks

For Mom, Dad, Jenéne, Linda, Bill, Amie, and Lance, and our extended family and neighbors. We couldn't have done it without you.

For Edward B. Arenson, M.D. and the entire dedicated, amazing, compassionate team of the Colorado Neurological Institute's Center for Brain & Spinal Tumors. You saved our lives.

For Janna Moll and Carol Komitor. Your Healing Touch and energy medicine was an integral part of more than survival, but healing.

For the women, husbands, and families of the Highlands Ranch/Littleton chapter of Mothers & More, then known as Formerly Employed Mothers at the Leading Edge (FEMALE). We couldn't have done it without you.

For every "Dear Everyone" mentioned herein. You saved our lives.

For Elizabeth L. Clark, Ann Leadbetter, and the women of the Grand Junction affiliate of Women Writing for (a) Change. I couldn't have done this without you.

If I could dedicate *Damocles' Wife* to every person who generously sent us encouragement and sustenance, everyone who lifted up prayers without having ever met us, every patient and caregiver who crossed our path in person or through email during all these years since 1998, I would need a hundred more pages. I hope you know how much your presence mattered.

Thank you!

Shelly L. Francis
Colorado, May 2012

About Two Louise Press

Two Louise Press is a small, virtual publishing house dedicated to making books that start a creative conversation and have a part in changing the world for the better.

Inquiries invited at twolouise@gmail.com.

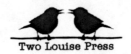

Two Louise Press

CPSIA information can be obtained at www.ICGtesting.com
Printed in the USA
LVOW051459120812

293983LV00008B/26/P